American Holistic Nurses' Association

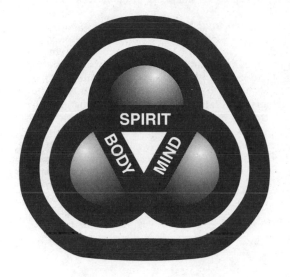

Core Curriculum for Holistic Nursing

Barbara Montgomery Dossey, RN, MS, HNC, FAAN
Editor

Director, Holistic Nursing Consultants
Santa Fe, New Mexico
and
Co-Director, Bodymind Systems
Temple, Texas

AN ASPEN PUBLICATION®
Aspen Publishers, Inc.
Gaithersburg, Maryland
1997

Library of Congress Cataloging-in-Publication Data

Core curriculum for holistic nursing/edited by Barbara Montgomery
Dossey.
    p. cm.
At head of title: American Holistic Nurses' Association.
Includes bibliographical references and index.
ISBN 0-8342-0870-9
1. Holistic nursing.   2. Holistic nursing—Examinations,
questions, etc.   I. Dossey, Barbara Montgomery.   II. American
Holistic Nurses' Association.
[DNLM: 1. Holistic Nursing.   2. Holistic Nursing—examination
questions.   WY 86 C797 1997]
RT42.C63   1997
610.73—dc20
DNLM/DLC
for Library of Congress
96-36535
CIP

Aspen Publishers, Inc., grants permission for photocopying for limited personal or internal use. This consent does not extend to other kinds of copying, such as copying for general distribution, for advertising or promotional purposes, for creating new collective works, or for resale. For information, address Aspen Publishers, Inc., Permissions Department, 200 Orchard Ridge Drive, Suite 200, Gaithersburg, Maryland 20878.

Orders: (800) 638-8437
Customer Service: (800) 234-1660

About Aspen Publishers • For more than 35 years, Aspen has been a leading professional publisher in a variety of disciplines. Aspen's vast information resources are available in both print and electronic formats. We are committed to providing the highest quality information available in the most appropriate format for our customers. Visit Aspen's Internet site for more information resources, directories, articles, and a searchable version of Aspen's full catalog, including the most recent publications: **http://www.aspenpub.com**

Aspen Publishers, Inc. • The hallmark of quality in publishing
Member of the worldwide Wolters Kluwer group

The author have made every effort to ensure the accuracy of the information herein. However, appropriate information sources should be consulted, especially for new or unfamiliar procedures. It is the responsibility of every practitioner to evaluate the appropriateness of a particular opinion in the context of actual clinical situations and with due considerations to new developments. Authors, editors, and the publisher cannot be held responsible for any typographical or other errors found in this book.

Editorial Resources: Ruth Bloom
Library of Congress Catalog Card Number: 96-36535
ISBN: 0-8342-0870-9

Printed in the United States of America

2   3   4   5

This book is dedicated to nurses who hold the common vision of a unified holistic profession and who actualize the essence of modern nursing—of being nurse healers—blending the knowledge of technology and the healing arts.

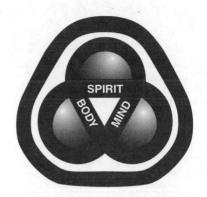

Table of Contents

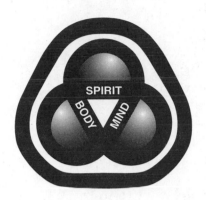

Contributors

Veda L. Andrus, RN, EdD, HNC
Co-Developer/Core Faculty
American Holistic Nurses' Association
Certificate Program in Holistic Nursing
American Holistic Nurses' Association
Raleigh, North Carolina

Elizabeth Ann Manhart Barrett, RN, PhD, FAAN
Private Practice, Health Patterning
Professor and Coordinator, Center for Nursing
  Research
Hunter-Bellevue School of Nursing
Hunter College of the City University of New York
New York, New York

Genevieve M. Bartol, RN, EdD
Professor
University of North Carolina at Greensboro
School of Nursing
Greensboro, North Carolina

Margaret A. Burkhardt, RN-C, PhD
Associate Professor
Robert C. Byrd Health Sciences Center of West
  Virginia University
School of Nursing
Charleston, West Virginia

Nancy Fleming Courts, RN, PhD, NCC
Associate Professor and Chair
Adult Health Division
School of Nursing
University of North Carolina at Greensboro
Greensboro, North Carolina
Eloise R. Lewis Professor

Barbara Montgomery Dossey, RN, MS, HNC, FAAN
Director
Holistic Nursing Consultants
Santa Fe, New Mexico
Co-Director
Body Mind Systems
Temple, Texas

Joan Engebretson, RN, DrPH
Associate Professor
University of Texas Houston Health Science
  Center
School of Nursing
Houston, Texas

Noreen Cavan Frisch, RN, PhD, FAAN
Professor and Chair
Department of Nursing
Humboldt State University
Arcata, California

H. Lea Barbato Gaydos, RN, MSN, CS
Clinical Specialist
Assistant Professor
Director, Graduate Holistic Nursing Tract
Beth-El College of Nursing and Health Sciences
Colorado Springs, Colorado

Cathie E. Guzzetta, RN, PhD, FAAN
Director
Holistic Nursing Consultants
Dallas, Texas
Nursing Research Consultant
Parkland Memorial Hospital and Children's
  Medical Center
Dallas, Texas

Dorothea Hover-Kramer, RN, EdD
Licensed Clinical Psychologist
Advisory Council and Editorial Board
American Holistic Nurses' Association
Director Behavioral Health Consultants
Poway, California

Pamela Potter Hughes, RN, MA, MSN, CS, CHTP
Healing Touch Practitioner and Instructor
Nurse Therapist
Director
New Mexico Center for Nursing Therapeutics
Albuquerque, New Mexico

Lynette W. Jack, RN, PhD, CARN
Assistant Professor
Health and Community Systems Department
University of Pittsburgh
School of Nursing
Pittsburgh, Pennsylvania

Lynn Keegan, RN, PhD, FAAN, HNC
Associate Professor
University of Texas Health Science Center
School of Nursing
San Antonio, Texas

Leslie Gooding Kolkmeier, RN, BS, MEd
Private Practice
Celeste, Texas

Susan Luck, RN, MA
Health Educator
Holistic Nurse Consultant
Holistic Nursing Associates
New York, New York

Jane Yetter Lunt, RN, MEd, HNC
Co-Developer/Core Faculty
Certificate Program in Holistic Nursing
American Holistic Nurses' Association
Raleigh, North Carolina

E. Jane Martin, RN, PhD, FAAN
Dean and Professor
West Virginia University
School of Nursing
Morgantown, West Virginia

Charlotte McGuire, MA, RNC, HNC
Founder, Past President
American Holistic Nurses' Association
Co-Founder, Director
Southwest Institute for Women's Healing
  Journeys
Flagstaff, Arizona

Maggie McKivergin, RN, MS
The Center: A Resource for Lifelong Learning
  and Healing
Columbus, Ohio

Mary Gail Nagai-Jacobson, RN, MSN
Community Health Consultant
San Marcos, Texas

Melodie Olson, RN, PhD
Associate Professor
College of Nursing
Medical University of South Carolina
Charleston, South Carolina

Sue Popkess-Vawter, RN, PhD
Professor of Nursing
University of Kansas School of Nursing
Kansas City, Kansas

Janet F. Quinn, RN, PhD, FAAN
Associate Professor and Senior Scholar
Center for Human Caring
University of Colorado Health Sciences Center
School of Nursing
Denver, Colorado

Lynn Rew, BSN, MSN, EdD
Associate Professor
School of Nursing
The University of Texas at Austin
Austin, Texas

Sharon Scandrett-Hibdon, RN, PhD, CS, FNP
Family Nurse Practitioner
Professor
University of Tennessee-Memphis
Primary Care
Memphis, Tennessee

Eleanor A. Schuster, RN, DNSc
Associate Professor
College of Nursing
Florida Atlantic University
Boca Raton, Florida

Karilee Halo Shames, RN, PhD, HNC
Healing Touch Practitioner and Instructor
Director
Nurse Empowerment Workshops and Service
Mill Valley, California

Victoria E. Slater, RN, PhD, CHTI, HNC
Private Practitioner
Energetic Healing
Clarksville, Tennessee

Eileen M. Stuart, RN, MS, CS
Project Director, CAD Prevention Program,
Deaconess Hospital
Senior Scientist, Mind/Body Medical Institute,
Deaconess Hospital
Lecturer in Nursing, Boston College and
Simmons College
Associate in Medicine, Harvard Medical School
Boston, Massachusetts

Carol L. Wells-Federman, RN, MEd, MS
Clinical Specialist, Co-Director, Chronic Pain
Program, Deaconess Hospital
Adjunct Clinical Instructor, Graduate School for
Health Studies, Simmons College
Adjunct Instructor, School of Public Health,
Boston University
Associate in Medicine, Harvard Medical School
Boston, Massachusetts

Patty Wooten, RN, BSN
Nurse Humorist
President
Jest for the Health of It!
Davis, California

Christine A. Wynd, PhD, RN, CNAA
Associate Professor
Director of Nursing Research
University of Akron College of Nursing
Akron, Ohio

Anneke Young, RN, BSN, CNAT
Co-director, Wholistic Health Center
Academic Dean, School for Wholistic Nursing
Director, Wholistic Nursing Registry
The New Center for Wholistic Health Education
and Research
Syosset, New York

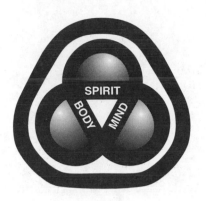

Reviewers

Gayle J. Acton, RN, PhD, CS
Clinical Specialty: Gerontological Nursing
Assistant Professor
The University of Texas at Austin, School of
Nursing
Austin, Texas

Karen Ahijevych, RN, PhD
Clinical Specialty: Adult Nursing
Assistant Professor
The Ohio State University College of Nursing
Columbus, Ohio

Sarah Jane H. Anderson, MSN, RNCS, CHTP
Clinical Specialty: Gerontological Nursing
Clinician/Owner
Nurturing Visions Holistic Nursing Practice
Albuquerque, New Mexico

Barbara C. Banonis, RN, MSN
Clinical Specialty: Health Promotion
Wellbeing Consultant
LifeQuest International
Charleston, West Virginia

Anne Boykin, RN, PhD
Clinical Specialty: Adult and Community Nursing
Professor and Dean
Florida Atlantic University College of Nursing
Boca Raton, Florida

Julia Byrd, RN, BA, CNAT
Clinical Specialty: Wholistic Nursing
Assistant Director of Wholistic Nursing
The New Center for Wholistic Health Education
and Research
Huntington, New York

Ruth Rosnick Carlson, MSN, RN
Clinical Specialty: Psychiatric-Mental Health
Nursing
Instructor
University of Akron College of Nursing
Akron, Ohio

Janet Cipkala-Gaffin, MSN, RN, CS
Clinical Specialty: Psychiatric Consultation/
Liaison Nursing
Clinical Nurse Specialist
University of Pittsburgh Medical Center
Pittsburgh, Pennsylvania

Jeanne Dorsey Colbath, RN, C, MS, ANP
Clinical Specialty: Cardiovascular Rehabilitation
Director
Cardiac Rehabilitation
St. Elizabeth's Medical Center
Boston, Massachusetts

Colleen Duggan, RN, MSN
Clinical Specialty: Medical-Surgical Nursing
Nursing Instructor
Johnson County Community College
Overland Park, Kansas

Helen L. Erickson, RN, PhD, FAAN
Clinical Specialty: Holistic Nursing
Professor and Chair
Holistic Adult Health Nursing
Special Assistant to the Dean, Graduate Studies
The University of Texas at Austin
Austin, Texas

Susan Ezra, RN
Clinical Specialty: Guided Imagery, Stress
  Management, Interactive Imagery^SM and
  Hospice Care
Co-Director
Nurses Certificate Program in Interactive
  Imagery^SM
San Rafael, California

Joan Furman, RN, MSN, HNC
Clinical Specialty: Holistic Nursing
Private Practice
Lecturer Community Health School of Nursing
Vanderbilt University
Nashville, Tennessee

Patricia W. George, RN, MSN
Clinical Specialty: Gerontology/Primary Care
Nurse Practitioner
ARH/Southern West Virginia Clinic
Beckley, West Virginia

Cathie E. Guzzetta, RN, PhD, FAAN
Clinical Specialty: Holistic Nursing/Research
Director
Holistic Nursing Consultants
Nurse Research Consultant
Parkland Memorial Hospital and Children's
  Medical Center
Dallas, Texas

Mary Enzman Hagedorn, RN, PhD, CNS, CPNP
Clinical Specialty: Pediatrics, Holistic Health
  Nursing
Associate Professor and Director
Graduate Family Nurse Practitioner Program
Beth-El College of Nursing and Health Sciences
Colorado Springs, Colorado

Elizabeth Heitman, PhD
Clinical Specialty: Ethics
Assistant Professor
University of Texas School of Public Health
Houston, Texas

Dorothy M. Johnson, EdD, RN
Clinical Specialty: Psychiatric-Mental Health
  Nursing
Assistant Professor
Department of Health Systems
West Virginia University School of Nursing
Morgantown, West Virginia

Mary B. Johnson, RN, PhD, OCN
Clinical Specialty: Oncology, Education
Associate Professor
St. Olaf College
Northfield, Minnesota

Lynn Keegan, RN, PhD, FAAN
Clinical Specialty: Holistic Nursing
Associate Professor
University of Texas Health Science Center at San
  Antonio
San Antonio, Texas

Katharine Kolcaba, RN, MSN, C
Clinical Specialty: Acute Care for Elders/Holistic
  Comfort Care
Instructor
Gerontological Nursing
The University of Akron College of Nursing
Akron, Ohio

Susan Lange, RN, BS
Clinical Specialty: Hospice
Home Care Hospice Nurse
Sharp Home Care and Hospice
Vista, California

Phyllis Mabbett, RN, PhD
Clinical Specialty: Mental Health
Acting Director
Behavioral Health Care Center
Scripps Memorial Hospital
La Jolla, California

Mary Madrid, RN, PhD
Clinical Specialty: Neuroscience Nursing
Clinical Nurse Associate
Neurointerventional Radiology
New York University Medical Center
New York, New York

Carol Lynn Mandle, PhD, RN
Clinical Specialty: Adult Health
Co-Director
Symptom Reduction Program
Scientist
Associate Professor
Boston College Graduate School of Nursing
Chestnut Hill, Massachusetts

Terry Miller, RN, MS
Clinical Specialty: Interactive Imagery^SM, Stress
  Management, Clinical Pathways
Co-Director
Nurses Certificate Program in Interactive
  Imagery^SM
Foster City, California

Ann Mitchell, RN, PhD
Clinical Specialty: Psychiatric/Mental Health
  Nursing
Assistant Professor
University of Pittsburgh School of Nursing
Pittsburgh, Pennsylvania

Darimell Mitchell-Waugh, RN, EdD
Clinical Specialty: Pediatrics/Adolescent
Associate Professor of Nursing
University of Texas Health Science Center
Houston, Texas

Susan Neary, MS, RNCS
Clinical Specialty: Gerontology/Home Care
Assistant Professor
Simmons College
Boston, Massachusetts

Marilyn Parker, RN, PhD
Clinical Specialty: Nursing in the Community
Professor and Associate Dean
Florida Atlantic University College of Nursing
Boca Raton, Florida

MaryAnn Ruffing-Rahal, PhD, RNC
Clinical Specialty: Community Health
Promotion
Associate Professor
Ohio State University College of Nursing
Columbus, Ohio

Liz Schaeffer-Teichler, MSN, RN-C, FNP
Clinical Specialty: Primary Care—Families and
Individuals
Senior Instructor
University of Colorado Health Sciences School
of Nursing
Denver, Colorado

Carole Schoffstall, RN, PhD
Clinical Specialty: Psychiatric/Mental Health
President and Dean
Beth-El College of Nursing and Health Sciences
Colorado Springs, Colorado

Mary K. Shannahan, RN, PhD, CPHN
Clinical Specialty: Women's Health/Nursing
Education
Associate Professor

Florida State University
Tallahassee, Florida

Aron Skrypeck, RN, MSN
Clinical Specialty: Child and Adolescent
Psychiatric Nursing
Independent Practice/Nurse Therapist
New Mexico Center for Nursing Therapeutics
Albuquerque, New Mexico

Nancy Telford, MSN, RN
Clinical Specialty: Holistic Nursing
Private Practitioner
Home Health Hospice Nurse
Clarksville Memorial Hospital Home Health and
Hospice
Clarksville, Tennessee

Kathleen Tovar, RN, MN
Clinical Specialty: Medical-Surgical Nursing
Nursing Instructor
MidAmerica Nazarene College
Kansas City, Missouri

Patricia C. Walsh, MA, RN, C, CNAA
Clinical Specialty: Mental Health/Community
Health/Administration
Nursing Instructor
Dominican College
Orangeburg, New York

Denise C. Webster, RN, PhD, CS
Clinical Specialty: Psychiatric-Mental Health
Nursing
Professor
University of Colorado Health Sciences School
of Nursing
Denver, Colorado

Pamela O. Werstlein, PhD, MN, RN, LPC
Clinical Specialty: Psychiatric/Mental Health
Assistant Professor
University of North Carolina
Greensboro, North Carolina

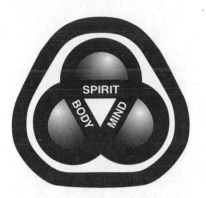

Foreword

When I started the American Holistic Nurses' Association in 1980, my vision was that all nurses would be holistic nurses. If Florence Nightingale could speak to us today, I believe she would say that this was her vision for nurses, too. The *American Holistic Nurses' Association (AHNA) Core Curriculum for Holistic Nursing* has been developed to further establish the discipline and foundation of holistic nursing practice and to assist nurses in their healing journey.

Many people ask what motivated me to start the AHNA. They are usually surprised when I say it was from a place of frustration and anger. I had an opportunity in the 1970s to observe a large number of health care facilities, first as a Medicare Program consultant and surveyor for the Texas Health Department and later as a corporate Vice President of Patient Care Services for 19 hospitals. In this capacity, I had unlimited opportunities to witness the lack of caring, compassion, support, and respect among nurses, physicians, and other health care providers. Many nurses were "burned out" with their jobs and with their profession. Most nurses had little or no focus on their own health and well-being. Health care administrators were focusing mostly on bottom line profits rather than quality of patient care or concern for the nursing staff. It was a sick health care system with sick health care providers. I was frustrated and angry because I believed that it did not have to be this way. Unfortunately, this is still the scenario in most acute care hospitals today.

In the late 1970s, I began to hear about holism, an ancient concept being re-introduced at a time when it was greatly needed in our world. It was an idea that struck a familiar cord. I knew immediately it would become a new paradigm for nursing and health care.

Wanting to learn quickly, I began to find books on the subject, and pioneering people simply appeared in my life. It was a fated meeting with Dr. C. Norman Shealy, Founder of the American Holistic Medical Association in La Crosse, Wisconsin in June 1980 that triggered the idea for me. An organization was needed for nurses to facilitate the healing of nurses and, ultimately, the healing of the nursing profession. It was a profound realization for me that healers need to heal themselves in order to change an ailing and failing health care system.

The founding meeting of the AHNA on January 17, 1981 in Houston, Texas, brought together 78 nurses from eight states. Nurses stood and told their stories of working in a health care system that did not value or respect them. Many expressed their hopes and visions of a nursing profession and a health care system that nurtured the nurturers and focused on "wellness" rather than "illness." That meeting clarified for me the idea that the AHNA was the vehicle for nurses to unite in support of each other as they learn to heal themselves. The challenge was to help nurses recognize and empower themselves as nurse healers and as nurse leaders.

With the new paradigm for the nursing profession, nurses are embracing and integrating holism into their nursing practice and their lives. This paradigm recognizes that we are all whole unitary beings that are interconnected with all that is called life. Now, many years later, holistic nurses are claiming their role in this emerging consciousness as nurse healers and are affecting both the nursing profession and the health care system.

The AHNA is taking bold and historic steps to enhance the discipline of holistic nursing. We are exploring and integrating holistic philosophy, holistic foundation, holistic ethics, holistic nursing and related research, and holistic nursing process with a focus on relationship-centered caring. Relationship-centered care involves three aspects of interactions: client–practitioner, community–practitioner, and practitioner–practitioner.

The AHNA intention is to realize the dream that one day all nurses will be holistic in both their personal lives and in their nursing practice.

Imagine your dream.

Hold it expectantly in your consciousness.

Watch it unfold.

Holistic nurses are walking the journey together, hand in hand, heart to heart, to manifest the common vision of caring and healing. The greater the number holding a unified vision, the more powerful the manifestation of that vision; therefore, let us unite to realize a healing health care system.

Charlotte McGuire, MA, RNC, HNC
Founder and Past President
American Holistic Nurses' Association
and
Co-Founder and Director
Southwest Institute for Women's Healing Journeys

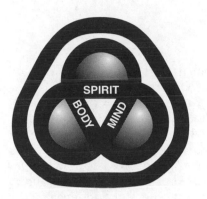

Preface

The *American Holistic Nurses' Association (AHNA) Core Curriculum for Holistic Nursing* has been developed to delineate the knowledge base for holistic nursing. The *AHNA Core Curriculum* not only will assist nurses interested in passing the holistic nursing certification (HNC) examination, but also will serve as a major reference for clinicians, educators, students, and researchers.

The scope of holistic nursing practice embraces the nurse, client, and various practice environments in which holistic nursing is provided. Radical changes are occurring in health care that are very dynamic. These changes provide holistic nurses with a greater opportunity to integrate caring and healing in their work and lives.

The AHNA has as its foundation the philosophy that nursing is an art and a science. The primary AHNA mission is to assist others toward the wholeness inherent within them. Holistic nursing is based on a broad and eclectic academic background that integrates artistic, scientific, analytic, and intuitive skills. The AHNA believes that health and disease are part of the human experience. Health involves the harmonious balance of body, mind, and spirit in an ever-changing environment. Disease and distress can be viewed as opportunities for increased awareness of the interconnectedness of body, mind, and spirit. The teaching–learning process enables nurses to assist people to assume personal responsibility for achieving health.

The AHNA has as its purpose the education of nurses and the public in the concepts and practice of health of the whole person. The AHNA objectives are as follows:

1. To encourage nurses to be models of wellness.
2. To improve the quality of health care by
   a. promoting education, participation, and self-responsibility for wellness.
   b. interacting with other health-related organizations.
   c. encouraging and reporting the research of holistic concepts and practice in nursing.
3. To function as an empowering network for persons interested in holistic nursing.
4. To explore, anticipate, and influence new directions and dimensions of health care, especially within the practice of nursing.

To operationalize the AHNA Standards of Holistic Nursing Practice (see Appendix A), the holistic nurse must possess knowledge of the standards of care and the standards of practice. The AHNA Standards of Holistic Nursing Practice provide the framework for the *AHNA Core Curriculum*. The AHNA Standards of

Holistic Nursing Practice has two major parts and addresses nine concepts as follows:

Part I: **Discipline of Holistic Nursing Practice**
Concept I.   Holistic Philosophy
Concept II.   Holistic Foundation
Concept III.   Holistic Ethics
Concept IV.   Holistic Nursing Theories
Concept V.   Holistic Nursing and Related Research
Concept VI.   Holistic Nursing Process

Part II: **Caring and Healing of Clients and Significant Others**
Concept VII.   Meaning and Wholeness
Concept VIII.   Client/Self-Care
Concept IX.   Health Promotion

Each of the 30 chapters within the *AHNA Core Curriculum* is organized by knowledge competencies, definitions, theories, and research. The nursing process is used to organize those chapters that develop specific caring–healing interventions. There is some replication of concepts, particularly in those chapters that have healing as part of the title. Each contributor was asked to conceptualize the chapter and to integrate the concepts of healing with the proposed topic. This replication will only enhance the learning, articulating, and integrating of the concepts, knowledge base, and holistic skills in clinical practice and holistic living. In Section I and Section II, the AHNA logo is inserted with a suggestion to *Pause for a moment . . .* to remind you to relax and affirm your HNC goal and mission in holistic nursing and holistic living.

The AHNA has established the knowledge and clinical competency in holistic nursing through its certification process. In 1997, the AHNA Certification Board completed the *IPAKHN Survey* (Inventory of Professional Activities and Knowledge of a Holistic Nurse) that defined and validated the professional activities statements and knowledge statements requisite for competent holistic nursing practice in various practice environments (see Appendix B). The *IPAKHN Survey* data analysis ensured adequate content validity for the HNC examination blueprint and revealed the percentage of HNC examination questions that should be apportioned for each content area.

The successful completion of the HNC examination offered by the AHNA is both a personal and a professional mark of achievement. Nurses who have passed the examination have the honor of listing the prized HNC after their name. Certification indicates excellence in the area of holistic nursing.

This is a remarkable time in the history of the AHNA and holistic nursing. Nurses are emerging on the doorsteps of the twenty-first century as nurse healers as they reclaim what has always been at the core of nursing and healing. Best wishes in your healing journey and in achieving your goal of holistic nursing certification.

* For more information on the application for the HNC examination, AHNA Certificate Program, and related programs, contact the AHNA:
American Holistic Nurses' Association (AHNA)
4101 Lake Boone Trail, Suite #200
Raleigh, North Carolina 27607
(919) 787-5181 or toll free (800) 278-AHNA
FAX (919) 787-4916

Barbara Montgomery Dossey, RN, MS, HNC, FAAN
Editor

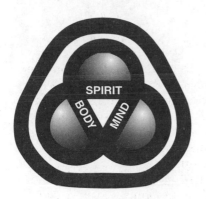

Acknowledgments

The *American Holistic Nurses' Association (AHNA) Core Curriculum for Holistic Nursing* represents the work of many people. From its inception as a proposal, the *AHNA Core Curriculum* was guided by the visionary AHNA Leadership Council, the AHNA Core Curriculum Committee, and the AHNA Certification Board. These dedicated nurse healers and nurse leaders provided encouragement, assistance, and advice.

The AHNA is indebted to the chapter contributors for their content expertise, their wisdom in holistic nursing and the healing arts, and their commitment to the development of the *AHNA Core Curriculum for Holistic Nursing.* Expert holistic nurses served as reviewers and offered their recommendations for improvements.

Special thanks are due to Jane Garwood, acquisitions editor at Aspen Publishers, Inc., who believed in the project from the beginning; to Ruth Bloom for her attention to editorial details; to Laura Smith for cover and book design, and production details; and to Gail Martin for her superb editing.

On a personal level, I would like to thank Larry Dossey—fellow writer, physician, colleague, and husband—for his love and healing presence in my life, and for his encouragement and support during this exciting project.

AHNA Core Curriculum Content

PART I

Discipline of
Holistic Nursing Practice

CONCEPT I

Holistic Philosophy

CHAPTER 1

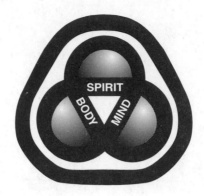

Holistic Nursing Practice

Barbara Montgomery Dossey

KNOWLEDGE COMPETENCIES

- Analyze the concept of holism.
- Contrast the allopathic model and the holistic model of care.
- Analyze the American Holistic Nurses' Association (AHNA) Description of Holistic Nursing.
- List the concepts addressed in the AHNA Standards of Holistic Nursing Practice.
- Discuss the mind/body dilemma.
- State the role and purpose of the Office of Complementary and Alternative Medicine (OCAM) at the National Institutes of Health (NIH).
- Contrast Era I medicine, Era II medicine, and Era III medicine and the states and manifestations of consciousness (local and nonlocal) in each era.
- Contrast the bio-psycho-social model and the bio-psycho-social-spiritual model.
- Describe the impact of meaning on an individual's perception of well-being and illness.
- List the three components of relationship-centered care.
- List four strategies for creating relationship-centered care.

DEFINITIONS

Allopathic Approach: a term erroneously used for the traditional practice of Western medicine to differentiate it from homeopathy; a system of treating by inducing a pathogenic reaction that is antagonistic to the disease being treated.

Alternative/Complementary Therapies: nontraditional therapies that can interface with traditional medical and surgical therapies; they may be used as complements to conventional medical treatments (see OCAM, pp. 6, 7).

Bio-Psycho-Social-Spiritual Model: the biologic, psychologic, sociologic, and spiritual elements that give meaning to a person's existence.

Healing: a process of integrating and balancing the parts of oneself at a deep level of inner knowledge in a way that gives each part equal importance and value; sometimes referred to as self-healing or wholeness.

Holism: the view that an integrated whole has a reality independent of and greater than the sum of its parts.

Process: the continual changing and evolution of one's self through life; the reflection of meaning and purpose in living.

Spirituality: values, meaning, and purpose; a turning inward to the human traits of honesty, love, caring, wisdom, imagination, and compassion; existence of a quality of a higher authority, guiding spirit, or transcendence that is mystical; a flowing dynamic balance that allows and creates healing of body-mind-spirit; sometimes involves organized religion.

Transpersonal: the quality of transcending or going beyond personal and individual identity to broader purposes, meanings, values, and unification with universal principles.

Pause for a moment . . .

❏ *I am studying the **AHNA Core Curriculum for Holistic Nursing** to enhance my ability to enunciate the knowledge base for holistic nursing.*

❏ *I am studying the **AHNA Core Curriculum for Holistic Nursing** to accomplish my personal goal of successfully completing the holistic nursing certification (HNC) examination.*

❏ *I am proud of the goal that I have set for myself.*

THEORIES AND RESEARCH

Holism

1. As a way of viewing everything in terms of patterns and processes that combine to form a whole, instead of seeing things as fragments, pieces, or parts,[1] holism has important implications for views of health-wellness-disease-illness. (See Chapters 4 and 5.)

2. Current focus in health care is on technology and allopathy. (See Table 1–1 for a comparison of the allopathic model and the holistic model of care.)

3. In the holistic model, primary assertions are that consciousness is real and that it is related to all matters of health-wellness-disease-illness.

4. Holistic nursing is the most complete way to conceptualize and practice professional nursing.
   a. The purpose of the AHNA is to promote the education of nurses and the public in the concepts and practice of health of the whole person.
      1) The AHNA Description of Holistic Nursing is seen in Exhibit 1–1.
      2) The AHNA Standards of Holistic Nursing Practice define and establish the scope of holistic practice. (See Appendix A, AHNA Standards of Holistic Nursing Practice.)
   b. The concepts of holistic nursing are based on broad and eclectic academic principles (Exhibit 1–2). Holistic concepts incorporate a sensitive balance between art and science,

Table 1–1 Assumptions of Allopathic and Holistic Models of Care

Allopathic Model	Holistic Model
Treatment of symptoms	Search for patterns, causes
Specialized	Integrated; concerned with the whole patient
Emphasis on efficiency	Emphasis on human values
Professional should be emotionally neutral	Professional's caring is a component of healing
Pain and disease are wholly negative	Pain and disease may be valuable signals of internal conflicts
Primary intervention with drugs, surgery	Minimal intervention with appropriate technology, complemented with a range of noninvasive techniques (psychotechnologies, diet, exercise)
Body seen as a machine in good or bad repair	Body seen as a dynamic system, a complex energy field within fields (family, workplace, environment, culture, life history)
Disease or disability seen as an entity	Disease or disability seen as a process
Emphasis on eliminating symptoms and disease	Emphasis on achieving maximum bodymind health
Patient is dependent	Patient is autonomous
Professional is authority	Professional is therapeutic partner
Body and mind are separate; psychosomatic illnesses seen as mental; may refer (patient) to psychiatrist	Bodymind perspective, psychosomatic illness is the province of all health care professionals
Mind is secondary factor in organic illness	Mind is primary or co-equal factor in all illness
Placebo effect is evidence of power of suggestion	Placebo effect is evidence of mind's role in disease and healing
Primary reliance on quantitative information (charts, tests, and dates)	Primary reliance on qualitative information, including patient reports and professional's intuition; quantitative data an adjunct
"Prevention" seen as largely environmental; vitamins, rest, exercise, immunization, not smoking	"Prevention" synonymous with wholeness: in work, relationships, goals, body-mind-spirit

Source: Reprinted by permission of J.P. Tarcher, Inc., a division of The Putnam Publishing Group from THE AQUARIAN CONSPIRACY by Marilyn Ferguson. Copyright © 1980 by Marilyn Ferguson.

Exhibit 1–1 American Holistic Nurses' Association Description of Holistic Nursing

Holistic nursing embraces all nursing practice which has healing the whole person as its goal. Holistic nursing recognizes that there are two views regarding holism: that holism involves studying and understanding the interrelationships of the bio-psycho-social-spiritual dimensions of the person, recognizing that the whole is greater than the sum of its parts; and that holism involves understanding the individual as an integrated whole interacting with and being acted upon by both internal and external environments. Holistic nursing accepts both views, believing that the goals of nursing can be achieved within either framework.

Holistic practice draws on nursing knowledge, theories, expertise, and intuition to guide nurses in becoming therapeutic partners with clients in strengthening the clients' responses to facilitate the healing process and achieve wholeness.

Practicing holistic nursing requires nurses to integrate self-care in their own lives. Self-responsibility leads the nurse to a greater awareness of the interconnectedness of all individuals and their relationships to the human and global community, and permits nurses to use this awareness to facilitate healing.

Source: Reprinted with permission from The American Holistic Nurses' Association, 4101 Lake Boone Trail, Suite 201, Raleigh, NC 27607, Phone: 1-800-278-AHNA, Fax: 919-787-4916.

analytic and intuitive skills, self-care skills, and the ability and interconnectedness of body, mind, and spirit.

  c. Holistic nursing concepts can be integrated into the care provided in any setting: hospital, clinic, community agency, and home.

  d. The AHNA Networker Guidelines provide information on how a nurse can start a local AHNA network in the community.

    1) A local AHNA network is an excellent way to explore holistic nursing in professional and personal domains.

    2) Within hospitals, clinics, or community agencies, staff members may find that brown bag lunch sessions, in-service education, and videos on holistic nursing are useful ways to explore caring–healing modalities and their implementation.

  e. There are two mechanisms to achieve AHNA certification (for details of each program, write AHNA):

    1) AHNA Holistic Nursing Certificate Program.

    2) AHNA Certification Examination is based on the AHNA Core Curriculum for Holistic Nursing and the IPAKHN Survey, The Inventory of Professional Activities and Knowledge of a Holistic Nurse (IPAKHN; see Appendix B).

The Mind/Body Dilemma

1. The relationship between mind and body has been called one of the most difficult philosophical problems in the history of Western medicine.

2. The mind–body split is a reductionistic view that rejects any consideration of the relationship between mind and body.

3. Medical science has focused on the anatomic, physiologic, cellular, molecular, genetic, and pharmacologic methods of decreasing, stabilizing, or reversing disease. This focus has concentrated solely on the body.

  a. Western medicine can no longer ignore the potent forms of physical, psychologic, social, and spiritual interventions that have surfaced outside mainstream medicine.

  b. The Office of Complementary and Alternative Medicine (OCAM) at the NIH has been established to evaluate complementary and alternative therapies. These therapies fall into seven fields of practice:[2]

Exhibit 1–2 Concepts Addressed in Holistic Nursing Practice

PART I: DISCIPLINE OF HOLISTIC NURSING PRACTICE

Concept I.	Holistic Philosophy
Concept II.	Holistic Foundation
Concept III.	Holistic Ethics
Concept IV.	Holistic Nursing Theories
Concept V.	Holistic Nursing and Related Research
Concept VI.	Holistic Nursing Process

PART II: CARING AND HEALING OF CLIENTS AND SIGNIFICANT OTHERS

Concept VII.	Meaning and Wholeness
Concept VIII.	Client Self-Care
Concept IX.	Health Promotion

Source: Reprinted with permission from a working document of the American Holistic Nurses' Association. Copyright © June 1996, The American Holistic Nurses' Association, 4101 Lake Boone Trail, Suite 201, Raleigh, NC 27607. Phone 1-800-278-AHNA; Fax (919) 787-4916.

1) mind/body or biobehavioral interventions (biofeedback, relaxation, imagery, meditation, hypnosis, psychotherapy, prayer, art, dance, music therapy, yoga)
2) bioelectromagnetics (BEM) application in medicine (study of various BEM devices and eight new applications of nonthermal, nonionizing EM fields for bone repairs, nerve stimulation, wound healing, osteoarthritis, electroacupuncture, immune system stimulation, neuroendocrine modulation)
3) alternative systems of healing (traditional oriental medicine, acupuncture, ayurvedic medicine, homeopathic medicine, anthroposophically extended medicine, naturopathic medicine, environmental medicine, community-based health care practice [shamans, Native American Indian, AA programs])
4) manual healing methods (osteopathy, massage, cranial-sacral, chiropractic, physical therapy, biofield therapeutics [therapeutic touch, healing touch, Huna, Qigong, Mar-iel, Reiki, kinesiology, polarity])
5) pharmacological and biologic treatments (antineoplastons, cartilage products, EDTA Chelation Therapy, ozone, immunoaugmentative therapy, 714-X, Hoxsey methods, Essiac, Coley's toxins, MTH-68, neural therapy, apitherapy, mistletoe)
6) herbal medicine (various herbs from Europe, China, Asia, India, and Native American Herbal Medicine)
7) diet and nutrition in the prevention of chronic disease (study of various food groups, vitamins, minerals on acute and chronic disease)

It is essential that nurses understand the nurse practice act in their state, however. Because each state nurse practice act is different, the permitted practice of alternative/complementary therapies may vary.

Eras of Medicine

1. Three eras of medicine are operational in Western medicine (Table 1–2).[3]
   a. Era I medicine focuses on combining drugs, medical treatments, and technology. A person's consciousness is considered a by-product of the chemical, anatomic, and physiologic aspects of the brain and is not perceived as a major factor in the origins of health or disease.
   b. Era II medicine involves therapies based on the principle that the actions of a person's mind or consciousness—thoughts, emotions, beliefs, meaning, and attitudes—exert important effects on the behavior of the physical body. In both Era I medicine and Era II medicine, a person's consciousness is said to be "local" in nature; that is, he or she is confined to a specific location in space (the body itself), and in time (the present moment and a single lifetime).
   c. Era III medicine has emerged from science. It is said to be a "nonlocal" era, which implies that consciousness is not bound to individual bodies. Rather, minds of individuals are spread throughout space and time; they are infinite, immortal, omnipresent, and ultimately one.
2. Era II medicine and Era III medicine take into account the transpersonal healing and caring (see Chapter 2), psychophysiology of body-mind healing (see Chapter 5), spirituality and healing (see Chapter 6), energetic healing (see Chapter 7), and all concepts addressed in the *AHNA Core Curriculum for Holistic Nursing.*

The Bio-Psycho-Social Model versus the Bio-Psycho-Social-Spiritual Model

1. The bio-psycho-social model has been generally accepted and represents the most comprehensive model available in mainstream health care.
   a. The bio-psycho-social model suggests that all disease has a psychosomatic component.
   b. Biologic, psychologic, and social factors are always involved in a patient's symptoms, disease, or illness.
   c. Various states of consciousness and spirituality are secondary factors in this model.
2. The bio-psycho-social-spiritual model provides a more complete and holistic understanding of human function; it is the most comprehensive model for holistic clinical practice, education, and research.[4,5]
   a. The bio-psycho-social-spiritual model illustrates that all four parameters are interdependent and interrelated (Figure 1–1).
   b. The advocates of this model assert that all these components must be addressed for optimal therapeutic results.

Table 1–2 Eras of Medicine

	Era I	Era II	Era III
Space–time characteristic	Local	Local	Nonlocal
Synonym	Mechanical, material, or physical medicine	Mind–body medicine	Nonlocal or transpersonal medicine
Description	Casual, deterministic, describable by classical concepts of space–time and matter–energy. Mind not a factor; "mind" a result of brain mechanisms.	Mind a major factor in healing *within* the single person. Mind has causal power; is thus not fully explainable by classical concepts in physics. Includes but goes beyond Era I.	Mind a major factor in healing both *within* and *between* persons. Mind not completely localized to points in space (brains or bodies) or time (present moment or single lifetimes). Mind is unbounded and infinite in space and time—thus omnipresent, eternal, and ultimately unitary or one. Healing at a distance is possible. Not describable by classical concepts of space–time or matter–energy.
Examples	Any form of therapy focusing solely on the effects of things on the body are Era I approaches—including techniques such as accupuncture and homeopathy, the use of herbs, etc. Almost all forms of "modern" medicine—drugs, surgery, irradiation, CPR, etc.—are included.	Any therapy emphasizing the effects of consciousness solely within the individual body is an Era II approach. Psychoneuroimmunology, counseling, hypnosis biofeedback, relaxation therapies, and most types of imagery-based "alternative" therapies are included.	Any therapy in which effects of consciousness bridge between different persons is an Era III approach. All forms of distant healing, intercessory prayer, some types of shamanic healing, diagnosis at a distance, telesomatic events, and probably noncontact therapeutic touch are included.

Source: Reprinted from *Healing Words: The Power of Prayer and the Practice of Medicine* by Larry Dossey, pp. 40–41, Harper San Francisco, with permission of Larry Dossey, © 1993.

c. Regardless of the technology, therapy, or treatment used, the human spirit must be addressed as a major healing force in reversing, stabilizing, and producing remission in diseases and illnesses.[6]

d. The human spirit becomes enfolded in a person's being, and the perceptions of meaning can make the difference between life and death.

e. The spiritual dimension incorporates a person's values, meaning, and purpose in life. (See Chapter 6.)

f. The individual's perception of meaning is related to all factors in health-wellness-disease-illness.

Exploration of Meaning

1. Phenomenology is a philosophy that focuses primarily on the question, "What does it mean to be human?"[7]

2. Meaning involves differences, contrasts, novelty, and heterogeneity; it is necessary for the healthy function of human beings.

3. Life is fuller and richer when it means something positive; it is not worth living without important meaning.

4. Meaning makes it possible to recognize more effective ways to cope with life and to work on life issues.

5. Meaning allows caregivers to be more effective guides when helping others search for the meanings in their lives.

6. The meanings that a person attaches to symptoms or illness are probably the most important influences on that person's journey through a life crisis. Human beings can view illness from at least eight frames of references:
   a. As a challenge.
   b. As an enemy.
   c. As a punishment.
   d. As a weakness.

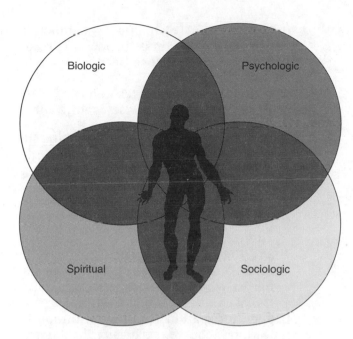

Figure 1–1 The Bio-Psycho-Social-Spiritual Model. *Source:* Reprinted from *Cardiovascular Nursing: Holistic Practice* by C.E. Guzzetta and B.M. Dossey, p. 6, with permission of Mosby–Year Book, © 1992.

e. As a relief.

f. As a strategy.

g. As an irreparable loss or damage.

h. As a value.[8]

7. Because they are individual and personal, meanings must have congruence with the person's experience, belief systems, rationality, expectations, and the context of the event. Context involves a person's past and present life story, as well as his or her beliefs about future events.

8. Interpretation and meaning are part of the syntactic category of learning. In syntax, one finds or seeks meanings through wholes, broad relationships, insights, and patterns. Only when some meaning is found can an experience become a paradigm experience. A person seldom retains meaningless experiences to form a foundation for future reference.[9]

9. Meaning is directly linked with mind modulation of all the body systems that influence states of health-wellness-disease-illness.

10. Recognizing that meanings in wellness and illness are vastly complex, that wellness is not a matter of considering simply the physical state, places much more responsibility on the individual and less on the physician for that individual's health.

11. Individual meanings are very personal; individuals must attend to their own meanings in the way that is best for them.

12. Meanings are never "all physical" or "all mental." It is no longer possible to defend these simplistic statements in modern medical and nursing science. Those who make such claims cannot even define "the physical" or "the mental," for there is no dividing line between them.

13. All other factors being equal, meanings and positive perceptions can actually increase the level of a person's health. Meanings can be as therapeutic as a medication or a surgical procedure.

 Pause for a moment . . .

❑ *The **AHNA Core Curriculum for Holistic Nursing** serves me as a major reference in my work and life.*

❑ *My study of the **AHNA Core Curriculum for Holistic Nursing** has significant value beyond the HNC examination.*

❑ *Practicing holistic nursing and living a holistic lifestyle bring me joy.*

Relationship-Centered Care

1. The Pew Health Professions Commission on Education for Health Care Professionals has described three essential components of relationship-centered care, each involving a unique set of tasks and responsibilities in the areas of knowledge, values, and skills:[10]

a. Patient–practitioner relationship.*

1) Reflection on skills and practice of increasing self-awareness of caring, healing, values, ethics, and ways to enhance and preserve the dignity and integrity of the patient and the family are required.

2) The practitioner collects data about the patient's symptoms and individual needs, and then incorporates the information into comprehensive biotechnologic care.

3) Active collaboration with the patient and the family in the decision-making process, including activities to promote health and

---

*The word *client* is interchangeable with the word *patient* in this model.

prevent stress/illness within the family, is also part of the relationship.

4) Listening actively and communicating effectively reduce the power inequalities with regard to race, sex, education, occupation, and socioeconomic status (Table 1–3).

b. Community–practitioner relationship.

1) Nurses are developing an increased awareness of the range of relationships and cultural diversity in the care of individuals. (See Chapter 13.)

2) Patients, their families, and their significant others simultaneously belong to many types of communities, such as the hospital community, immediate family, relatives, friends, co-workers, neighborhoods, and religious organizations.

3) Practitioners must be sensitive to the various communities and develop a sense of cooperation as these communities interact with the patient and the family.

4) The harmful elements that block a person's healing must be identified and improved to enhance health and well-being (Table 1–4).

c. Practitioner–practitioner relationship.

1) There are many diverse practitioner–practitioner relationships.

2) Practitioners should be aware of the diversity of healing modalities and the many different types of practitioners, as well as the range of healing modalities that they use.

3) Practitioners must be willing to integrate alternative/complementary practices and therapies (e.g., relaxation, imagery, music and touch therapies, folk healers, herbs) when appropriate in the traditional clinic and hospital setting.

4) Such integration requires continuously learning about the experiences of different healers, appreciating different modalities, and valuing cultural diversity (Table 1–5).

Table 1–3 Patient–Practitioner Relationship: Areas of Knowledge, Skills, and Values

Area	Knowledge	Skills	Values
Self-awareness	Knowledge of self Understanding self as a resource to others	Reflect on self and work	Importance of self-awareness, self-care, self-growth
Patient experience of health and illness	Role of family, culture, community in development Multiple components of health Multiple threats and contributors to health as dimensions of one reality	Recognize patient's life story and its meaning View health and illness as part of human development	Appreciation of the patient as a whole person Appreciation of the patient's life story and the meaning of the health-illness condition
Developing and maintaining caring relationships	Understanding of threats to the integrity of the relationship (e.g., power inequalities) Understanding of potential for conflict and abuse	Attend fully to the patient Accept and respond to distress in patient and self Respond to moral and ethical challenges Facilitate hope, trust, and faith	Respect for patient's dignity, uniqueness, and integrity (mind-body-spirit unity) Respect for self-determination Respect for person's own power and self-healing processes
Effective communication	Elements of effective communication	Listen Impart information Learn Facilitate the learning of others Promote and accept patient's emotions	Importance of being open and nonjudgmental

Source: PEW Health Professions Commission at the Center for the Health Professions, University of California, San Francisco, 1388 Sutter Street, Suite 805, San Francisco, California 94109, (415) 476-8181.

Table 1–4 Community–Practitioner Relationship: Areas of Knowledge, Skills, and Values

Area	Knowledge	Skills	Values
Meaning of community	Various models of community Myths and misperceptions about community Perspectives from the social sciences, humanities, and systems theory Dynamic change—demographic, political, industrial	Learn continuously Participate actively in community development and dialogue	Respect for the integrity of the community Respect for cultural diversity
Multiple contributors to health within the community	History of community, land use, migration, occupations, and their effect on health Physical, social, and occupational environments and their effects on health External and internal forces influencing community health	Critically assess the relationship of health care providers to community health Assess community and environmental health Assess implications of community policy affecting health	Affirmation of relevance of all determinants of health Affirmation of the value of health policy in community services Recognition of the presence of values that are destructive to health
Developing and maintaining community relationships	History of practitioner–community relationships Isolation of the health care community from the community-at-large	Communicate ideas Listen openly Empower others Learn Facilitate the learning of others Participate appropriately in community development and activism	Importance of being open-minded Honesty regarding the limits of health science Responsibility to contribute health expertise
Effective community-based care	Various types of care, both formal and informal Effects of institutional scale on care Positive effects of continuity of care	Collaborate with other individuals and organizations Work as member of a team or healing community Implement change strategies	Respect for community leadership Commitment to work for change

Source: PEW Health Professions Commission at the Center for the Health Professions, University of California, San Francisco, 1388 Sutter Street, Suite 805, San Francisco, California 94109, (415) 476-8181.

2. Many strategies are available for creating relationship-centered care.
   a. Holistic nurses must become more engaged in educational and clinical strategies to assist students, practitioners, and educators.
   b. It is essential to approach these strategies not as competencies or skills to be learned, but as a new way of being, seeing, and experiencing the healing capacities within oneself.
   c. Four strategies are crucial to the process.
      1) Through mentorship, holistic nurses can share and explore the scientific principles as well as the intuitive hunches that guide their practice and the coordination of care; they can model caring–healing practices. Mentorees will experience enhanced self-awareness, values, skills, and open communication about new possibilities.
      2) Noncompetitive assessment of individuals' educational attainments is an empowering process that reinforces relationship-building between faculty, clinicians, and students; numerous

Table 1–5 Practitioner–Practitioner Relationship: Areas of Knowledge, Skills, and Values

Area	Knowledge	Skills	Values
Self-awareness	Knowledge of self	Reflect on self and needs	Importance of self-aware-
		Learn continuously	ness
Traditions of knowledge in health professions	Healing approaches of various professions	Derive meaning from others' work	Affirmation and value of diversity
	Healing approaches across cultures	Learn from experience within healing community	
	Historical power inequities across professions		
Building teams and communities	Perspectives on team-building from the social sciences	Communicate effectively	Affirmation of mission
		Listen openly	Affirmation of diversity
		Learn cooperatively	
Working dynamics of teams, groups, and organizations	Perspectives on team dynamics from the social sciences	Share responsibility responsibly	Openness to others' ideas
			Humility
		Collaborate with others	Mutual trust, empathy, support
		Work cooperatively	
		Resolve conflicts	Capacity for grace

Source: PEW Health Professions Commission at the Center for the Health Professions, University of California, San Francisco, 1388 Sutter Street, Suite 805, San Francisco, California 94109, (415) 476-8181.

quantitative and qualitative approaches can be used to evaluate the depth of attitudes, knowledge, and skills.

3) An ongoing educational strategy of support for practitioners and faculty development is essential to the learning and development of the skills to be integrated into the healing process; participation in an evolving process of healing relationships enhances the creativity and the ability of students, practitioners, and faculty.

4) Information management and dissemination systems incorporate computer-based learning programs, support groups, audiovisual self-paced programs,[11,12] role playing, sharing stories, and cultural diversity; clarify the meaning of data related to the many factors that influence health-wellness-disease-illness; and reveal patterns of practice, established outcomes, the origins of care, and the need for quality improvement activities for patient, communities, and practitioners.

REFERENCES

1. L. von Bertalanffy, *General Systems Theory* (New York: George Braziller, 1972).

2. *Alternative Medicine: Expanding Medical Horizons* (Chantilly, VA: NIH Report No. 94-066, 1994).

3. L. Dossey, *Healing Words: The Power of Prayer and the Practice of Medicine* (San Francisco, CA: Harper San Francisco, 1993).

4. B.M. Dossey et al., *Holistic Nursing: A Handbook for Practice,* 2nd ed. (Gaithersburg, MD: Aspen Publishers, 1995).

5. B.M. Dossey and C.E. Guzzetta, Holistic Cardiovascular Nursing, in *Cardiovascular Nursing: Holistic Practice,* ed. C.E. Guzzetta and B.M. Dossey (St. Louis: Mosby–Year Book, 1992), p. 6.

6. L. Dossey, *Prayer Is Good Medicine* (San Francisco, CA: Harper San Francisco, 1996).

7. P. Munhall, *Revisioning Phenomenology: Nursing and Health Science Research* (New York: National League for Nursing, 1994).

8. Z.J. Lipowski, Physical Illness, the Individual and the Coping Process, *Psychiatric Medicine* 1 (1970): 90.

9. E.O. Bevis, Accessing Learning: Determining Worth or Developing Excellence—From a Behaviorist toward an Interpretative–Criticism Model, *Toward a Caring Curriculum: A New Pedagogy for Nursing,* ed. E.O. Bevis and J. Watson (New York: National League for Nursing, 1990).

10. C.P. Tresolini and the Pew–Fetzer Task Force, *Health Professions Education and Relationship-Centered Care* (San Francisco: Pew Health Professions Commission, 1994).

11. *Holistic Nursing* (Raleigh, NC: American Holistic Nurses' Association, 1996). Video available through 1-800-278-AHNA.

12. *At the Heart of Healing: Experiencing Holistic Nursing* (Woodstock, NY: Kineholistic Foundation, 1994). Video available through 1-800-255-1914, ext 277.

CHAPTER 2

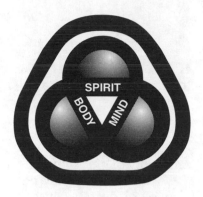

Transpersonal Human Caring and Healing

Janet F. Quinn

KNOWLEDGE COMPETENCIES

- Identify the elements of a "caring occasion."
- Compare and contrast the processes of healing and curing.
- Discuss the nature of "right relationship" as it applies to healing.
- Discuss examples of healing at the body, mind, and spirit levels of human experience.
- Analyze the nature of control and prediction in the healing process.
- Describe a healing health care system.
- Identify ways in which the nurse is the healing environment.
- Discuss the concept of the "wounded healer," and apply it to holistic nursing practice.

DEFINITIONS

Healing: the emergence of "right relationship" at one or more levels of the body-mind-spirit system.[1]

Healing System: a true health care system in which people can receive adequate, nontoxic, and noninvasive assistance in maintaining wellness and in healing for body, mind, and spirit, as well as benefit from the most sophisticated, aggressive curing technologies in the world, when necessary. Such a system has not yet been created; only half the healing system—the allopathic, curing half—is currently available.

Human Caring: the moral ideal of nursing in which the whole self of the nurse is brought into relationship with the whole self of the patient/client to protect the vulnerability and preserve the humanity and dignity of the patient/client.[2]

Right Relationship: a process of connection among or between parts of the whole that increases energy, coherence, and creativity in the whole body-mind-spirit system.

Transpersonal: that which transcends the limits and boundaries of individual ego identities and possibilities to include acknowledgment and appreciation of something greater. Transpersonal may refer to consciousness, intrapersonal dynamics, interpersonal relationships and lived experiences of connection, unity and oneness with the larger environment, cosmos, and/or Spirit.

THEORIES AND RESEARCH

Transpersonal Human Caring

1. Nurses who enter into caring–healing relationships with patients, bringing with them an acknowledgment and appreciation of the body, mind, and spirit dimensions of human existence, are engaged in a transpersonal human caring process.
2. In this type of relationship, the nurse feels interconnected with the patient and with the larger environment and cosmos. Nurses know that they are walking on sacred ground when they walk this path with their patients, and they recognize that neither will be the same afterward. Watson called these healing encounters "caring occasions,"[3] which actually transcend the bounds of space and time.
3. The field of consciousness created in and through the caring–healing relationship has the potential to continue healing the patient

long after the physical separation of nurse and patient.

Healing: The Emergence of "Right Relationship"

1. The origin of the word *heal* is the Anglo-Saxon word "haelan," which means to be or to become whole.
2. Wholeness is frequently understood to mean harmony of body, mind, and spirit, while harmony may be defined as an esthetically pleasing set of relationships among the elements of the whole.
3. Wholeness is not just about the structure and function of the physical body, nor is it a state of being in perfect balance at every level. Rather, wholeness is fundamentally about relationship.
4. Healing is a process rather than a state. It is the emergence of "right relationship" at any one or more levels of the human body-mind-spirit system.
5. "Right relationship," in this context, refers to a process that maximizes the energy in the body-mind-spirit system to do the work of the system. Right relationship increases coherence and decreases chaos in the system, thus gaining for the system maximum freedom, choice, and capacity to creatively unfold.
6. For this reason, true healing is always a process of emergence into something new, rather than a simple returning to a prior state of being.
7. Healing occurs at different levels:
   a. Body: the bonding together, the new relationship, of cells and tissues as wounds close or fractures knit.
   b. Mind/emotion: a shift from resentment to forgiveness in relation to an event in the past, releasing energy for new growth and an expanded consciousness.
   c. Spirit: the experience of being loved unconditionally and for all time, allowing the person to transcend the sense of separateness and feel at one with God and all of creation.

 Pause for a moment . . .

❏ *I am visualizing successful completion of the holistic nursing certification (HNC) examination as a mark of achievement and proficiency.*

❏ *I am preparing for successful completion of the HNC examination as defined by the AHNA Certification Board.*

Healing vs. Curing

1. Curing is the elimination of the signs and symptoms of disease, which may or may not end the patient's disease or distress, since it involves only one dimension of the body-mind-spirit system.
2. Empirics, that is, the use of the five senses and their technologic extensions (e.g., X-ray and laboratory data) make curing measurable.
3. Healing is harder to measure empirically and requires the use of the whole self, both of nurse and of the patient, in other ways of knowing such as personal/intuitive knowing, esthetic knowing, and/or ethical knowing[4] (see Chapter 3).
4. Sometimes a healing moment is noticed as a felt sense of awe, surprise, or peacefulness in the nurse and/or the patient. The nurse healer pays attention to these subtle cues of healing and reflects them back to the patient when appropriate.
5. Curing may occur without healing; for example, the patient who returns to her unhealthy preoperative lifestyle following successful bypass surgery is cured, but may not be healed.
6. Conversely, healing may occur without curing; for example, the person who is living with AIDS may find that his relationship to long-hidden or rejected parts of the self, estranged family members, or God is shifting. In this context, the dying process may be a healing process.
7. Healing is always possible, while curing is not. Healing, the emergence of "right relationship," may occur up to and including the moment of death. In fact, some spiritual traditions call death "the ultimate healing." In this context, a healing model is always optimistic, always hopeful.
8. There is no way to predict the outcome of any individual's healing process or the length of time that it will take. Healing is completely unique and may not be coerced, manipulated, or controlled—by the one healing or by anyone else. The nurse healer facilitates this process as a sort of midwife but does not carry out the healing.

9. All healing emerges from within the unique body-mind-spirit of the patient. Sometimes, but not always, therapeutics (i.e., drugs, surgery, complementary therapies) provide assistance, but they are not sufficient alone.

10. The assumption that the patient accomplishes all healing and curing does not mean that all healing and curing are controlled by the patient. The causes of illness and cure are so complex and multifaceted that no simple statement of cause and effect is appropriate.

11. One can participate knowledgeably in the healing process, formulating a healing intention and doing what he or she believes is best in this situation, but the outcome of that process is a mystery even to the one healing. If we accept the premise that we are indeed body-mind-spirit, we must also accept that at least part of the healing process will always be a mystery unfolding. Suggesting otherwise to patients may contribute to their sense of failure when they are unable to cure themselves of disease. Nurses must remember that caring is a moral commitment to protect the vulnerability of another, not add to it.

A True Healing System: Integrating the Masculine and the Feminine

1. The Western sick-care/medical system is the best in the world. Because men have created that system and continue to be the dominant culture of the system, it is characterized almost exclusively by attributes usually considered masculine. These attributes include an emphasis on decisive intervention, curing, fixing, precision, "power over," and goal/outcome-oriented approaches. This approach is extremely useful in the treatment of acute injury and illness, but is incomplete.

2. To facilitate true healing, it is essential to walk in the unknown, using all ways of knowing and following the lead of the patient. These qualities are usually associated with the feminine principles of receptivity, intuition, nurturing, caring, tending, "shared power," and process-oriented approaches.

3. The current health care system is characterized by the masculine principle and focuses almost exclusively on curing. Thus, all patients and providers alike are denied the healing potential inherent within the feminine principle.

4. The true health care system will finally emerge when both sets of attributes, masculine and feminine, are equally valued and available to guide the work of all men and women.

 Pause for a moment . . .

❑ *My studying of the **AHNA Core Curriculum for Holistic Nursing** is satisfying.*
❑ *I am preparing for successful completion of the HNC examination to prepare for my present and future role as a holistic nurse.*

The Nurse As Healing Environment

1. One of the most powerful tools for healing is the presence of the nurse in the patient's environment. Simply by virtue of the role, a nurse has all the ritual power of the shaman of other cultures. The nurse is guardian of the patient's journey through illness and healing.

2. In a model of the universe that includes the nonlocal nature of consciousness[5] or the possibility for the existence of a human energy field that extends beyond the skin,[6] the nurse is not simply part of the patient's environment—the nurse *is* the patient's environment. As Newman noted, "In the case of a nurse interacting with a patient, the energy fields of the two interact and form a new pattern of interpenetration, spirit within spirit."[7]

3. The nurse's intentional shift of consciousness into a centered or meditative state may maximize the healing environment of the patient. The interconnectedness of the energy fields of the nurse and the patient can facilitate relaxation, rest, and/or healing.[8]

4. When the nurse is centered in the present moment, the nurse's intention to be a healing environment may be carried in the energy field and also manifested in the voice, the eyes, and the quality of touching.

   a. The voice of a relaxed and centered person carries a different vibration than the voice of someone who is stressed, hurried, or angry. In considering the use of voice, nurses should ask themselves:
      1) Do patients hear in my voice that I care?
      2) That I have time for them?
      3) That they are safe with me?

b. In considering the impact of the way that they look at the patient, nurses should ask themselves:
   1) What is the quality of my facial expression?
   2) Of my eyes?
   3) Do they communicate care and compassion, or are they perfunctory and distant?
   4) Does the patient feel seen or overlooked?
   5) If the eyes are the windows of the soul, what is my soul saying to the soul of my patient?
   6) What is the patient's soul saying to me?
c. In considering the use of touch, nurses should ask themselves:
   1) Am I focused on the task at hand and simply touching the patient to get the job done?
   2) Does my touch convey care, support, nurture and competence? (See Chapter 26.)

5. Learning to shift consciousness into a healing state is a basic skill for the holistic nurse. We are not separate selves "doing to" the patient, but an integral part of the patient's healing journey. The quality of the energy with which the patient is interacting is part of what we attend to, and this means attending to our own state of consciousness and well-being before, during, and after our interactions with patients.

6. Taking time to learn and practice relaxation, meditation, centering, or other self-care strategies becomes essential to provide optimal care for patients and avoid burnout for nurses.

The Wounded Healer

1. Everyone is wounded. Life does not allow any one to slide under its radar and escape its trials. Thus, being wounded is not optional. (See Chapter 3.)

2. In doing the work of healing that their own woundedness requires, nurses have the capacity to become "wounded healers" for others.

3. Having undertaken to become healed themselves, wounded healers are unafraid of the healing journey and are courageous companions on the healing journey of others. They know the territory of healing from the inside and can guide others at one moment and console them the next, for the journey is always shifting.

4. Conversely, wounded healers know their limitations and can make sure that another staff member is assigned to a patient who touches them in an unhealed place so that the patient's care will not be compromised by a wounded healer's inability to provide a caring presence.

5. The more that nurses become healed and whole themselves, the more they have to offer patients. As nurses grow and develop in self-love and compassion, their well of compassion and mercy for others expands. Vaughan, a transpersonal psychologist, put it this way: "Healing happens more easily through us when we allow it to happen in us. In this way the wounded healer who, at the existential level, identifies with the pain and suffering of those he or she attempts to heal, becomes the healed healer who, being grounded in emptiness and compassion, can facilitate healing more effectively."[9]

6. As they heal, nurses become more and more aware of the sacred trust and privilege of participating in another person's healing journey. They accept the privilege and its demands and responsibilities willingly.

REFERENCES

1. J. Quinn, On Healing, Wholeness and the Haelan Effect, *Nursing and Health Care* 10, no. 10 (1989): 553–556.

2. J. Watson, *Nursing: Human Science and Human Care* (New York: National League for Nursing, 1988), 54.

3. Watson, *Nursing: Human Science and Human Care,* 59.

4. B. Carper, Fundamental Patterns of Knowing, *Advances in Nursing Science* 1, no. 1 (1978): 13–28.

5. L. Dossey, *Healing Words: The Power of Prayer and the Practice of Medicine* (San Francisco, CA: Harper San Francisco, 1993), 43.

6. M. Rogers, Nursing: Science of Unitary, Irreducible, Human Beings: Update 1990, in *Visions of Rogers Science-Based Nursing,* ed. E.A.M. Barrett (New York: National League for Nursing, 1990).

7. M. Newman, The Spirit of Nursing, *Holistic Nursing Practice* 3, no. 3 (1989): 6.

8. J.F. Quinn, Holding Sacred Space: The Nurse As Healing Environment, *Holistic Nursing Practice* 6, no. 4 (1992): 26–36.

9. F. Vaughan, *The Inward Arc* (Boston: Shambala, 1985), 70.

CHAPTER 3

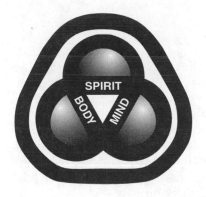

The Nurse As an Instrument of Healing

Maggie McKivergin

KNOWLEDGE COMPETENCIES

- Discuss the importance of presence as a foundation of care on which to build nursing interventions.
- Explain the four dimensions of presence and their application to experiencing wholeness.
- Identify barriers to the practice of presence.
- Describe the characteristics of nurse healers.
- Discuss ways to create sacred space.
- Define the alignment of self as an instrument of healing.
- Describe theoretical perspectives related to the process of healing.
- Perform a whole person assessment.
- Identify appropriate methods of intervention that will reach the individual's inner healer/teacher.
- Co-create a dynamic of healing with the client.
- Define outcomes of a healing intervention.
- Design a team of support with the client when indicated.

DEFINITIONS

Healing: the return of the integrity and wholeness of the natural state of an individual;[1] the emergence of the right relationship at, between, and among all levels of the human being;[2] the process of bringing together parts of oneself (i.e., physical, mental, emotional, spiritual, relational) at deeper levels of inner knowing, leading to an integration and balance, with each part having equal importance and value.[3]

Healing Environment: surroundings that facilitate the emergence of the Haelen effect, that is, the synergistic, organismic, multidimensional response of the whole person in the direction of healing and wholeness;[4] the physical, emotional, social, kinesthetic, and energetic properties of the surroundings/field that can provide a climate of support for the individual and aid in the healing process.

Nurse As Instrument of Healing: one who offers unconditional presence and helps remove the barriers to the healing process; one who creates the space and opportunity for another to feel safe and bring into alignment that which has been painful and out of harmony with self, Creator, others, and creation.[5]

Presence: a multidimensional state of being available in a situation with the wholeness of one's individual being; relational style and quality of "being with" rather than "doing to."[6]

Whole Person Assessment: an intellectual, emotional, kinetic, and intuitive interpretation of another individual in relation to himself or herself, others, Creator, and creation.[7]

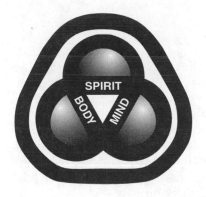 ***Pause for a moment . . .***

I have made a study plan.

❏ *I will study in (quiet environment and location):* _____ .

❏ *I will commit to study at (times and dates):* _____ .

❏ *I will assemble all the materials that I need to study:* _____ .

THEORIES AND RESEARCH

Nursing Theories

1. The essence of healing is phenomenologic in nature: it is intersubjective in the lived experience.
2. All nurse theorists have an important perspective regarding the nature of health, disease, healing, and the dynamics of caring for another. The following nurse theorists provide insights into the dynamics of healing:
   a. Florence Nightingale: natural healing.[8,9]
      1) The nurse places the individual in the best condition for nature to act, particularly by providing an environment conducive to the reparative process.
      2) The client is viewed as having vital, natural, reparative powers that can be reached by creating the right environmental circumstances.
   b. Helen Erickson, Evelyn Tomlin, and Mary Ann Swain: modeling and role modeling.[10]
      1) Through unconditional acceptance, the nurse puts himself or herself in the client's position and addresses the client's foremost need at hand, building trust and the basis for a healing relationship.
      2) The client's locus of perceived need and agenda is the priority.
   c. Madeleine Leininger: transcultural nursing.[11]
      1) The nurse's professional caring includes behaviors, techniques, processes, and patterns that enhance or maintain healthy conditions or lifestyles.
      2) Each client represents a unique expression of needs determined by background and culture; thus, the approach of care should encompass the diversity of caring responses.
   d. Betty Neuman: systems theory.[12]
      1) The nurse approaches the client as an open system composed of physical, psychologic, social, developmental, and spiritual dimensions and focuses on stressors with the goal of impeding or arresting an entropic or disorganized state.
      2) Health is a movement of free energy flow between the client and the environment.
   e. Margaret Newman: health as expanding consciousness.[13]
      1) With an understanding of the pattern of a person's life, the nurse can facilitate access to deeper meaning.
      2) Health involves developing an awareness of self and environment, coupled with an increased ability to perceive and respond to alternatives.
   f. Dorothea Orem: self-care.[14]
      1) the nurse's actions focus on human developmental processes and the enhancement of self-care ability, with the goal being optimal wellness.
      2) The client has the capacity for self-knowledge; the extent of this knowledge determines his or her ability to engage in self-care, with the benefit of maintaining life, health, and well-being.
   g. Rosemary Rizzo Parse: human-living-health.[15]
      1) The nurse's recognition of the multidimensional nature of the human process supports and guides the co-creation of health with the individual.
      2) The client chooses the meaning established in co-created situations and is responsible for the choices made in the open process of becoming.
   h. Martha Rogers: human energy fields.[16]
      1) The nurse studies the nature of human development by observing the patterns that emerge from the client, revealing the flow and organization of energy within the client's field. The nurse can help to interpret his or her own energy field as well as the client's.
      2) The environment influences the wholeness of the client, which, in turn, influences the openness and pattern of the person. Qualities of energy become a key indicator of healthy or nonhealthy ways of living.
   i. Sr. Callista Roy: adaptation model.[17]
      1) The nurse supports the client by educating and promoting adaptive responses to life's stressors.
      2) The client adapts to stimuli in the environment that are focal, contextual, or residual in nature and achieves health in the process.
   j. Jean Watson: caring.[18]
      1) The nurse makes contact with the person's emotional and subjective world as the route to the inner self.
      2) The human care process engages the mind-body-soul with another in a lived moment, which increases harmony and leads to self-knowledge, self-reverence, self-healing, and self-care.

Concepts of Presence[19]

1. The essence of presence—"being with"—implies a conscious intention to appreciate the connection of the moment.
   a. A moment in time, the reality of the shared experience in the "now," creates an open container through which life, energy, and healing can flow.
   b. Letting go of past concerns or future fears, even for a moment, can create the space and opportunity for the system to open up and reveal what is needed to make it more whole.
   c. Caregivers can encourage this presence and help to focus and bring forth the deepest desires for wholeness from another, creating the safe container and nurturing that allows another to open up.
   d. The practice of presence does not depend on physical proximity, but can take place through indirect, long-distance communication.
2. Presence to self: focuses attention and care on that which brings energy to or drains energy from one's life.
   a. Conscious intent, sensitivity, and awareness to what it takes to be aligned with one's personal process of healing and unfolding.
   b. This process makes it possible to achieve deeper meaning, to recognize the unique gift of one's life, and to nurture one's growth to the fullest capacity.
3. Presence with Creator requires openness to the unfolding of one's life in any moment, co-creating the unique expression of the gift of one's life with the Creator/Spirit (as defined by the individual) in the essence of a loving nature.
   a. When brought forth into the many dimensions of life (e.g., physical, emotional), the presence of the Creator can bring a deeper understanding of wholeness, integrity, meaning, and truth of the moment/situation/self. Respect for the individual's belief system is essential so as not to impose the caregiver's agenda on another.
   b. The recognition of the self as sacred integrates the essence in this life through inspiration, transcendence, truth, grace, hope, and forgiveness.
4. Presence to others provides the multidimensional gift of interpersonal connection with another at any moment in life.
   a. Presence implies relating to another person in the moment at hand in a way that the other person defines as meaningful. Presence to others is more powerful when connected with self, Creator, and creation.
   b. The connection with another can be physical, emotional, psychologic, intuitive, spiritual, kinetic, or therapeutic in nature, with varying levels of depth and transcendence.
   c. The vibration that occurs between two people who are aligned in intention and open to the rhythm of healing produces a resonant vibration called entrainment; the mutuality of vibration helps to remove the barriers that inhibit the flow of energy.[20]
5. Presence to creation involves the relationship of individuals with the inherent healing rhythm of nature and all of creation.
   a. With a sensitivity to the essence of life, its seasons, and its rhythms, it is possible to recognize the message, meaning, and life-giving energy inherent in all of creation that heals.
   b. There are several avenues for natural healing:
      1) Traditions of native peoples.
      2) Florence Nightingale's philosophy of nursing.
      3) The natural healing rhythm of the earth.
      4) Natural elements of sound, color, light, temperature, earth, water.
      5) Seasonal themes relating to creation, new life, blossoming, fullness of life, letting go, changing, re-creation.
      6) Metaphors of growth (e.g., the seed, planting, nurturing, harvesting, renewal).
      7) Metaphors found within creation (e.g., flow, flexibility, rootedness).
6. Levels of presence are the dimensions of care that the nurse uses in providing a whole person approach:
   a. Physical presence. The nurse performs many interventions while physically with the client, including the routine tasks that are prescribed for the client. This level of presence includes the skills and knowledge to provide client care in a safe environment.
   b. Psychologic presence. The nurse is with the client in a therapeutic milieu that meets the client's needs for help, comfort, and support.
   c. Therapeutic presence. The nurse relates to the client as one whole being to another, using all the resources of body, mind, emotions, and spirit (Table 3–1).[21]
7. Presence evolves as the nurse develops the skill of being present to others as meaning unfolds in their lives.

Table 3–1 Levels of Healing Presence

Level of Interaction	Type of Contact	Skills
Physical presence	Body to body	Seeing, examining, touching, doing, hearing, hugging
Psychologic presence	Mind to mind	Assessing, communicating, listening actively, writing, reflecting, counseling, attending to, caring, empathizing, remaining nonjudgmental, accepting
Therapeutic presence	Spirit to spirit Whole being to whole being Centered self to centered self	Centering, meditating, demonstrating intentionality, and "at-one-ment," imaging, keeping open and intuitive, communing, loving, connecting

    a. Basic nursing care includes the skill to provide safe care.

    b. The nurse evolves in the recognition of the connection between a person's life and health.

    c. An understanding of the connections between life and health expands a nurse's perception to the essence of health and enhances the nurse's ability to offer a healing presence to the different dimensions of an individual in any moment/situation in time.

    d. With each level of understanding, the nurse's attitude shifts from "What can I do?" to "How can I be with the person in this moment?" to provide the best possible outcome.

    e. Presence may be uncomfortable because remaining with the person exposes one's humanness and vulnerability in offering comfort and healing support.[22]

    f. Being present to one's self allows for a greater capacity to understand others.

8. Barriers to presence may be either intentional or unintentional.

    a. At times, it may seem unrealistic to spend the time with self, Creator, another person, or creation, but even a few seconds of present attention can help modulate an unfolding pattern. The breath can inspire presence in the moment, for example.

    b. Barriers to presence include the following:

       1) Busyness/task focus.

       2) Fear.

       3) Concern over what other people will think.

       4) Feelings of inadequacy (e.g., I'm not ____ enough).

       5) Lack of desire/intent to be present.

       6) Distractions.

       7) Need to be in control.

       8) Goal direction; responsibilities.

       9) Lack of patience.

      10) Lack of openness.

9. Outcomes of presence include the following:

    a. Increased coping strength, even in the midst of unchanged circumstances.

    b. Sense of well-being/more being.

    c. Lessened sense of isolation; more connections.

    d. Decreased sense of vulnerability.

    e. Neutralization of the intimidating atmosphere of the health care system or the moment.

 Pause for a moment . . .

❑ *I am preparing for the holistic nursing certification (HNC) examination to meet my personal and professional goals.*

❑ *I am imaging successful completion of the HNC examination.*

Creation of Sacred Space

1. To create a sacred space in which healing can occur, the nurse not only can shape the physical environment (external), but also can provide a personal environment (relationship-focused) to evoke the healing process.

    a. The healing environment (external)

       1) The physical properties of natural light, running water, plants, earth elements, fresh air, pleasant sounds, music, healing smells, and neatness contribute to an ex-

ternal environment that promotes healing.

2) The emotional, social, and energetic properties of the surroundings/field have a profound effect on the individual.
3) A sense of order in the environment can support the individual's alignment with healing and wholeness.
4) The energy of the space can be cleansed and protected through a variety of blessings and rituals:
   - Holy water.
   - Epsom salts and alcohol.
   - Smudging with sage.
   - Prayer.

The Nurse As a Healing Environment

1. By connecting with the sacred within each person and accessing the person's inner healer, the nurse enhances and guides the healing process in a powerful way.
2. The process of expanding consciousness and creating a sacred space for healing benefits the nurse as well as the client.
3. The immense power evoked in the relationship between the nurse and the client is instrumental in the therapeutic process of healing.
   a. Through unconditional presence, the nurse patterns an environment of support and healing.
   b. With attention and intention, the environment can become one in which the client can feel safe and explore the dimensions of self in the healing moment.
   c. Not only is the nurse in the healing environment, but also the nurse becomes part of the environment in which the individual can dwell.[23]
   d. The following build one's capacity to hold the unfolding of the whole person and, therefore, develop greater depth, breadth, and height in the dynamic of healing:[24]
      1) Self-care.
      2) Personal interpretation of life's lessons and meaning.
      3) Rootedness and expansiveness; an understanding of the balance between a grounded approach and the intuitive inspiration that creates a vision of health and wholeness.
      4) Core dynamics; recognition of the holographic nature and metaphor of systems and the essential nature of life, health, and healing.
      5) Expansion of consciousness; the ability to broaden one's thinking, shift perspectives, and encompass a new approach to life.
      6) Growth in love; the ability to grow more and more in loving presence to self, others, and the world, thus creating the highest level of healing.
      7) Courage; the ability to overcome the fear encountered in the healing process as one passes through the barrier/pain.
      8) Alignment with the Divine.
      9) Openness to being an instrument of the Creator's healing grace.
      10) The ability to detach oneself from the outcomes.
      11) Groundedness and reliability.
      12) Patience.
      13) Authenticity.
      14) Mindfulness.
   e. Nurse healers share a broad range of characteristics:[25]
      1) Awareness that self-healing is a continual process.
      2) Familiarity with the terrain of self-development.
      3) Recognition of personal strengths and weaknesses.
      4) Openness to self-discovery.
      5) Willingness to make continued efforts to learn about life's purposes and to avoid mechanical behavior.
      6) Awareness of present and future steps in personal growth.
      7) Ability to model self-care in order to help self and clients with inward process.
      8) Awareness that a nurse's presence is as important as his or her technical skills.
      9) Respect and love for clients, regardless of who and how they are.
      10) Willingness to offer the client methods for working on life issues.
      11) Ability to guide the client in discovering creative options.
      12) Recognition that clients know the best life choices for themselves.
      13) Active listening.
      14) Empowerment of clients to recognize that they can cope with life processes.
      15) Sharing of insights without imposing personal values and beliefs.

16) Nonjudgmental acceptance of what clients say.
17) Perception of time with clients as an opportunity to serve and share with them.
f. A part of every nurse healer needs healing.[26] Despite the temptation to ignore this woundedness, embracing perceived limitations (as teachers) guides nurse healers to increased wholeness.
   1) Making one's wounds a source of healing does not call for a sharing of superficial pains, but for a constant willingness to see the pain and suffering as rising from the depth of the human condition.
   2) Acknowledging vulnerability and oneness with another in the human condition provides a synchrony and common ground from which healing can begin at a deeper level.
   3) Peak experiences are reference points from which to share and are as much a celebration of life's unfolding as other opportunities from which one grows.
g. Approaching a situation with the "beginner's mind" provides openness, freshness, and the opportunity to respect mutual knowing.[27]
   1) Unknowing is a necessary foundation for openness within the dynamic of healing.[28]
   2) This state evokes a mutual response rather than placing the patient in a dependent position; thus, it provides access to the inner healer, teacher, and guide.
   3) The healing power of vulnerability originates in the nurse's willingness to be open in the midst of the moment to co-create the outcome rather than impose a preconceived agenda for the moment.
h. Four patterns of knowing are a necessary foundation for healing:[29]
   1) Empirical knowledge.
   2) Personal knowledge.
   3) Ethical knowledge.
   4) Aesthetic knowledge.
i. Inherent in life are threats to the integrity of one's system, either actual or perceived; both types require protective measures.
   1) Understanding the protective options available makes it possible to choose an appropriate response to life's challenges.
   2) The system protects itself by closing down to varying degrees.

3) A completely closed system does not have a healthy intake of life-giving energy and release of that which is toxic to the system, resulting in patterns of disease, pain, negative energy, and disconnection.
4) To avoid absorbing the others' negative energy or patterns, nurse healers need to develop healthy ways in which to protect themselves in the midst of a healing intervention.
5) Healthy ways for nurse healers to protect themselves include
   a) Giving and receiving only love.
   b) Praying for protection of the Creator.
   c) Visualizing white light surrounding self and other.
   d) Establishing healthy boundaries.
   e) Being in a healthy, centered, energetic place themselves so that they have enough personal energy to serve as an instrument of healing to another.

The Process of Healing

1. Healing can occur across the continuum of illness through reaching one's highest potential at any moment in time.
2. A barrier to energy flow that is a response to the patterns of life or an imbalance in the dimensions that encompass the human experience can produce disease.
3. The nurse who serves as an instrument of healing goes through the steps of the nursing process to achieve desired client outcomes and to facilitate the healing process.
4. Assessment includes the following:
   a. Whole person well-being.
   b. Openness or closure of the person as a system, with identification of possible places for an intervention.
   c. Scanning of the person's energy field.
   d. Interview and interpretation of responses to life's events, ranging from self-destructive to life-affirming.
   e. Functional capacity.
   f. Health risk indicators.
   g. Quality-of-life indicators.
   h. Process analysis/personal goals.
5. Nursing diagnoses could cover many categories as appropriate, particularly that of "energy field disturbance."
6. Interventions can occur in many ways on many levels in many dimensions (e.g., pres-

ence, environment), guided by the individual's need and response in the moment.

7. It is important to address physical pain as a first priority in providing comfort, as pain relief allows the individual to relax and be receptive to additional interventions and healing.

Energy Field Healing

1. Dolores Krieger and Dora Kunz first described and researched the procedure of energy field intervention known as Therapeutic Touch.[30]
2. Many schools of healing have emerged worldwide with healers focusing on the diverse aspects of healing.
3. Assessment and modulation of the human energy field and its flow is a mindful process that requires deliberation and attention to the many levels of being.
4. As the source of pattern disturbance comes into awareness, the nurse helps the client reach his or her inner healer so as to co-create a conscious repatterning of thought, memories, pain, anxiety, tension, and energy flow.
5. The release of chaotic patterns or the bringing of awareness and energy into formerly stagnant areas yields a variety of outcomes as reported by the client.
6. Five recurring elements of self-involvement appear to be aspects of the natural healing process of the client:
   a. Awareness.
   b. Appraisal.
   c. Intention.
   d. Alignment.
   e. Acceptance.[31]
7. The nurse healer may find the following techniques particularly important:
   a. Center, align, and focus attention.
   b. Focus on achieving the highest good for the client without considering personal ego needs and outcomes.
   c. Be present and create an environment within which the client feels safe and healing can emerge. Be conscious of giving and receiving only love.
   d. Assess the energy field by using intuition, as well as by running hands over the different levels of the aura.
   e. Note areas of energy congestion or stagnation; provide feedback to the client in order to enhance synchrony and to make the process one of conscious awareness.
   f. Be present to the many levels of the client's being as energy is modulated, barriers to flow removed, and congestion dissipated.
   g. Encourage open communication to enhance the depth of the healing experience.
   h. Provide grounding by continuing to reflect truth as the client explores new dimensions to his or her being.
   i. Help the client reframe experiences and memories in the removal of barriers that surface within the healing dynamic.
   j. Apply different techniques as appropriate to help drain pain, chelate the energy, relax and smooth the area while helping the client to breathe into the area and release patterns that do not serve the client's well-being.
   k. Be aware of the levels and patterns of energy within the client's aura and field, and facilitate the flow of energy as the healing takes place.
   l. Smooth out the whole field at the completion of the session, and help the client become grounded, conscious to the present, and oriented with the change.
   m. Ritualize the closure of the session by honoring the process as sacred (e.g., blow out the candle, give a gift of a flower).

Evaluation of a Healing Intervention

1. In a debriefing after the session, the nurse healer
   a. Notes significant areas of assessment, change, and energy balance.
   b. Asks the client to report the significance of this experience and examines the implications for next steps.
   c. Supports the shift of consciousness within the client by discussing the nature of the changes and insights gained, as well as possible different approaches to life and health.
   d. Affirms positive self-care initiatives.
2. The nurse assists the client with next steps and follows up as appropriate.
   a. The client may schedule a personal daily time of reflection in which to be present to the process of self-unfolding through journal keeping, art therapy, music therapy, and meditation.
   b. The client may need access to a team of support:
      1) Therapeutic/pastoral counselor.
      2) Physical fitness coach, body worker, chiropractor, physician.

3) Significant family member or friend who can help nurture.

3. Follow-up with the client determines the need for continuation of process and care. Clients should have the nurse healer's telephone number and backup number should there be any lingering effects or additional needs.

Outcomes of Healing

1. Outcomes reflect a change in a person's awareness, perception, behavior, and relationship to self, Creator, other, and creation.
2. Outcome assessment may focus on a variety of factors:
    a. Whole person outcomes.
        1) Physical: decreased pain, enhanced wound healing, increased energy.
        2) Emotional: enhanced ability to feel, to name feelings, and to express oneself.
        3) Intellectual: perceptual reframing of an experience that influences the belief structure, attitudes, and ways of thinking about life; healing of a painful memory; increased enthusiasm and expression of self; expansion of consciousness.
        4) Social: improved relationship with self, self-esteem, improved self-concept; deeper connection with others and understanding of the reciprocal nature of relationships.
        5) Spiritual: deeper sense of connectedness with all of life, self, Creator, creation; enhanced meaning regarding a life event; forgiveness of self or others.
        6) Vocational: identification of and alignment with life's purpose and path of expression; improved excitement and creativity in work.
        7) Environmental: harmony with nature and inherent healing rhythms; recognition of meaning and metaphor in the symbols of the earth.
    b. Ability to cope: enhanced recognition of the impact of stress on life, access to relaxation response, ability to maintain a flow state; decreased exhibition of self-destructive behavior.
    c. Sense of well-being/quality of life: increased happiness, life satisfaction, sense of security.
    d. Functional capacity: increased ability to care for self, move, have less pain.
    e. Systemness: greater sense of freedom and openness; establishment of healthy boundaries; connectedness; willingness to change and become less defined by external parameters.

Conclusion

1. The phenomenon of healing does not occur in a vacuum. There is a stimulus to move, grow, and change beyond the current state of being into a direction that makes one more whole.
2. The healing phenomenon can occur at any point on the spectrum from illness to health, from pain to potentiation, affecting many dimensions of well-being.
3. The nurse has the opportunity to give the gift of self freely, providing the foundation from which all healing and interventions can be based.
4. The privilege of conscious and intentional involvement with another is celebrated by the exchange of presence in any particular moment in time.
5. It is possible to cultivate the skill of becoming an instrument and sensing the open door through which healing can emerge.
6. The ability to assess the multidimensional nature of another person in reference to that person's life experience is complex and requires an intuitive, spiritual, and skilled approach.
7. The process of healing is one in which the nurse exchanges energy, truth, and communication with clients to help them attune to their own healing capacities.
8. The nurse mirrors the client's essence to the client, who reflects on past, present, and future perceptions in the process of becoming more whole.
9. The healing process often involves facing that which has been avoided, buried, or blocked because of the painful nature of the incident.
10. As nurses offer partnership in the journey of healing, they offer new insights, ways of coping, and a release from the bondage of fear and pain.
11. Nurses offer the gift of walking with a person so that he or she is not alone at the crossroads of healing.
12. Life and health become a celebration of the unfolding of the essence and beauty of the human spirit within the natural flow of healing.

REFERENCES

1. M.J. McKivergin, *The Essence of Presence* (In press).

2. J.F. Quinn, Holding Sacred Space: The Nurse As Healing Environment, *Holistic Nursing Practice* 6, no. 4 (1992): 26–36.

3. B.M. Dossey et al., *Holistic Nursing: A Handbook for Practice*, 2nd ed. (Gaithersburg, MD: Aspen Publishers, 1995).

4. Quinn, Holding Sacred Space.

5. McKivergin, *The Essence of Presence*.

6. J.G. Paterson and L.T. Zderad, *Humanistic Nursing* (New York: John Wiley & Sons, 1976).

7. McKivergin, *The Essence of Presence*.

8. F. Nightingale, *Notes on Nursing* (Philadelphia: J.B. Lippincott, 1992).

9. L. Selanders, *Florence Nightingale: An Environmental Adaptation Theory* (Newbury Park, CA: Sage Publishers, 1993).

10. H. Erickson et al., *Modeling and Role-Modeling: A Theory and Paradigm for Nursing* (Lexington, SC: Pine Press, 1983).

11. M. Leininger, *Cultural Care Diversity and Universality: A Theory of Nursing* (New York: National League for Nursing Press, 1991).

12. B. Neuman, *The Neuman Systems Model* (Norwalk, CT: Appleton-Century-Crofts, 1982).

13. M.A. Newman, *Health As Expanding Consciousness*, 2nd ed. (New York: National League for Nursing Press, 1994).

14. D.E. Orem, *Nursing: Concepts of Practice*, 3rd ed. (New York: McGraw-Hill Publishing Co., 1985).

15. R.R. Parse, Human Becoming: Parse's Theory of Nursing, *Nursing Science Quarterly* 5 (1992): 35–42.

16. M. Rogers, *The Theoretical Basis of Nursing* (Philadelphia: F.A. Davis Co., 1970).

17. C. Roy and H.A. Andrews, *The Roy Adaptation Model: The Definitive Statement* (Norwalk, CT: Appleton & Lange, 1991).

18. J. Watson, *Nursing: Human Science and Human Care* (New York: National League for Nursing, 1988).

19. McKivergin, *The Essence of Presence*.

20. E.L. Rossi, *The Symptom Path to Enlightenment: The New Dynamics of Self Organization in Hypnotherapy: An Advanced Manual for Beginners* (Pacific Palisades, CA: Palisades Gateway Publishing, 1996).

21. M.J. McKivergin and M.J. Daubenmire, The Healing Process of Presence, *Journal of Holistic Nursing* 1 (1994): 65–81.

22. J. Pettigrew, The Ministry of Presence, *Critical Care Nursing* 2 (1990): 503–508.

23. Quinn, Holding Sacred Space.

24. McKivergin, *The Essence of Presence*.

25. Dossey et al., *Holistic Nursing: A Handbook for Practice*.

26. H.J.M. Nouwen, *The Wounded Healer* (Garden City, NJ: Image Books, 1979).

27. McKivergin, *The Essence of Presence*.

28. P. Munhall, Unknowing Toward a New Pattern of Knowing in Nursing, *Nursing Outlook* 41 (1993): 125–128.

29. B. Carper, Fundamental Patterns of Knowing, *Advances in Nursing Science* 1 (1978): 13–28.

30. D. Krieger, *Accepting Your Power To Heal: The Personal Practice of Therapeutic Touch* (Santa Fe, NM: Bear & Company Publishing, 1993).

31. S. Scandrett-Hibdon and M.I. Freel, The Endogenous Healing Process: A Conceptual Analysis, *Journal of Holistic Nursing* 1 (1989): 66–71.

Holistic Foundation

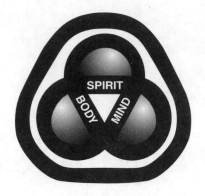

CHAPTER 4

Concepts of Health-Wellness-Disease-Illness

H. Lea Barbato Gaydos

KNOWLEDGE COMPETENCIES

- Contrast the concepts of compliance and non-compliance with the concepts of engagement and lack of engagement.
- Describe the health belief model in relation to the process of engagement.
- Discuss change theory as it relates to addictive behaviors.
- Explore the dialectic relationship of health-wellness-disease-illness.
- Examine the importance of values.
- Discuss the effect of culture on definitions of health and illness and the development of values.
- Recognize the rights of individuals to receive holistic and value-consistent care.
- Explain the values clarification process.
- Discuss motivation and wellness in the workplace.

DEFINITIONS

Attitudes: feelings arising out of thoughts, emotions, and behaviors associated with a particular person, idea, or object.

Beliefs: a subset of attitudes that indicate faith in a particular person, idea, or object.

Dialectic: the art of discourse, implying a relationship in which there is a synthesis of objective and subjective perspectives.[1,2]

Disease: a discrete entity causing specific symptoms; more broadly, a phenomenon causing a deviation from normal state or an imbalance.[3]

Engagement: the process of commitment, involvement, and performance of value-consistent health behaviors.

Health: a state or process in which the individual experiences a sense of well-being and the integration of body, mind, and spirit interacting harmoniously with the environment; harmony and unity (Watson, Leininger); a process of becoming (Parse); expanding consciousness (Neuman).[4]

Illness: a subjective experience of symptoms and suffering to which the individual ascribes meaning and significance; not synonymous with disease.[5]

Self-Responsibility: the desire, will, and ability to choose and act on one's own behalf.

Values: endow a particular person, idea, object, or behavior with worth, truth, or beauty.

Wellness: integrated, congruent functioning aimed toward reaching one's highest potential.[6,7]

 Pause for a moment . . .

- ❏ *My successful completion of the holistic nursing certification (HNC) examination allows me to place HNC after my name.*
- ❏ *I will be proud to have the distinction of excellence in the area of holistic nursing.*

THEORIES AND RESEARCH

Health Behaviors: Engagement and Lack of Engagement

1. Compliance denotes behaviors of clients that are consistent with the prescriptions of health care providers.

a. The concept of compliance originates in the paternalistic belief that the care provider is responsible for the client's behavior.

b. People who modify or do not follow prescribed treatment or care plans are labeled noncompliant.

2. In holistic care, individuals are responsible for their own health choices and behaviors.

a. The provider and the client collaborate regarding treatment and care plans appropriate to the attitudes, values, beliefs, and lifestyle of the client; the client is engaged in making value-congruent choices.

b. When individuals choose not to follow collaborative plans, it is an indication of lack of engagement.

c. Lack of engagement is not a failure, although it may signal the need for reassessment and further collaboration.

3. Because the terms *engagement* and *lack of engagement* indicate collaboration and self-responsibility for health choices, they are preferred over the terms *compliance* and *noncompliance*.[8]

The Health Belief Model

1. An individual's perceptions of the seriousness and personal susceptibility to a disease moderated by demographic factors, social factors, and the perceived threat of the disease can predict the likelihood that the individual will take preventive health care action.[9]

2. Individuals take preventive health care action when the perceived benefits of the action outweigh the perceived costs and barriers to action.

3. Strong feelings of belonging, sources of emotional and material support, and the attention of others can indicate, to some degree, the potential of the person to engage in health-promoting behaviors.[10]

4. An understanding of the relationship of attitudes, beliefs, and social support to engagement has indicated four categories of individual circumstances that can be used to identify appropriate intervention strategies (Table 4–1).[11]

5. The nurse determines the category that reflects the client's circumstances by evaluating the following:

a. Beliefs about health.

b. Willingness to seek health advice.

c. Willingness to accept health advice.

d. Perception of the seriousness of high-risk behaviors.

e. Perception of susceptibility and vulnerability as a result of risk behaviors.

f. Perception of the risk:benefit ratio of new behaviors.

g. Perception of the degree of interference that the new behavior will have on current social role function.[12]

6. The Health Belief Model has certain limitations.

a. It focuses on cognition and does not explicitly integrate affect.[13]

Table 4–1 Assessment and Facilitation of Engagement

	Clients			
	Category 1	*Category 2*	*Category 3*	*Category 4*
Attitudes, beliefs	Positive health beliefs and attitudes	Negative health beliefs and attitudes	Positive health beliefs and attitudes	Negative health beliefs and attitudes
Social support	Adequate social support	Adequate social support	Little or inadequate social support	Little or inadequate social support
Intervention strategies to facilitate engagement	Address affective, cognitive, and psychomotor domains; match information to coping style and locus of control.	Focus on consciousness raising, self-help groups, values clarification; behavior modification techniques may be helpful.	Strengthen social support system; promote involvement in community agencies, self-help groups, and cognitive strengthening programs.	Use a "foot-in-the-door" strategy that requires little change; simplify care regimens; establish basic goals; written contracts are recommended.

Source: Reprinted from Dossey et al., *Holistic Nursing: Handbook for Practice*, 2nd ed., pp. 125–126, © 1995, Aspen Publishers, Inc.

b. It places the burden of action entirely on the client and does not address the larger forces impinging on clients, such as the health care system.

7. Because governmental and organizational policy shapes an individual's range of health choices, nursing interventions aimed at increasing health and wellness must extend beyond the individual to regional and national policy making.[14]

Application of Change Theory (Addictive Behaviors)

1. Change occurs in several stages.[15]
   a. Precontemplation. Although unaware of the need for change, the individual may agree to make changes under pressure of family and friends. Changes are usually minimal and last only as long as pressure is applied.
   b. Contemplation. The individual is aware of the need to make changes, but is not committed to action. This stage can last as long as 2 or more years as the person thinks about the problem behavior and the risks and rewards of changing.
   c. Preparation. Despite beginning efforts toward change in the past year, the individual has not yet reached the goal and is preparing to act again within the next month.
   d. Action. During the action stage individuals change their behaviors and the context of the behavior (environment, experience), making significant effort to reach goals. The individual is considered to be in the action stage if the behavior has been changed for 1 day to 6 months. This stage offers the most external recognition as others become aware of the effort that the individual is making toward change.
   e. Maintenance. In this stage, the healthy behaviors have replaced addictive behaviors for longer than 6 months. The individual directs efforts toward preventing relapse.

2. Individuals usually go through the stages several times before conquering an addiction, even if they have professional help.

3. Movement through the stages occurs in a spiral pattern as the individual moves backward into previous stages and forward through succeeding stages.

   a. This upward and forward spiral movement toward elimination of the behavior occurs as the individual learns from previous experience.
   b. The greater the number of successes the individual has over time in this spiral movement, the greater the possibility of sustained change.

4. The processes of change are varied.
   a. Consciousness raising: increasing awareness through cognitive and affective domains.
   b. Self-reevaluation: determining one's feelings, attitudes, beliefs, values in regard to a problem behavior.
   c. Self-liberation: commitment to act, belief in one's potential to change; use of decision-making therapy, logotherapy, and commitment enhancing techniques.
   d. Counterconditioning: substitution of alternative behaviors for problem behaviors.
   e. Stimulus control: avoidance of stimuli that provoke the problem behavior.
   f. Reinforcement: use of rewards for changed behaviors, either self-rewards or rewards by others.
   g. Helping relationships: development of trusting, caring relationships, both therapeutic and social.
   h. Dramatic relief: use of the affective domain to experience and express feelings (e.g., psychodrama).
   i. Environmental reevaluation: analysis of the relationship of the problem behavior to one's physical environment.
   j. Social liberation: exploration of alternative, nonproblem behaviors.

5. Integration of the stages and processes of change
   a. There are processes appropriate to each stage of change, and the use of stage-inappropriate processes may be detrimental to progress.
   b. Individuals in the precontemplation stage expend little time or energy on the problem and experience less negative reactions to the behavior, but as they move into contemplation, the processes of consciousness raising, dramatic relief, and environmental reevaluation are helpful.
   c. People in the contemplation stage moving into the preparation stage benefit from self re-evaluation.

d. Individuals in the preparation stage moving into the action stage benefit from self liberation processes.

e. Individuals in the action and maintenance stages benefit from reinforcement management, helping relationships, counterconditioning, and stimulus control.

 Pause for a moment . . .

❑ *I can do relaxation (primarily deep breathing) exercises to manage my test-taking anxiety.*

❑ *I am preparing to be alert, relaxed, and calm while taking the HNC examination.*

Dynamics of Health-Wellness-Disease-Illness

1. Culture determines the definition of health.[16,17]
2. Definitions of health in nursing literature fall into four groups:
   a. Health as the absence of disease or injury.
   b. Health as the ability to perform role functions.
   c. Health as adaptation.
   d. Health as the expression of the maximum potential of the individual.[18]
3. From the holistic perspective, health, wellness, illness, and disease are distinct parts of the whole human health experience best understood in interaction rather than as discrete entities.[19]
   a. There are four possible relationships of health, wellness, disease, and illness:
      1) Health-wellness as the polar opposite of disease-illness.
      2) Health-wellness as a different dimension of the human experience from disease-illness.
      3) Health-wellness on a graduated continuum with disease-illness.
      4) Holistic health as a totality of experience encompassing wellness, disease, and illness.[20]
   b. The dialectic relationship of health-wellness-disease-illness is a natural, ever changing, temporal process.
   c. Wellness-illness and health-disease have both cognitive and affective dimensions through which individuals ascribe meaning and significance to their health experience.

1) Health-disease may be cognitively experienced as comprehensible/incomprehensible, manageable/unmanageable, meaningful/meaningless.
2) Themes of the affective domain of health-disease are joy/despair, acceptance/resentment, power/fear, anticipation/confusion.

4. Effects of the Dialectic Relationship of Health-Wellness-Disease-Illness
   a. Health-disease can alter wellness-illness through the impact of changes in the body.
   b. The dialectic of wellness-illness involves conflict and contradiction.
   c. The dynamic, dialectic interrelationship of health-disease-wellness-illness is a process that creates a pattern of meaning in everyday life.

5. Among the factors affecting health-wellness-disease-illness dynamics are intrapersonal factors (e.g., personality, past experience, emotional state), interpersonal factors (e.g., social supports and relationships), health-disease factors (e.g., severity and prognosis of the disease), and extrapersonal factors (e.g., cultural orientation).

6. People have a right to culturally congruent, value-sensitive care.[21]

7. Providing culturally congruent nursing care requires knowledge of cultural attitudes, beliefs, values, and norms integral to the health experience.

Importance of Values

1. Values influence and guide behavior while providing a framework for understanding and integrating human experience.
2. Values are not inherently right or wrong.
3. A state of uncertainty is produced when an individual holds opposing values; this state of uncertainty is termed a value conflict.
4. When conflicts arise in personal and professional values, nurses have the right to not participate in behaviors contrary to personal values.
5. Values are more dynamic and motivational than attitudes because they possess cognitive, affective, and behavioral dimensions.
6. Five questions about the nature of reality reveal the dominant values in a culture.[22]
   a. What is the inherent nature of human beings? Are humans good, evil, or a combination?

b. What is the relationship of human beings to nature? Does nature dominate human beings, do humans dominate nature, or do humans coexist in harmony with nature?

c. What is the temporal focus of human experience? Is the perception of time predominantly focused on the past, present, or future?

d. What is the human mode of activity? Is human potential to be found in being (spontaneity is valued), growing (personal control and self actualization are valued), or doing (action is valued)?

e. What is the pattern of human relationships? Are significant relationships linear and hereditary, collateral and group-oriented, individual-oriented with emphasis on independence and autonomy?

7. Nurses can explore their own dominant value orientation by answering these questions on a personal level.

Values Clarification

1. A "strategy of discovery," values clarification makes one consciously aware of cherished values held by an individual or group.[23]

2. Being clear about one's values makes value-congruent behavior possible and, thus, leads to a greater experience of personal authenticity and genuineness.

3. The process of values clarification has three steps:[24]

a. Choosing. The individual considers the range of possible options and freely chooses the most desirable option.

b. Prizing. The individual cherishes the chosen value and affirms the choice publicly.

c. Acting. The individual incorporates the value into action.

4. Clarification of values has a myriad of uses:[25]

a. To help the nurse avoid imposing cultural values on clients.

b. To reduce anxiety and emotional reactivity in situations involving personal risk.

c. To identify and solve moral and ethical dilemmas.

d. To facilitate behavior change.

e. To validate a person's readiness or unreadiness for behavior change.

f. To help clients manage difficult emotions in the face of behavior changes.

g. To empower individuals to work toward realizing their visions and achieving their goals.

Workplace Programs for Wellness and Motivation[26]

1. Effective workplace wellness programs decrease the costs of unhealthy employee behaviors.

2. Such programs focus on stress management; nutrition and weight management, including fitness and exercise; hypertension management; control of drug and alcohol use; smoking cessation; prevention of accidents; and screening programs for early detection of diseases such as cancer and glaucoma.

3. To develop wellness programs, nurses should be knowledgeable about successful programs, current health practices, research and evaluation methods for individuals and groups, marketing, health care reimbursement, and needs assessment techniques.

4. Successful workplace wellness programs motivate workers to engage in new behaviors.

5. Imagination, determination, discipline, and creativity are essential to creating and implementing individual wellness plans that are personally congruent and satisfying.

6. Barriers to motivational efforts include the following:

a. Self-doubt and fear of the unknown.

b. Belief that higher priority projects leave too little time for learning or implementing new behaviors.

c. Dislike on the part of the learner for the new behavior.

d. Previously unsuccessful attempts to change behavior.

e. Lack of confidence in implementing new behaviors.

f. Cultural beliefs in conflict with the proposed change or behavior.

g. Lack of social support.

REFERENCES

1. R. Barnhart, ed., *The Barnhart Concise Dictionary of Etymology* (New York: HarperCollins Publishers, 1995).

2. L. Jensen and M. Allen, Wellness: The Dialectic of Illness, *Image* 25, no. 3 (1993): 220–224.

3. Ibid.

4. S. Leddy and J.M. Pepper, *Conceptual Bases of Professional Nursing Practice,* 3rd ed. (Philadelphia: J.B. Lippincott, 1995).

5. B.M. Dossey et al., *Holistic Nursing: A Handbook for Practice,* 2nd ed. (Gaithersburg, MD: Aspen Publishers, 1995), 115–134.

6. H.L. Dunn, *High Level Wellness* (Arlington, VA: R.W. Beatty, 1961).

7. P. Benner and J. Wrubel, *The Primacy of Caring: Stress and Coping in Health and Illness* (Reading, MA: Addison-Wesley Publishing Co., 1989).

8. D. Lauver, A Theory of Care Seeking Behavior, *Image* 24, no. 4 (1992): 56–63.

9. M.H. Becker, ed., *The Health Belief Model and Personal Behavior* (Thorofare, NJ: Charles B. Slack, 1974), 1–8.

10. Dossey et al., *Holistic Nursing: A Handbook for Practice,* 124.

11. Ibid., 125–126.

12. J. Prochaska et al., In Search of How People Change, *American Psychologist* 47, no. 9 (1992): 1102–1114.

13. Lauver, A Theory of Care Seeking Behavior.

14. P. Butterfield, Thinking Upstream: Conceptualizing Health from a Population Perspective, in *Community Health Nursing: Promoting the Health of Aggregates,* eds. J.M. Swanson and M. Albrecht (Philadelphia: W.B. Saunders, 1993), 67–71.

15. Prochaska et al., In Search of How People Change.

16. J. Achterberg, *Woman As Healer* (Boston: Shambhala Publications, 1990).

17. R. Spector, *Cultural Diversity in Health and Illness,* 4th ed. (Norwalk, CT: Appleton & Lange, 1996).

18. J.A. Smith, The Idea of Health: A Philosophical Inquiry, *Advances in Nursing Science* 3 (1981): 43–50.

19. Lauver, A Theory of Care Seeking Behavior.

20. Leddy and Pepper, *Conceptual Bases of Professional Nursing Practice,* 122.

21. Joint Commission on Accreditation of Healthcare Organizations, Patient Rights, *Accreditation Manual for Hospitals* (Chicago: 1992).

22. M.M. Andrews, Cultural Diversity and Community Health Nursing, in *Community Health Nursing: Promoting the Health of Aggregates,* eds. J.M. Swanson and M. Albrecht (Philadelphia: W.B. Saunders, 1993), 371–403.

23. K.H. Kavanaugh, Values Clarification for Change and Empowerment, in *Community Health Nursing,* eds., C.M. Smith and F.A. Maurer (Philadelphia: W.B. Saunders, 1995).

24. Dossey et al., *Holistic Nursing: A Handbook for Practice,* 121.

25. Kavanaugh, Values Clarification for Change and Empowerment.

26. Dossey et al., *Holistic Nursing: A Handbook for Practice,* 131–133.

CHAPTER 5

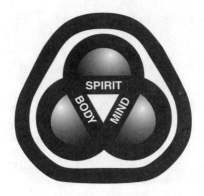

Psychophysiology of Bodymind Healing

Genevieve M. Bartol and Nancy Fleming Courts

KNOWLEDGE COMPETENCIES

- Discuss the meaning of bodymind.
- Describe the implications of the theories for bodymind healing.
- Explain the concept of autopoiesis.
- Explain Reiser's proposed theory of mind (spirit), body, and environment.
- Explore the cognitive, emotional, spiritual, and biochemical responses to selected images and information as suggested by self-regulation theory.
- Analyze the role of natural biologic rhythms in maintaining and promoting healing.
- Analyze state-dependent learning and memory.
- Discuss mind modulation.
- Diagram the physiologic reactions of the autonomic, endocrine, immune, and neuropeptide systems.
- Explain the interrelationships of the autonomic, endocrine, immune, and neuropeptide systems and mind modulation.
- Examine the relationship between psychophysiology and stress disorders.
- Identify theories of pain.
- Differentiate experiences of acute and chronic pain.

DEFINITIONS

Autopoiesis: the self-organizing force in living systems.

Bodymind: a state of integration that includes body, mind, and spirit.[1]

Cardiovascular Reactivity: a relatively rapid and acute change in cardiovascular functioning as a result of a stressor. Cardiovascular reactivity is an individual phenomenon, but differences are consistent within an individual and tend to remain consistent over time.[2]

Mind Modulation: the bidirectional interrelationships of thoughts and feelings with neurohormonal messengers of the nervous, endocrine, immune, and neuropeptide systems that support bodymind connections.[3]

Psychoneuroimmunology: a branch of science that strives to show the connections among psychology, neuroendocrinology, and immunology.

Psychophysiology: the study of the continuous relationship of mind, spirit, and body within the framework of psychologic and physiologic components.

Self-Regulation Theory: an explanation for a person's ability to effect positive changes at the biochemical level within the cells through cognitive processing of information.

State-Dependent Learning and Memory: enhancement or inhibition of learning and memory according to the psychophysiologic state at the time of the learning.[4]

Ultradian Performance Rhythms: varying biologic patterns in humans alternating 90 to 120 minutes of activity with 20 minutes of rest and rejuvenation.

Ultradian Stress Syndrome: the physical, psychologic, and spiritual stress that results from failure to respond appropriately to one's natural, biologic rhythms.

Pause for a moment . . .

❑ *I have begun to study the content areas that I find most challenging and know the least about.*

❑ *I am taking the practice examination to determine the areas on which I need to concentrate.*

❑ *I am gaining confidence in these areas early in my study plan.*

❑ *I am receiving great satisfaction from my progress toward holistic nursing certification (HNC).*

THEORIES AND RESEARCH

Conceptualizations with Implications for Immune System Functioning[5]

1. Einstein's relativity theory suggests that all things and events connect and are relative.
   a. The mind and body are one.
   b. All happenings in one's life are interconnected.
   c. Immunity interacts with everything and everyone.
   d. Bodymind systems are a form of energy interacting both internally and externally.
2. Plank's Quantum Mechanics suggests many worlds are operating with many levels of functioning, as well as many rules and concepts.
   a. The world and a person make up an interconnected dynamic system.
   b. One set of rules cannot explain immunity. Mechanical and Newtonian laws cannot adequately explain the quantum and universal nature of immunity.
3. Bohr's Complementarity suggests all parts of the world are unified and complement one another.
   a. All parts of the body function together as one.
   b. Wellness and illness are both natural and necessary; the human immune system allows for both.
   c. Humans are dynamic and adaptive.
   d. The body and the mind are in continuous interaction; it is not possible to establish either the body or the mind as the single causal site of any state of wellness or illness.
4. Bell's Theorem maintains the whole determines the actions of the parts and changes occur instanteously. Even a passing feeling or a fleeting thought can effect changes in the system.

a. There are no limits on wellness and healing.
   b. Healing does not take time; it depends on hope and belief beyond time.
   c. Belief is as important as thought in respect to the immune system.
5. Prigogine's Dissipative Structures asserts the world and persons evolve through change.
   a. Stability is not balance, but change.
   b. Symptoms are signals of stability.
   c. Symptoms represent the intrinsic organization and adaptability of the body.
   d. All development is due to breakdown and self-renewal.
   e. Hope and a positive viewpoint are essential factors in wellness and illness.
6. Von Bertalanffy's Systems Theory states the world and a person make up an interconnected dynamic system.
   a. A change on any level effects a change at all other levels and in the whole system.
   b. Feedback, integration, rhythm, and dynamic equilibrium are all part of the biodance.
7. Heisenberg's Uncertainty Principle holds every explanation has limits.
   a. Even one additional piece of data will change the whole configuration.
   b. All diagnosis is provisional; it is important to remain open to all possibilities.
   c. Emphasizing one aspect makes everything else more uncertain.

Applications of Biologic Principles to Human Health and Illness[6]

1. Autopoiesis refers to a fundamental self-organizing force that exists in living systems but remains unexplained by physical principles. In humans, for example
   a. Homeostatic mechanisms maintain body temperature.
   b. Repair of body tissues in response to a wound preserves integrity of the body.
   c. Complex instinctual patterns for protection and reproduction ensure survival of the individual and the species.
2. Organisms appear to be under the direction of an overall design or purpose, not just functioning mechanically. Humans create, and their activity is purposeful.
3. Evolution has not been a steady and uniform progression from simple to more complex organisms.

4. There have been periods of quiescence in which relatively few new forms appeared and brief periods during which there was an utter explosion of new forms.
5. The novelty in evolution is akin to the creativity in humans that may foster adaptation in the face of myriad challenges in all states of wellness and illness.
6. No mechanistic model explains the functioning of the human "immune-healing-regeneration system," which seems to involve communication and creative problem-solving processes.

Reiser's Proposed Theory of Mind (Spirit), Body, and Environment[7]

1. Wellness and illness are multicausal and complex human responses that represent the interaction of innumerable physiologic, psychologic, social, and physical environmental factors.
2. Perceptions registered in the cortex of the brain may later be recalled in the presence of new stimuli. In this way, perceptions in the cortex acquire new meaning.
3. Meanings influence responses and set enduring patterns that may lead to changes in structure and function.
4. The individual's physiologic and psychologic responses to multiple factors may predispose to particular states of wellness and illness.
5. There are three main phases in the natural history of disease.
   a. In the preclinical phase, genetic (genotype), intrauterine, perinatal, and postnatal (phenotype) influences may predispose a person to a particular state of health or disease condition.
   b. In the precipitation phase, a certain combination of events triggers the disease process.
   c. In the established disease phase, the person manifests a constellation of symptoms (known as disease) that represent the body's attempt to reorganize in response to a threat.
6. The complexity of human responses to the innumerable physiologic, psychologic, social, and environmental factors in all states of wellness and illness provides an opportunity for all types of interventions, ranging from the simple to the elaborate.[8]
7. Emotional, instrumental, and informational social supports, in their many manifestations, are important factors in promoting health and healing. Appropriate touch, presence, prayer, and community may promote the trust and foster the communication that supports health and healing.
8. Healing rituals are founded on a shared world view and embedded in culture. Interventions must be in tune with the individual's Gestalt; otherwise, they may increase stress and impede health and healing.

Self-Regulation Theory[9]

1. When an individual experiences an event, the perception of that event elicits mental and emotional responses that are stored in the bodymind at the cellular level.
2. Specifically, the mental and emotional responses generate limbic, hypothalmic, and pituitary biochemical responses, which in turn effect physiologic changes that are also perceived and responded to, creating a cybernetic feedback loop that is stored in the bodymind.
3. A subsequent event can arouse a stored schema of mental and physiologic responses generated by a prior event. The retrieval of this stored information can also provoke thought, images, and behavior associated with the prior event. All these responses are considered the raw material of a perception of an event.
4. Self-regulation theory centers on accessing the raw material of these inner schema and promotes internal healing by modulating positive imagery patterns (the combined cognitive and emotional responses) to effect positive changes at the biochemical level within the cells to promote healing and elicit a desired behavioral response.
5. For example, by attending to the objective features of a procedure instead of the subjective emotional responses, individuals can access their internal healing resources by reconfiguring the original schema and creating a positive response.

Ultradian Stress Syndrome and Performance Rhythm

1. Humans have various natural, biologic rhythms.[10]
   a. Infradian rhythms are those that take longer than a day, such as a woman's menstrual cycle.
   b. Circadian rhythms are those that rise and fall each day, such as sleep and wake patterns.
   c. Ultradian rhythms refer to the cyclic pattern of activity and rest in which periods of 90 to 120 minutes of activity alternate with peri-

ods of 20 minutes of rest in less than a 24-hour period. Individual variations in the timing of this pattern often shift with changing demands.

2. The body's ultradian/circadian rhythms provide important psychologic and physiologic clues about staying well (e.g., hunger and fatigue).

3. Excessive disregard of clues distorts normal ultradian/circadian rhythms of activity and leads to ultradian stress syndrome.

4. Responding appropriately to clues allows the natural ultradian/circadian rhythms to normalize themselves and relieves ultradian stress syndrome.

5. Nurses can teach people to respect their natural ultradian/circadian rhythms in ways that promote health in the face of the constantly shifting and challenging events of daily life.

 Pause for a moment . . .

❑ *I can integrate the **AHNA Core Curriculum for Holistic Nursing** information in my current practice environment.*

❑ *I know the content areas where I am strong and those where I need more study time.*

Principles of Psychophysiology

1. Higher brain centers regulate both skeletal and visceral activities because nearly all spinal nerves and many cranial nerves contain both somatic and autonomic fibers. The brain interprets and responds to stimuli (messages) based on past experiences, current conditions, and reflexes.

2. Adaptation to internal and external changes involves both skeletal muscles and enhanced responses from visceral organs. For example, running challenges the skeletal muscles so that they require additional oxygen and glucose; to supply the oxygen and glucose, autonomic control mechanisms increase heart rate and breathing to maintain dynamic equilibrium.

3. The nervous system is composed of the central nervous system (CNS), the brain and spinal cord, and the peripheral nervous system (PNS), all nerves outside the brain and spinal cord.

4. The PNS is divided into the somatic and the autonomic nervous systems.

    a. The somatic nervous system axons extend from the CNS to effectors (skeletal muscle),

release acetylcholine at the synapse, and stimulate muscle contraction. The somatic nervous system allows conscious muscle control and is known as the voluntary nervous system.

    b. The autonomic nervous system maintains internal dynamic equilibrium and consists of the sympathetic, parasympathetic, and enteric systems.

5. The sympathetic and parasympathetic fibers innervate the same organs, but stimulate opposite activity.

6. The sympathetic fibers originate in the thoracolumbar (T1–L2) spinal cord.

    a. A few sympathetic preganglionic axons synapse with the adrenal medulla, stimulating that gland to secrete epinephrine and norepinephrine.

    b. Most sympathetic postganglionic axons secrete norepinephrine at effectors (cardiac and smooth muscle fibers and glands).

    c. Sympathetic stimulation produces the following profound physiologic changes:

        1) Increase in heart rate.
        2) Dilation of bronchioles with rapid, deep breaths.
        3) Cold, sweaty skin.
        4) Dilated pupils.
        5) Shift of blood from visceral to peripheral circulation.
        6) Stimulation of liver to produce more glucose for cells.
        7) Slowing of gastric and urinary tract motility.
        8) Changing brain wave patterns.

7. The parasympathetic fibers originate in the craniosacral division (brain stem and sacrum).

    a. All parasympathetic postganglionic axons release acetylcholine.

    b. Preganglionic parasympathetic fibers of the oculomotor, facial, and glossopharyngeal nerves supply the parasympathetic innervation of the head. Postganglionic fibers synapse with the trigeminal nerve and "travel" with these fibers.

    c. The parasympathetic nervous system, active in calm, nonstressful conditions, is concerned with low energy use, digestion, and elimination of urine and feces.

8. The enteric nervous system is interconnected with the central and autonomic nervous systems.

    a. Enteric neurons form two intrinsic nerve plexuses (the submucosal and the myenteric) in the alimentary tract walls that communicate and regulate digestion.

    b. The submucosal nerve plexus regulates gland activity and smooth muscles.

    c. The myenteric plexus controls gastrointestinal tract motility.

    d. Afferent visceral fibers link the alimentary canal with the CNS.

    e. Motor fibers of sympathetic and parasympathetic branches of the autonomic nervous system are found in the enteric plexuses.

    f. Stimulation of the parasympathetic nervous system aids digestion by increasing mobility and enhancing secretory activity; stimulation of the sympathetic nervous system decreases digestion.

9. The limbic system, whose structures encircle the upper part of the brain stem, is known as the emotional or affective brain. It is biochemically interrelated with the rest of the body.

    a. The extensive connections between the limbic structures and higher regions of the brain promote response to and integration of environmental stimuli.

    b. The interaction with the prefrontal or thinking part of the brain permits integration of thinking and feelings. At times, logic may be stronger than emotion; at other times, emotion may override logic.

10. The hypothalamus, which lies deep within the brain and is the clearinghouse for both autonomic nervous system and emotional responses, maintains dynamic equilibrium.

    a. The hypothalamus regulates involuntary nervous system activity, such as blood pressure, rate and force of heart contraction, motility of digestive tract, respiratory rate, and pupil size.

    b. The connections of the hypothalamus with the cortical areas and the limbic structures control physical expressions of emotion.

    c. Osmoreceptors in the hypothalamus respond to the concentration of solutes in the extracellular fluid by releasing or inhibiting release of antidiuretic hormone.

    d. The hypothalamus links the CNS and the endocrine systems, produces and releases hormones, and is a neuroendocrine organ in its own right.

11. The thalamus, composed of many nuclei with special functions, is a communicating link to the cerebral cortex.

    a. Sensory afferent fibers converge in the thalamus where information is grouped and sent to appropriate areas of the sensory cortex.

    b. Almost all ascending inputs are funneled via the thalamic nuclei.

    c. The thalamus helps mediate sensation, cortical arousal, motor activities, and memory.

12. Neuropeptides are composed of amino acids that circulate widely in the body and have a broad spectrum of effects. They are considered messengers connecting mind and body.

    a. The neuropeptide substance P is a mediator of pain signals, while endorphins and enkephalins bind with the natural opiate receptors in the brain and produce even stronger effects than opiates. The neuropeptide endorphin is credited with producing the "runner's high," while enkephalins are at an especially high level during childbirth so that labor pain is reduced.

    b. The small intestine secretes the nonneural hormone cholecystokinin in response to food. The target organs are the liver, pancreas, and gall bladder, which, in turn, stimulate release of digestive factors.

    c. Somatostatin, secreted by the CNS, hypothalamus, and brain, inhibits the release of growth hormone.

Impact of Stress

1. Stress is a multidimensional concept with three interactive components:

    a. The stress stimuli or input.

    b. Systems to process stress, including the subjective experience; endocrine, autonomic, and immune systems; and neuropeptides.

    c. The stress response.[11]

2. Among the factors that affect response to stress are the following:

    a. Number and intensity of the stressors.

    b. Chronicity of stressors (acute or time limited).

    c. Stressor sequence.

    d. Intermittent occurrence (weekly or monthly) or permanence (disabilities, bad job situation) of stressors.

    e. Coping mechanisms and support systems available.

3. The brain's perception that something desired is missing or threatened; uncertainty or lack of information, and inability to secure positive

outcomes or prevent negative outcomes may stimulate the stress response.

4. The physiologic stress-response systems include the hypothalamic-pituitary-adrenal system, sympathetic-adrenal-medulla system, and the immune system.[12]

5. The hypothalamus-pituitary-adrenal axis includes secretion of corticotropin-releasing hormone from the hypothalamus. This hormone stimulates the anterior pituitary to secrete adrenocorticotropic hormone, which, in turn, stimulates the adrenal gland.

   a. The adrenal cortex secretes the glucocorticoids, which provide stress resistance through their effect on cellular metabolism. The normal circadian secretion of glucocorticoids maintains constant glucose levels and blood volume.

   b. During highly stressful times such as severe infections or hemorrhage, the output of the glucocorticoid cortisol (hydrocortisone) is increased significantly and acts on target cells to suppress the immune system, decreasing the individual's ability to resist infections and disease.

   c. Excessive levels of cortisol increase the vasoconstrictive effects of epinephrine by raising blood pressure; inhibit inflammation and delay healing; promote osteoporosis; and change cardiovascular, gastrointestinal, and neural function.

6. As part of the stress response, the sympathetic-adrenal-medulla nervous system stimulates the adrenal medulla to secrete the catecholamines that constrict blood vessels; raise blood pressure; increase heart rate; raise glucose levels; and divert blood from nonessential organs to large skeletal muscles, the heart, and the brain. This helps prepare the body for "fight or flight."

7. Chronically high levels of catecholamines dampen the immune system, while short exposure to high levels activate or suppress immune cell activity.

8. There is some evidence that the immune system sends feedback to the brain; for example, an infection can stimulate an increase in brain activity.

9. It is clear that the stress response supports adaptation to changing internal and external environments. Physiologically, the body is prepared for enhanced function. Although high levels of stress are incompatible with enhanced psychologic function, low levels enhance performance.

Stress-Induced Illness

1. Given the interrelationship of neuroendocrine and immunologic psychophysiologic changes stimulated by stress, it seems reasonable that prolonged stress and stressful environments could lead to structural and functional changes at the cellular and organ system levels.

2. The research on stress-induced illnesses is interesting, suggestive, but inconclusive. There are numerous research design issues.[13]

   a. It is easier to measure acute stress outcomes than chronic stress outcomes.

   b. Self-report of anxiety and depression may be skewed by social desirability issues.

   c. Chronic stress may be more important in the development of illness, since the physiologic reactions are more subtle.

   d. Variables of stress-induced illness include strength, number, severity, and length of stressors.

3. Conditions conducive to the development of stress-induced illness include the genetic vulnerability of the person, the hyperactivity of the body system, and the use of coping mechanisms.

4. Emotional stress and/or environmental challenges lead to visceral illnesses via the limbic structures to the hypothalamus and the adrenal cortex.

Pain and Its Effects

1. Cognitive and affective factors influence pain perception.

2. Pain stimulates the sympathetic nervous system. Therefore, it is a stressor and, as a stressor, affects the neuroendoimmunologic systems.

3. There are millions of sensory nerve endings throughout the body tissues and organs.

4. Pain is classified as somatic or visceral.

   a. Somatic pain originates in the muscles, joints, or skin. Superficial somatic pain is localized to skin and mucosa and is sharp, prickly, and brief. Deep somatic pain is burning, aching, or itching from stimulation of deep skin, joint, or muscle pain receptors; is more diffuse; and indicates tissue damage.

b. Visceral pain (dull, aching, gnawing) arises from tissue stretching, ischemia, and muscle spasms; because it follows the same pathways as somatic pain does, it can be perceived as somatic or referred pain.

5. Tissue damage releases pain-producing substances such as serotonin, histamine, bradykinin, and substance P at nerve endings.

6. The pain impulses travel along the peripheral pathways through the spinal cord to the reticular formation, thalamus, limbic structures, and the cortex.

7. It is the cortex that permits evaluation of location, nature, and intensity of pain. The pain experience, then, is dependent on interpretations, emotional state, and past experiences.

a. The individual's psychophysiologic state at the time shapes the pain experience; a recollection or anticipation of a second painful experience elicits the pain response even before the pain event (i.e., state-dependent learning).

b. Cognitive factors, such as the ability to solve problems and make decisions, give patients a sense of control (mind modulation) that affects pain perception, which, in turn, affects physiologic responses.

c. The significance of the pain or the message conveyed by the pain affects perception. For example, pain indicating that a condition is returning or worsening is generally more poorly tolerated.

d. Affective factors such as beliefs, values, goals, and emotions influence the meaning of pain; for example,
   1) A patient with a physical condition that will interfere with personal goals may experience higher levels of pain.
   2) People may view pain as a punishment for their past sins and believe that they should suffer.

e. Patients who feel like victims look for something or someone to blame and have difficulty managing pain. Even patients who are truly victims need to become "managers of recovery" to begin healing.[14]

f. Patients whose conditions contribute to a loss of hopes and dreams need to grieve their losses before they can begin to heal.

g. Both pain and fear of the unknown stimulate the hypothalamus to activate the sympathetic nervous system, which then stimulates the adrenal medulla to secrete epinephrine and norepinephrine mediating short-term stress and the adrenal cortex to secrete steroids for prolonged stress. This results in the physiologic state of heightened anxiety, preventing patients from attending to information and being able to make decisions.

h. Pain and anxiety are circuitous; that is, both pain and anxiety increase SNS stimulation with physiologic responses that, in turn, worsen the pain and increase anxiety.

Models of Pain

1. The gate control theory suggests that the substantia gelatinosa in the dorsal horn of the spinal cord, the dorsal column fibers, and the central transmission cells inhibit or stimulate nociceptive impulses.[15]

a. Stimulation of large-diameter fibers closes the "gate" and inhibits impulses. Stimulation of smaller fibers opens the gate, and the impulses continue to the cortex.

b. Psychologic factors open or close the gate. Loss of control and feelings of helplessness tend to open the gate for greater perception of pain, while feelings of control and concentration on problem solving tend to close the gate and reduce perception of pain.

2. The interpersonal influence model, a psychologic pain model, reflects the dramatic impact of "being with" a patient when one is powerless to relieve the suffering otherwise.[16]

a. Helping patients identify the need and then helping them to grieve their losses is an integral part of the interpersonal influence model.

b. It is important to avoid personalizing patients' strong emotions. The feelings are not directed at the caregiver or family.

c. The nurse's ability to listen to patients talk about painful events decreases suffering and supports healing.

3. The self-regulation model,[17] also a psychologic pain model, is designed to help patients manage their cognitive, affective, and physiologic responses to pain. Successful use of this model requires knowledgeable nurses to provide information, training, and follow-up. (See Chapters 23, 24, 25, and 26 for specific techniques.)

a. Cognitive processing of information and use of specific skills such as relaxation techniques and mental imagery can change physiology.

b. Interventions to reduce and control pain also provide affective changes, increase feelings of control, and decrease feelings of helplessness.

c. These changes occur on the cellular level.

d. Because the effective use of the self-regulation model requires an interpersonal relationship with the one teaching the skills, the two models overlap to some extent.

Acute vs. Chronic Pain

1. Pain that lasts longer than the time anticipated becomes chronic pain. The actual length of time for acute pain to become chronic pain varies.

2. Chronic pain may be ongoing, or it may have remissions and exacerbations (such as in rheumatoid arthritis, lupus erythematosus, or migraines).

   a. In chronic pain, the pain may become the disease or condition and may demand lifestyle changes that affect the whole family.

   b. Over time, chronic pain depletes sympathoadrenal responses, leading to irritability and depression.

3. Acute pain generally indicates an acute problem that requires diagnosis and treatment.

   a. Usually, acute pain is associated with an identifiable event and is accompanied by sympathetic stimulation that leads to physiologic changes and the experience of anxiety.

   b. The tissue injury releases pain-producing substances that stimulate nociceptors directly and causes them to send afferent impulses to the brain.

   c. Vasospasm, stimulated by the pain-producing substances and accompanied by muscle tension, increases pain perception.

d. Acute pain stimulates the SNS, inducing the stress response.

4. Interventions for pain control are consistent with holistic nursing practice. The interconnectedness and reciprocity of mind, body, and spirit make it possible to achieve patient outcomes through a variety of approaches.

REFERENCES

1. B.M. Dossey et al., *Holistic Nursing: A Handbook for Practice*, 2nd ed. (Gaithersburg, MD: Aspen Publishers, 1995), 88.
2. K. Hughahl, *Psychophysiology The Mind-Body Perspective* (Cambridge, MA: Harvard University Press, 1995).
3. Dossey et al., *Holistic Nursing: A Handbook for Practice*.
4. Ibid.
5. P. Pearsall, *Superimmunity* (New York: Fawcett Gold Metal, 1987), 280–281.
6. W.W. Harmon, Exploring the New Biology, *Noetic Sciences Review*, Summer, no. 34 (1995): 29–33.
7. M. Reiser, *Mind, Brain, Body: Toward a Convergence of Psychoanalysis and Neurobiology* (New York: Basic Books, 1984).
8. T.L. Rosenthal, To Soothe the Savage Beast, *Behavioral Research Therapy* 31, no. 5 (1993): 439–462.
9. Dossey et al., *Holistic Nursing: A Handbook for Practice*, 95.
10. Ibid., 95–97.
11. H. Ursin and M. Olff, The Stress Response, in *Stress from Synapse to Syndrome*, ed. S.C. Stanford and P. Salmon (New York: Academic Press, 1993), 3–22.
12. K. Hughahl, *Psychophysiology The Mind-Body Perspective*.
13. B.J. Lowery and A.D. Houldin, From Stressor to Illness: The Psychological-Biological Connections, in *Psychiatric-Mental Health Nursing*, ed. A.B. McBride and J.K. Austin (Philadelphia: W.B. Saunders, 1996), 11–29.
14. J.R. Dane and R.S. Kessler, A Matrix Model for the Psychological Assessment and Treatment of Acute Pain, in *Handbook of Critical Care Pain Management*, ed. R.J. Hamil and J.C. Rowlingson (New York: McGraw-Hill, 1994), 53–81.
15. R. Melzack and P.D. Wall, Pain Mechanisms: A New Theory, *Science*, 150 (1965): 971–979.
16. Dane and Kessler, A Matrix Model for the Psychological Assessment and Treatment of Acute Pain.
17. Ibid.

CHAPTER 6

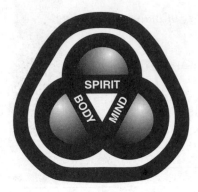

Spirituality and Healing

Margaret A. Burkhardt and Mary Gail Nagai-Jacobson

KNOWLEDGE COMPETENCIES

- Describe spirituality.
- Differentiate spirituality and religion.
- Discuss characteristics of spirituality.
- Discuss mystery, suffering, forgiveness, grace, hope, and love as spiritual issues.
- Explore the place of prayer in healing.
- Describe forms and expressions of prayer.
- Discuss the interplay of psychology and spirituality.
- Explore the need for nurses to nurture their own spirits and approaches for doing so.
- Explore spirituality and the nursing process.
- Discuss ways in which ritual, rest and leisure, play, and creativity relate to spirituality.
- Discuss listening as intentional presence.
- Explore ways of nurturing important connections.
- Discuss the relationship between spirituality and story.
- Describe approaches for responding to spiritual concerns, including assessment as an intervention.

DEFINITION

Spirituality: the unifying force of a person; the essence of being that shapes, gives meaning to, and is aware of one's self-becoming. It is characterized by unfolding mystery, interconnectedness, and inner strength. Spirituality permeates all of life and is manifested in one's being, knowing, and doing. It is expressed and experienced uniquely by each individual through and within connections to God/Life Force/the Absolute, the environment, nature, other people, and the self.

Pause for a moment . . .

❏ *I can visualize complete success in the holistic nursing certification (HNC) process.*
❏ *I can give myself positive affirmations and feedback.*

THEORIES AND RESEARCH

Differentiation of Spirituality and Religion[1-3]

1. Spirituality and religion are not synonymous.
   a. Spirituality is an integral dimension of all persons, an aspect of humanity that, as a manifestation of a person's wholeness, is not subject to choice, but simply is.
   b. Religion per se is not essential to existence and is chosen.
   c. Issues of spirituality may be described as "life issues" that are sometimes, but not always, related to religion.
2. Religion refers to a belief system and practices of worship related to that system.
   a. Religious beliefs can be shared and may relate to cultural perspectives.
   b. Spirituality may be expressed and experienced not only within a particular religion, but also in other ways.
   c. Information about religious practices may or may not relate to spiritual strength or health.
   d. Knowledge of the many religious traditions that a nurse may encounter, their histories, symbols, practices, beliefs, and languages,

increases the nurse's ability to hear and address religious needs of patients/clients.

Elements of Spirituality [4-6]

1. Spirituality is experienced as a unifying force, life principle, essence of being.
   a. This force of principle is a power greater than the self, both within and beyond the self.
   b. It is mystery, that which is beyond words.
   c. Individuals refer to the force or principle by many names, including Absolute, God, Higher Power, Goddess, Lord, Inner Light, Life Source, Allah, Tao, Spirit, The Way, Universal Love.
2. Spirituality is expressed and experienced in and through connectedness with nature, the earth, the environment, and the cosmos.
   a. It is essential to recognize and appreciate the interconnected web of all of life—what happens to the earth affects everyone, and everyone's behavior affects the earth.
   b. Spirituality may be experienced as a sense of awe, finding God/Absolute in all things.
   c. Spirituality may be experienced as one derives strength from and nurtures one's spirit through nature and remains aware of one's surroundings.
   d. Appreciating, respecting, caring for the earth and all its inhabitants are elements of spirituality.
3. People express and experience spirituality in and through connectedness with other people, such as the following:
   a. Loving and painful, supportive and difficult relationships with family, friends, and acquaintances.
   b. Caring for others and being cared for by others.
   c. Love, honesty, acceptance, support, and reconciliation.
   d. Sharing of everyday life experiences and significant life events, joys and sorrows, ritual, prayer, play, concerns.
   e. Appreciation of a common humanity and common bonding.
   f. Recognition of relationships as a source of growth and change.
4. Spirituality shapes the self-becoming and is reflected in one's being, knowing, and doing.
   a. Being is the art of stillness and presence with self, others, the Absolute, and nature; it includes

1) Experiencing the present moment more deeply.
2) Experiencing inner peace, synchrony and harmony, openness; paying attention to the quiet place inside; attuning to sources of inner strength.
3) Bringing one's whole self—alert, quiet, and aware—intentionally into an experience.
   b. Knowing is awareness about one's self (one's physical, mental, emotional, and spiritual natures), one's connections, and one's surroundings.
1) It flows from a stance of openness and a sense of inner knowing.
2) It involves actively seeking knowledge and insights.
3) It includes an attitude of gratitude.
   c. Doing is the outward, visible expression of spirituality.
1) Actions such as assisting others, participating in church or ritual, gardening, being involved in environmental activities, raising children, and visiting the sick demonstrate spirituality.
2) Doing reflects being and knowing.
5. Spirituality permeates life, providing purpose, meaning, strength, and guidance and shaping the journey.
   a. A state of being that does not go away, spirituality is the eternal form of the bodymind.
   b. Because it is practical and relevant to daily life, people experience spirituality in the mundane as well as the profound.
   c. Spirituality is connected to values, although it may or may not be related to religious beliefs.
   d. It provides a sense of place, a sense of how one fits in the world.
   e. Encountering obstacles, learning through experiences, and developing new awarenesses may change one's spirituality; reconciling new experiences with previously held values may result in new values and understandings.
   f. The pattern of the journey and the meaning of life events may become clear only in retrospect.
   g. It is necessary to trust that one has or is given the resources needed for dealing with the unexpected.

Spirituality and the Healing Process [7,8]

1. The words *healing, whole,* and *holy* all derive from the same roots—Old English hal and

Greek holos—suggesting that what is holy or spiritual is intimately connected with health.

2. Spiritual issues are core "life issues" that are not quantifiable and often have no clearly defined answers.

   a. Mystery, that which is not understood or explained, is sometimes described as a truth beyond understanding or explanation.

      1) Spirituality involves the questions of mystery that are part of life.
      2) Seeking and questioning are important aspects of the place of mystery in human life.
      3) In considering spiritual issues, accepting mystery is important.

   b. Suffering, in both its presence and its meaning, is one of the core issues and mysteries of life. Cultural and religious traditions have arisen as people throughout the ages have sought to understand the reason for apparently irrational suffering.

      1) Nurses' awareness of their own responses to and understanding of suffering will help them to be with those who are suffering in an intentional, healing way.
      2) Suffering wears many faces and occurs on many levels—body, mind, and spirit.
      3) Cultural, religious, environmental, and familial factors all influence an individual's response to suffering.
      4) Knowledge of personality, culture, religious traditions, and family background may assist the nurse in understanding the nature and meaning of suffering for a particular client.
      5) The nurse must discern whether honoring another's suffering requires action, presence, absence, or a combination of these.
      6) The nurse must be willing to confront suffering that cannot be alleviated and must simply be borne. In such situations, the nurse's ability to *be* with another is crucial.
      7) An important part of being with those who suffer is listening with one's whole being as they wonder aloud and express deep feelings regarding some of life's unanswerable questions.

   c. Forgiveness is a deep need and hunger of the human experience.

      1) Many religious traditions address the issue of forgiveness, both given and accepted.
      2) Forgiveness involves a person's conscious choice to release someone perceived to have wounded him or her from the sentence of judgment, regardless of whether that judgment seems justified.
      3) Problems around forgiveness include the following:
         a) The difficulty of forgiving another.
         b) The difficulty of accepting forgiveness.
         c) The difficulty of forgiving oneself.
         d) One's understanding of the nature of God or the Absolute.
         e) Specific beliefs of a particular religious tradition.

   d. Grace comes into one's life unearned, without regard to merit, and provides a blessing.

      1) Grace offers a measure of peace or acceptance.
      2) Grace provides a framework within which to understand those gifts of life that are sometimes attributed to providence.

   e. Hope is desire accompanied by expectation of fulfillment.

      1) Hope is a significant factor in overcoming illness and in living through difficult situations.
      2) It helps people deal with fear and uncertainty.
      3) There are two levels of hope: specific hope as a goal or desire and a more general sense that the future is somehow in safekeeping.
      4) Hoping goes beyond believing or wishing.

   f. Love, an acknowledged mystery that involves both choice and emotion, is experienced and expressed in caring given and received.

      1) Love includes dimensions of self-love and divine love, as well as love for others and all of life.
      2) Love often underlies acts of courage and compassion that defy explanation.
      3) Love heals, and its relationship to healing is a continuing source of exploration and wonder.
      4) Love is living from one's heart, one's center where the ego is detached from outcomes.

3. Prayer can affect healing.[9,10]

   a. Prayer has been described as
      1) A deep human instinct.
      2) An endeavor that starts and ends without words.
      3) The most fundamental, primordial, and important language that humans speak.

4) A representation of one's longing for communion or communication with God or the Absolute.

b. Prayer has many forms and expressions.

1) It is part of many religious traditions and rituals.

2) Prayer may be individual or communal, public or private.

3) At times, prayer is a conscious activity; other times, it is less conscious.

4) Speaking (sometimes silently), listening, waiting, and silence may be elements of prayer.

5) Prayer includes petition, intercession, confession, lamentation, adoration, invocation, and thanksgiving.

6) A reminder of our nonlocal, unbounded nature, prayer is infinite in space and time; it is Divine, the universe's affirmation that we are not alone.

c. Research on the efficacy of prayer in healing suggests the following:[11,12]

1) Prayer works, and both directed and nondirected methods are effective.

2) Nondirected prayer (no specific outcome prayed for) may be more effective than directed prayer.

3) Outcomes in nondirected prayer appear to be "what is best for the organism."

4) Prayer at a distance alters processes in a variety of organisms, including plants and people.

5) Observed effects of prayer do not depend on what the one prayed for thinks.

d. Varied techniques are used in prayer:

1) Relaxation, quieting, and breath awareness.

2) Attention training and focusing.

3) Imagery and visualization.

4) Intentionality.

5) Movement, such as dancing, walking, drumming.

4. Psychologic and spiritual elements are interconnected.

a. In a holistic paradigm, body-mind-spirit is an intertwined and interpenetrating unity, and every experience has body-mind-spirit components.

b. Before the time of Freud, phenomena of the sentient realm that could not be explained physically were often viewed in religious terms.

c. It is important to refrain from labeling an unfamiliar spiritual perspective as a psychologic aberration.

d. Psychologic concerns are identified and dealt with according to particular psychologic theories.

e. Spiritual issues are appreciated and experienced more broadly and are subject to unique personal interpretation.

 Pause for a moment . . .

❑ *I am learning the contents contained within the **AHNA Core Curriculum for Holistic Nursing**.*

❑ *I am learning how the HNC examination is constructed.*

❑ *I am identifying the areas that will need more study time than the others.*

Nurturing the Spirit[13]

1. The ability to care for and nurture oneself is basic to functioning in a healing role with another.

2. Attentiveness to one's spirit is a key component of living in a healing way.

a. Awareness of and care for one's own spirit are important components of integrating spirituality into clinical practice.

b. Care of the spirit/soul includes pausing, taking time, and paying attention.[14]

c. Approaches to nurturing the nurse's spirit are the same as those suggested for patients.

HOLISTIC NURSING PROCESS

Assessment

1. Attentive listening and focused presence are essential, because issues of spirituality come in many shapes and contexts.

2. Good therapeutic communication skills facilitate the exploration of spiritual issues, and broad, open-ended questions are often useful.

3. It is beneficial to create a space where spirituality can be expressed.

4. Nurses should be clear about their own spiritual perspective so as not to cloud their ability to hear a client's perspective.

5. It is important to listen for story and metaphor.
6. Spirituality assessment guides may be useful in the process of assessment (Exhibit 6–1).
   a. Guides help the nurse understand and know the unique client.
   b. They are openings or reference points for discussion of spirituality, not checklists or surveys in which all questions must have a response.

7. The nurse assesses the client's understandings of and ways of expressing spirituality, including
   a. Important connections and their role/influence in the present circumstances.
   b. Issues related to meaning and purpose.
   c. Important beliefs, values, and practices.
   d. Prayer or meditation styles.
   e. Desire for connection with religious groups or rituals.

Exhibit 6–1 Spiritual Assessment Tool

To facilitate the healing process in clients/patients, families, significant others, and yourself, the following reflective questions assist in assessing, evaluating, and increasing awareness of the spiritual process in yourself and others.

MEANING AND PURPOSE These questions assess a person's ability to seek meaning and fulfillment in life, manifest hope, and accept ambiguity and uncertainty.

• What gives your life meaning?
• Do you have a sense of purpose in life?
• Does your illness interfere with your life goals?
• Why do you want to get well?
• How hopeful are you about obtaining a better degree of health?
• Do you feel that you have a responsibility in maintaining your health?
• Will you be able to make changes in your life to maintain your health?
• Are you motivated to get well?
• What is the most important or powerful thing in your life?

INNER STRENGTHS These questions assess a person's ability to manifest joy and recognize strengths, choices, goals, and faith.

• What brings you joy and peace in your life?
• What can you do to feel alive and full of spirit?
• What traits do you like about yourself?
• What are your personal strengths?
• What choices are available to you to enhance your healing?
• What life goals have you set for yourself?
• Do you think that stress in any way caused your illness?
• How aware were you of your body before you became sick?
• What do you believe in?
• Is faith important in your life?
• How has your illness influenced your faith?
• Does faith play a role in regaining your health?

INTERCONNECTIONS These questions assess a person's positive self-concept, self-esteem, and sense of self; sense of belonging in the world with others; capacity to pursue personal interests; and ability to demonstrate love of self and self-forgiveness.

• How do you feel about yourself right now?
• How do you feel when you have a true sense of yourself?
• Do you pursue things of personal interest?
• What do you do to show love for yourself?
• Can you forgive yourself?
• What do you do to heal your spirit?

These questions assess a person's ability to connect in life-giving ways with family, friends, and social groups and to engage in the forgiveness of others.

• Who are the significant people in your life?
• Do you have friends or family in town who are available to help you?
• Who are the people to whom you are closest?
• Do you belong to any groups?
• Can you ask people for help when you need it?
• Can you share your feelings with others?
• What are some of the most loving things that others have done for you?
• What are the loving things that you do for other people?
• Are you able to forgive others?

These questions assess a person's capacity for finding meaning in worship or religious activities and a connectedness with a divinity or universe.

• Is worship important to you?
• What do you consider the most significant act of worship in your life?
• Do you participate in any religious activities?
• Do you believe in God or a higher power?
• Do you think that prayer is powerful?
• Have you ever tried to empty your mind of all thoughts to see what the experience might be like?

continues

Exhibit 6–1 continued

- Do you use relaxation or imagery skills?
- Do you meditate?
- Do you pray?
- What is your prayer?
- How are your prayers answered?
- Do you have a sense of belonging in this world?

These questions assess a person's ability to experience a sense of connection with all of life and nature, an awareness of the effects of the environment on life and well-being, and a capacity or concern for the health of the environment.

- Do you ever feel at some level a connection with the world or universe?

- How does your environment have an impact on your state of well-being?
- What are your environmental stressors at work and at home?
- Do you incorporate strategies to reduce your environmental stressors?
- Do you have any concerns for the state of your immediate environment?
- Are you involved with environmental issues such as recycling environmental resources at home, work, or in your community?
- Are you concerned about the survival of the planet?

Source: Based on Margaret Burkhardt: Spirituality: An Analysis of the Concept, *Holistic Nursing Practice* 3(3):69. 1989. Reprinted with permission from C.E. Guzzetta and B.M. Dossey, *Cardiovascular Nursing: Holistic Practice,* p. 9, © 1992, Mosby-Year Book.

Nursing Diagnoses

1. Although spirituality can be an important consideration with any health concern, nursing diagnoses regarding spirituality are still in the formative stage.
2. In addressing deep needs, it may be more useful to describe rather than to label. The fact that one is searching for or has needs in the area of spirituality does not mean there is an impairment.
3. Nursing diagnoses related to common human response patterns and compatible with spirituality interventions include the following:
   a. Relating: all current diagnoses.
   b. Valuing: all current diagnoses.
   c. Choosing: all current diagnoses.
   d. Perceiving: all except sensory-perceptual alterations.
   e. Feeling: all current diagnoses.

Client Outcomes

1. Establishing client outcomes requires assessment.
2. The client should participate in determining outcomes.

Plan and Intervention

1. Be aware of your own spiritual perspective and understand its impact on your interactions with a client.

2. Acknowledge when you are uncomfortable with a client's spiritual perspective and make arrangements for others to provide the needed care for that client.
3. Involve the client and family in developing the plan and organizing overall care to incorporate spiritual interventions.
4. Frame the plan within the client's spiritual perspective.
5. Promote an atmosphere accepting and encouraging of many forms of spiritual expression.
6. Identify the nurse's role in meeting spiritual needs, and bring in other resources as needed.

General Guidelines for Responding to Spiritual Concerns[15]

1. By remembering that persons are spiritual beings, the nurse remains attuned to spiritual concerns, which may be shared in a variety of ways, both verbally and nonverbally.
2. Assessment of spiritual concerns is often part of the intervention, because the questions provide an opportunity for clients/patients to become more aware of their spiritual journeys.
3. In responding to spiritual concerns, the nurse keeps in mind certain principles.
   a. An intentional healing presence provides a context for sharing concerns of the spirit.
   b. Awareness of and care for self as a spiritual being undergirds care for others.
   c. Several practices help the nurse be fully present to the client:

1) Centering and awareness as a regular personal practice, with each patient encounter.
2) Use of common activities (e.g., hand washing) as rituals for leaving behind what has gone before in order to be present now.

d. Some clients need verbal encouragement, along with healing presence, to share spiritual concerns.
   1) "You said you had been doing a lot of thinking. Is that anything you want to share?"
   2) "You said you didn't know why this was happening to you. Sometimes things are hard to understand, aren't they?" (Prepare to be fully present while waiting for an answer.)
   3) Sharing observations and recognizing that the person has "deep" concerns often facilitate sharing.

e. Important connections/relationships are the context for the client's lived experiences.

f. The nurse nurtures and facilitates important relationships.
   1) Some family members may need special encouragement to visit or call.
   2) Clients/patients may need some assistance in sharing certain aspects of the health care situation with others.
   3) Recognizing and affirming the support of significant others remind the patient of this network of care and support.
   4) Imagery, pictures, and stories help persons connect with important places, people, or experiences.
   5) Pets or special places may be as important as human relationships, and the nurse should encourage "visits."
   6) Times with friends or members of religious or social communities are beneficial when these are important connections for the person.

g. For some clients, themes or concerns are recurring.
   1) The nurse should reflect and validate these themes and concerns.
   2) It is also important to clarify with the person how these themes fit into the current situation and whether any specific resources are needed to deal with them at this time.

h. Clients have different understandings and experiences of the sacred.
   1) What is sacred for this person?
   2) What nurtures spirit for this person—particular music, books, objects, foods, rituals, prayers, places?
   3) Can the person's experience of the sacred be enhanced through things like rituals, contact with certain people, prayer, or music?

i. A nurse needs a willingness to be present with mystery, uncertainty, pain, or suffering, seeking not to "fix" or to "answer," but to be *in the mystery with another*. Responses such as: "This is beyond my understanding, too" or "It is understandable that you ask these questions, though I have no answer for them either" are appropriate.

Rituals to Nurture Spirit [16]

1. Rituals, either shared with others or highly personalized, are significant aspects of various religious traditions and cultures.
2. Anything done with awareness can be a ritual.
3. Rituals provide a rich resource in caring for the spirit, and intentionally setting aside time for rituals is an important aspect of care for self and others (Exhibit 6–2).
4. The nurse can facilitate and provide opportunities for the patient to consider and experience the place of rituals in his or her life.
   a. What are significant rituals for the patient?
   b. What areas of the patient's life might benefit from rituals?
   c. What resources can be used to increase the patient's understanding and practice of rituals?
   d. What is the significance of sacred space?
5. Ritual has three phases.
   a. The separation phase is a symbolic breaking away from everyday busyness.
   b. The transition phase requires identifying and focusing on areas of life that need attention.
   c. The return phase is the reentry into everyday life.

Centering, Mindfulness, Awareness

1. Processes in which one consciously pauses and seeks to pay attention are at the heart of many spiritual disciplines.
2. The nurse may help clients with several considerations:

Exhibit 6–2 The First Ritual Guide to Getting Well

This ritual helps you decide what to do if you are diagnosed with the unknowable, the unthinkable, the awful, or the so-called incurable. By doing this, you can better determine how to survive treatment, yourself, your friends and family, and life in general.

1. Find a quiet place, a healing place, and go there. This might be a corner of your favorite room where you have placed gifts, pictures, a candle, or other symbols that signal peace and inner reflection to you. Or it might be in a park, under an old tree, or in a special place known for its spirit, such as high on a sacred mountain or on the cliffs overlooking a coastline or in the quiet magnificence of a forest.

2. Ask questions of your inner self about what your diagnosis or treatment means in your life. How will life change? What are your resources, your strengths, your reasons for staying alive? These deeply philosophical or spiritual issues often come to mind when problems are diagnosed. Listen with as quiet a mind as possible for any answers or messages that come from within, or from your higher source of guidance.

3. Take this time, knowing that very few problems advance so quickly that you must rush into making decisions about them immediately, without first gaining some perspective.

4. Find at least one friend or advocate who can be level-headed when you think you are going crazy; who can be positive for you when you are absolutely certain you are doomed; who can listen when your head is buzzing with uncertainty.

5. Love yourself. Ask yourself moment by moment whether what surrounds you is nurturing and life-giving. If the answer is no, back off from it. Kindly tell all negative-thinking people that you will not be seeing them while you are going through this. You may need never to see them again, and this is your right and obligation to yourself.

6. Assess your belief system. What do you believe? How did you get to believe it in the first place? What is really happening inside you and outside you? How serious is it? What will it take to get you well?

7. Gather information, keeping an open mind. Everyone who offers to treat you or give you advice has their lives invested in what they tell you. Stand back and listen thoughtfully.

8. Now go and hire your healing team. Remember, you hired them—you can fire them. They are in the business of performing a service for you, and you are paying their salaries. Sometimes this relationship gets confused. Make sure they all talk to each other. You are in command. You are the captain of the healing team.

9. Don't let anyone talk you into treatment you don't believe in or don't understand. Keep asking questions. Replace anyone who acts too busy to answer your questions. Chances are, they're also too busy to do their best work for you.

10. Don't agree on any diagnostic or lab tests unless someone you trust can give you good reasons why they are being ordered. If the tests are not going to change your treatment, they are an expensive and dangerous waste of your time.

11. Sing your own song, write your own story, take your own spiritual journey through a journal or diary. A threat to health and well-being can be a trigger to becoming and doing all those things you've been putting off for the "right" time.

12. Consider these maxims in your journey:
    • Everything cures somebody, and nothing cures everybody.
    • There are no simple answers to complex issues, like why people get sick in the first place.
    • Sometimes disease is inexplicable to mortal minds.

13. You will not be intimidated by the overbearing world of medicine or alternative health know-it-alls but can thoughtfully take the best from several worlds.

14. You can teach gentleness and compassion to the most arrogant doctor and the crankiest nurse. Tell them that you need your mind and soul nurtured, as well as the best medical treatment possible in order to get well. If they are not up to it, you'll find someone someplace who is.

Source: From *Rituals of Healing: Using Imagery for Health and Wellness*, by Jeanne Achterberg, B. Dossey, and L. Kolkmeier. Copyright © 1994 by Jeanne Achterberg, Barbara Dossey, and Leslie Kolkmeier. Used by permission of Bantam Books, a division of Bantam Doubleday Dell Publishing Group, Inc.

a. Making intentional decisions to pause and be aware.
b. Observing, without judging, what is going on within the self—thoughts, feelings, hindrances to being quiet and mindful.
c. Observing what is going on in the environment—sensations.
d. Being fully present in the moment.

3. The processes of relaxation and imagery facilitate awareness and centering (see Chapters 23 and 24).

Prayer and Meditation

1. Because prayer and meditation take variable forms in many traditions, it is important to explore the patient's way of praying.

2. The nurse can help patients consider
   a. The place and meaning of prayer in their lives.
   b. Ways that they reach out to God/Absolute.
   c. Ways that they experience the presence of and communion with the Absolute.
   d. Changes that they want to make in their prayer life.
   e. Forms of prayer, including any desire for shared prayer or religious worship.
3. Imagery can facilitate access to environments that foster prayer for the person (e.g., church/temple or natural settings).
4. Inspirational or sacred readings, music, drumming, movement, and other practices may be part of the person's way of praying.

Rest and Leisure[17]

1. Because they contribute to growth, creativity, and spiritual renewal, rest and leisure are integral aspects of holistic living and ways to nurture spirit.
2. Nurses can assist persons in considering the place for rest and leisure in their lives by exploring several questions.
   a. How are rest and leisure incorporated into the person's life?
   b. What helps the person rest, and what are considered experiences of leisure?
   c. What changes are necessary, and how can the person plan for those changes?
   d. How can the person evaluate changes and continue to make conscious decisions about this area of life?
   e. What places, situations, or persons facilitate the experience of rest and leisure?
3. Techniques that may enhance times of rest and leisure include meditation, exercise, imagery, music, and commitment to incorporating this into one's life.

Power of Storytelling[18]

1. People often speak of spirituality and spiritual concerns through story and metaphor.
2. An understanding of the power of story in healing enhances the practice of holistic nursing.

3. Each person, including oneself, is an ongoing story.
   a. Knowing one's own story makes it possible to share stories of hope, encouragement, struggle, and other appropriate experiences.
   b. It is important to recognize the ongoing, unfinished nature of life stories.
4. Nurses and clients can share a variety of wonderings and questions.
   a. If your life is a story, what is the title?
   b. What is the title of the current chapter?
   c. Who are some of the heroines and heroes of your story?
   d. How would you like this chapter to turn out?
5. Clients need encouragement and space for the sharing of stories.
   a. The nurse should affirm the sharing of stories through statements (e.g., "Your sharing has helped me see things in a different light").
   b. The nurse should encourage significant people in the person's life to participate in the sharing of story.
6. Some exercises that may facilitate one's ability to be more attentive to story are included in Exhibit 6–3.

Intentional Listening

1. Listening actively and intentionally is necessary in caring for the spirit; one listens best when one listens with one's whole being.[19]
2. By listening well—being fully present with another—the nurse enables the client to understand and experience the present and thereby to move into the future with more awareness.
3. Exhibit 6–4 lists guidelines for listening in healing ways.

Evaluation

1. It is essential to establish whether patient outcomes were achieved.
2. The incorporation of ongoing assessment allows the nurse to determine whether other needs are emerging in the course of caring for the patient.

Exhibit 6–3 Exercises To Facilitate Awareness of Story

1. Take a few moments to become quiet, perhaps using some breath awareness. In this quiet space allow yourself to remember, in as much detail as possible, something about yourself, some event or incident which comes to mind. How has this experience or event become a part of who you are? What meaning does it have for your life at this moment?
2. Keep a journal in which you record events, feelings, experiences, insights, questions in your life. Periodically review your writings, noting themes flowing through your story. Reflect on your story as it is evolving.
3. Think about books, stories, songs, fairy tales, movies, plays, or works of art that have special meaning for you. Take time to consider why and how they hold that meaning for you. Think about the images, characters, colors, and sounds that are found in each of these and how they are reflective of your own story. What meanings do you find that provide insight into your own unfolding journey?
4. Write an autobiography for your eyes only. Take your time. Re-read and reflect on it. Are there parts you want to share? With whom would you share? What new awarenesses and learnings have come to you?
5. Look at some old family photos or photos of friends. What story do they tell? What memories and feelings come with these pictures? Do you want to tell someone else about them? What do you want to say? Would you like to hear someone else's story about these same photos?

Source: M. Burkhardt and M.G. Nagai-Jacobson, © 1997.

Exhibit 6–4 Listening in Healing Ways

- Be intentionally present.
- Maintain focus on the patient/client as a whole person.
- Set aside the need to "fix," "answer," or "correct."
- Learn to be with another in silence.
- Interrupt as little as possible, recognizing that even what is not said at a particular time has meaning and that the way and sequence in which a story is told are part of the story.
- Appreciate that the client is an embodied spirit, with an ongoing and unfinished story.
- Hear the journey, the relationships, the meanings in the story.
- Listen with all your senses.
- Do not prematurely diagnose.
- Let the conversation flow, being with silence as well as words.
- Breathe!

Source: M.G. Nagai-Jacobson and M. Burkhardt, © 1997.

REFERENCES

1. M.A. Burkhardt, Spirituality: An Analysis of the Concept, *Holistic Nursing Practice* 3 (1989): 69–77.
2. M.G. Nagai-Jacobson and M.A. Burkhardt, Spirituality: Cornerstone of Holistic Nursing Practice, *Holistic Nursing Practice* 3 (1989): 18–26.
3. J.D. Emblem, Religion and Spirituality Defined According to Current Use in Nursing Literature, *Journal of Professional Nursing* 8 (1992): 41–47.
4. M.A. Burkhardt, Becoming and Connecting: Elements of Spirituality for Women, *Holistic Nursing Practice* 8 (1994): 12–21.
5. P.G. Reed, An Emerging Paradigm for the Investigation of Spirituality in Nursing, *Research in Nursing and Health* 15 (1992): 349–357.
6. M.G. Nagai-Jacobson and M.A. Burkhardt, Awareness and Relatedness: Elements of Spirituality for Men (Unpublished data).
7. M.A. Burkhardt and M.G. Nagai-Jacobson, Reawakening Spirit in Clinical Practice, *Journal of Holistic Nursing* 12 (1994): 9–21.
8. Nagai-Jacobson and Burkhardt, Spirituality: Cornerstone of Holistic Nursing Practice.
9. L. Dossey, *Healing Words: The Power of Prayer and the Practice of Medicine* (San Francisco, CA: Harper San Francisco, 1993).
10. L. Dossey, *Prayer Is Good Medicine* (San Francisco, CA: Harper San Francisco, 1996).
11. L. Dossey, *Healing Words*.
12. L. Dossey, *Prayer Is Good Medicine*.
13. Burkhardt and Nagai-Jacobson, Reawakening Spirit.
14. T. Moore, *Care of the Soul* (New York: HarperCollins Publishers, 1992).
15. Burkhardt and Nagai-Jacobson, Reawakening Spirit.
16. B.M. Dossey et al., *Holistic Nursing: A Handbook for Practice*, 2nd ed. (Gaithersburg, MD: Aspen Publishers, 1995), 78–80.
17. L. Doohan, *Leisure: A Spiritual Need* (Notre Dame, IN: Ave Maria Press, 1990).
18. M.G. Nagai-Jacobson and M.A. Burkhardt, Viewing Persons As Stories: A Perspective for Holistic Care, *Alternative Therapies in Health and Medicine* 2 (1996): 54–57.
19. B.M. Dossey et al., *Holistic Nursing: A Handbook for Practice*, 71–72.

CHAPTER 7

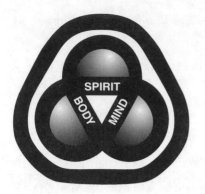

Energetic Healing

Victoria E. Slater

KNOWLEDGE COMPETENCIES

- List three components of human energetic anatomy.
- Describe two characteristics of an electromagnet.
- Apply electromagnet characteristics to the human.
- Describe one traditional portrayal of an aura.
- Describe the very low amplitude direct electric current that Becker associates with meridians.
- Describe one traditional understanding of chakras.
- Describe a Fourier analyzer and L-C circuits.
- Compare a Fourier analyzer to the chakra system and L-C circuits to individual chakras.
- Discuss the quantum theory of consciousness-created reality.
- Describe Assagioli's theory of psychosynthesis and his model of the dimensions of the psyche.
- Apply consciousness-created reality and psychosynthesis to holistic healing.
- Apply the Energetic Healing Modalities Model.

DEFINITIONS

Aura: an atmosphere; a vague, luminous glow surrounding something.

Chakra: an energy center in the subtle body that resembles a whirling vortex.

Consciousness-Created Reality: a quantum theory that the universe acts like a wave and is in a state of potentia, that no reality exists until a wave (potentiality) "collapses" into a particle (an actuality), and that the collapse of an actuality from quanta waveforms of potentiality requires a conscious observer.

Energetic: having a capacity for work; active, showing great physical or mental energy.

Energetic Healing: healing that occurs through the medium of energy; a metaphoric term used to mean healing that occurs at the quantum and electromagnetic levels of a person, plant, or animal.

Healing: becoming well or whole again; restoring to health; causing something, such as an emotion, to be no longer grievous.

Meridian: parallel pathways that are conduits of ch'i, an invisible nutritive energy. (Ch'i is called qi, prana, or ki in various cultures.) In Chinese philosophy, there are 12 pairs of meridians.

Psychosynthesis: Assagioli's psychologic theory that proposes a multidimensional human psyche.

 Pause for a moment . . .

- ❏ *The **AHNA Core Curriculum for Holistic Nursing** that is most challenging for me is _____.*
- ❏ *I am having great success at learning these more challenging areas.*

THEORIES AND RESEARCH

[*Note:* All theories and relationships used here are metaphorical and speculative. They are presented as images from which to work, not as fact. The human is portrayed as a conscious information-processing body. Electric, electromagnetic, and computer images are analogous to the waveforms that transmit information to and throughout the human being for interpretation.]

The Electromagnetic Human

1. An electromagnetics acts like an electromagnet with fields and variable strength (e.g., electricity flowing around an iron core), produces heat, magnetism, and/or phosphorescent light.[1] It is surrounded by layers of magnetic density that diminish in step-wise fashion as distance from the core increases.
    a. A magnetic field has field lines that curve from top to bottom. One magnet will pull the field of a second magnet toward it (Figure 7–1).
    b. An electromagnet's strength varies with changes in electric input, and changing the current's direction reverses its polarity.
2. The human has an iron core (hemaglobin) that is surrounded by an electric flow (neuronal activity) and produces heat, light, and magnetism, and possibly phosphorescent light.
3. The human being, and all living matter, is understood in many cultures to be surrounded by a field of nonvisible light, called an aura, that changes incrementally as the distance from the core increases.[2]
4. The human aura resembles an electromagnetic or magnetic field. Figure 7–1B suggests that, as

two magnets affect each other, two humans may affect each other's magnetic or electromagnetic field.

The Electric Human[3]

1. Direct electric currents flow in one direction and lose power if there is resistance along the line.
    a. Routing electric current along parallel (alternate) pathways and periodically boosting the current's strength reduces resistance.
    b. The flow of direct electric current can be reversed.
2. Human beings have a very low amplitude direct electric current (less than 1 millionth of an ampere), the strength of which is periodically boosted. The current flows along multiple parallel pathways thus reducing resistance and maintaining strength.
    a. In the human being, meridians correspond to the parallel paths of the very low amplitude direct current; acupuncture points have the electrical and distance requirements of a direct current booster.
    b. Meridians in a human being are like telephone lines in a city. They carry information throughout the entity along parallel lines.
3. The direct current system also resembles a computer that carries energy and information in slow wavelike fluctuations along parallel pathways.

A

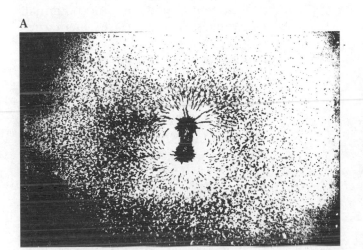

B

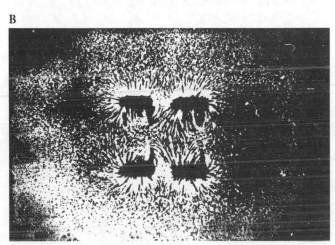

Figure 7–1 A. Magnetic field lines surrounding one magnet. **B.** Magnetic field line interaction between two magnets.

The Frequency Analyzing Human

1. Fourier Analyzers and L-C Circuits[4] act on components of electromagnetic waves.
   a. Fourier analyzers detect electromagnetic wave characteristics and separate the wave into its electromagnetic frequencies, called sine waves (repetitive undulating wave patterns).
   b. An L-C circuit acts on a particular frequency. It also protects a system from violent surges of current, enabling a direct current to be constant rather than fluctuating. The electromagnetic frequency of a current that a coil will moderate depends on the coil's construction.
2. Chakras are described as vortices of whirling energy (light) that detect and process frequencies in the human internal and external environment.
   a. Their characteristics, such as color and tone, have differing frequencies.
   b. The entire chakra system has characteristics of a Fourier analyzer; that is, the entire system detects waves and separates them into their various frequencies.
   c. Each individual chakra acts like an L-C circuit; each chakra acts on a specific frequency range (sine wave) of the entire wave.[5]
   d. Chakras are associated with different emotions, needs, drives, and organs; the specific frequency of a particular chakra may modulate a particular emotion, need, drive, and/or organ (Figure 7–2).
   e. Chakras are like radio and television sets (Fourier analyzers). One can obtain different information (programs) by tuning to different frequencies, but each station (L-C circuits) analyzes only one.

Pause for a moment . . .

❑ *When I think about taking the holistic nursing certification examination, I feel _____.*
❑ *I possess the knowledge and skills to evoke deep relaxation to study the requirements and to develop my study plan.*

Physical Theories[6]

1. Newton proposed a mechanistic universe in which matter is stable and constructed of fundamental, indivisible units called atoms that move in absolute space and absolute time.
   a. The theory is valid only for objects larger than a few atoms.
   b. Electric and magnetic phenomena are not included in Newtonian theory.
2. Quantum theory is really a collection of theories about subatomic structure and interactions, such as the wave/particle theory of light.
   a. The fundamental aspect of the universe is called a quantum, or energy packet that is dynamic.
   b. Space and time are not absolute, but form the fourth dimension of space-time.
   c. Matter is not stable, but has a potential to exist and events have potentials to occur.
   d. The space (field) around a particle (matter) is dynamic, such as an electric or a magnetic field; particles and fields vibrate and can travel through space.
   e. The quantum view of nature is that matter (subatomic particles) and fields (energy) interact randomly. There are various quantum theories about activity in the quantum realm, but no dispute that matter as known in Newtonian physics does not exist at the quantum level.
3. Consciousness-created reality[7] is one quantum theory that looks at how actuality comes into being.
   a. According to the wave/particle theory, no actuality (particle) exists until a measurement (observation) is made of a quantum waveform (a quantum tendency to exist, a potentiality). Until an observation is made, there is no actual particle, only potentialities of particles. Prior to measurement, there are only waveforms.
   b. Two quantum theories address the questions, "What is an observation, and who/what does the observing?"
      1) In observer-created reality, the observer does not have to be conscious, but may be a machine, an experiment, or a photograph, for example.
      2) In consciousness-created reality, the observer must be an aware consciousness.
   c. Another popular quantum theory implies that there are parallel universes or many worlds. Reality consists of a number of universes that are created with each observation of a potentiality. All potential outcomes actually occur; only one is perceived.

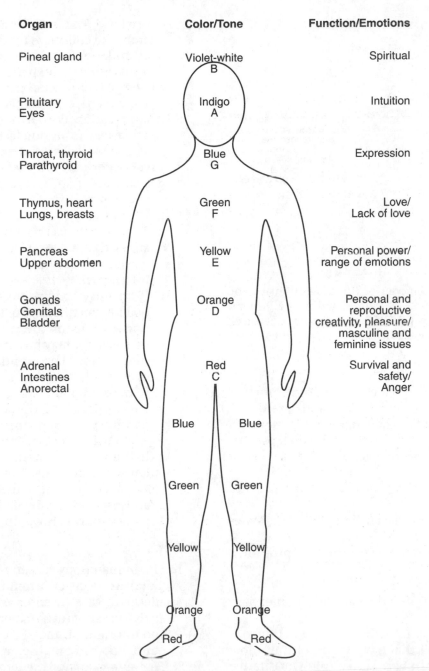

Organ	Color/Tone	Function/Emotions
Pineal gland	Violet-white B	Spiritual
Pituitary Eyes	Indigo A	Intuition
Throat, thyroid Parathyroid	Blue G	Expression
Thymus, heart Lungs, breasts	Green F	Love/ Lack of love
Pancreas Upper abdomen	Yellow E	Personal power/ range of emotions
Gonads Genitals Bladder	Orange D	Personal and reproductive creativity, pleasure/ masculine and feminine issues
Adrenal Intestines Anorectal	Red C	Survival and safety/ Anger

Figure 7–2 Major chakra locations and characteristics. *Sources:* V. Slater, "Toward an Understanding of Energetic Healing, Part 1, Energetic Structures," *Journal of Holistic Nursing* 13, no. 3 (1995): 216; J. Mentgen and M.J. Bulbrook, *Healing Touch Level I Notebook* (Lakewood, CO: Healing Touch, 1994); Copyright © 1997, Victoria E. Slater.

d. Others suggest that the universe is a hologram in which each part contains the whole.

A Theory of Consciousness[8]

1. If an observing consciousness is required before a potentiality can become an actuality, the consciousness must be active in the quantum world. If such a consciousness is a human, that consciousness must also be an aware, experiencing one, such as a conscious self.

2. Psychosynthesis is a theory in which the psyche has six dimensions, including one that has access to the quantum realm. Three dimensions hold and process emotional and psychologic experiences (see Figure 7–3). One dimen-

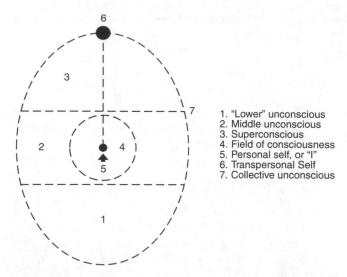

1. "Lower" unconscious
2. Middle unconscious
3. Superconscious
4. Field of consciousness
5. Personal self, or "I"
6. Transpersonal Self
7. Collective unconscious

Figure 7–3 Assagioli's model of the dimensions of the psyche. *Source:* Reprinted by permission of The Putnam Publishing Group/Jeremy P. Tarcher, Inc. from P. Ferrucci, WHAT WE MAY BE, by Piero Ferrucci. Copyright © 1992 by Piero Ferrucci.

sion is the field on which events and emotions are perceived, and two dimensions are different aspects of the experiencing self. A seventh dimension is external to the individual psyche.

a. These dimensions include three levels of unconscious:
   1) Lower: earliest, most immature psychological self.
   2) Middle: on-call current skills and states of mind.
   3) Superconscious: intuition, aspirations, ethics.
b. The two selves are:
   1) Personal self, I: the part of us that experiences.
   2) Transpersonal Self: the aspect of our conscious Self that has a vision of the whole psyche; can be accessed using meditative and other techniques, but is not part of one's obvious aware state; may be one's soul.
c. Field of consciousness is the perceptual field—our alert moment-to-moment awareness.
d. Jung termed a pool of unconscious universal archetypes and species memories the collective unconscious.[9,10] The collective unconscious is not part of an individual's psyche but is like an impersonal psychological ocean in which the individual psyche

"swims." The individual psyche is separated from the collective unconscious by a porous boundary; thus, it is separate from, but one with, universal experience.
   e. The goal of psychosynthesis therapy is to integrate the dimensions of the psyche. The supposition is that a person can use consciousness-exploring techniques to heal his or her emotional and mental (conscious) pain.
3. Psychosynthesis implies that unsynthesized dimensions of one's psyche produce a different conscious reality than does a synthesized psyche.
   a. The theory of consciousness-created reality states that an aware consciousness acts on waveforms of potentia to bring an actuality into being.
   b. If an unsynthesized consciousness acts on quanta potentia, any of the three levels of the unconscious or the personal self or Transpersonal Self may be the actor. They may take turns acting. The resulting conscious experience will range from immature to altruistic, from self-centered I to transpersonal.
   c. If a synthesized consciousness acts upon quanta potentia, one's conscious experiences will reflect an integrated Self.
   d. If the quanta potentia upon which one's consciousness acts results in physical, as well as conscious actualities, then physical and psychologic healing may occur in the process of psychosynthesis.

Synopsis

1. The human body has an electromagnetic field (aura), an electric current that flows along parallel pathways (meridians), and information-analyzing structures (chakras). Electric energy and information may be transmitted throughout the body along the meridians.
2. The aura also stores energy and information. Chakras may receive and sort information from the aura or from the external environment.
3. One's body uses the energy; one's consciousness gives meaning to the information. When the flow of electricity and information ceases, death results.
4. One's consciousness may interact with the energy and information in both current and field.
   a. One may alter one's electric characteristics (the current), such as one's polarity, at will as during meditation. Centering may be the act of altering one's electromagnetic charac-

teristics through a type of self-referencing meditative-type biofeedback.

  b. One may learn to reach the information carried in the field through meditation and related consciousness-exploring techniques.

5. With access to information in the human electric current and electromagnetic field, as well as access to the quantum realm, it may be possible to alter the information in the current and field. Healing may result.

6. Any of the dimensions of the psyche, whether synthesized or unsynthesized, presumably may act on an individual's electromagnetic state and/or the quanta potentia to adjust physical and psychologic experiences. An individual's experiences may be a function of which dimension(s) of the psyche is(are) acting.

7. *Energetic* healing implies that both dysfunction and healing can occur at the electromagnetic levels of the physical body, as well as at the abstract level of the *quantum* energetic being.

Holistic healing involves the use of all possible avenues for healing.

IMPLICATIONS FOR HOLISTIC NURSING PRACTICE

1. Holistic nurses perceive the body-mind-spirit as a unity, a whole.

2. Each person is his or her only healer; only the individual has access to his or her own consciousness to synthesize it or to use it to further personal healing.

3. A holistic nurse's priority is to establish a physical and psychologic environment that enhances an individual's ability to act as his or her own healer.

4. Holistic healing is approached from both consciousness and physical avenues.

5. The Energetic Healing Modalities Model, which may guide holistic nursing interven-

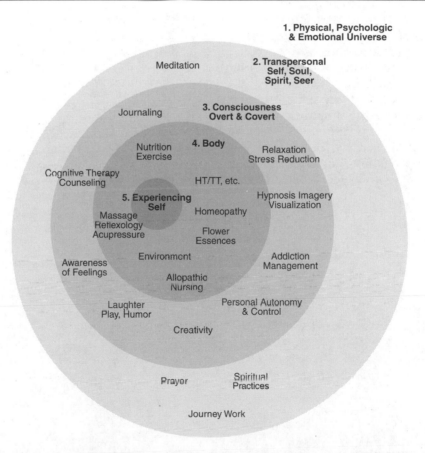

Figure 7–4 Energetic Healing Modalities Model. Copyright © Victoria E. Slater. *Note:* HT/TT refers to all hand-mediated energetic healing modalities such as healing touch, therapeutic touch, Reiki, polarity, touch for health, pranic healing, and others.

tions, has five levels of experience, three of which are active (Figure 7–4).

a. The physical, psychologic, and emotional universe.
1) Quantum physics applies at this level.
2) No energetic interventions are directed specifically to this level; the results of healing interventions may or may not be reflected in the universe.

b. Transpersonal Self, soul, spirit, seer.
1) The dimension of the being that is beyond everyday awareness, is eternal, and may be responsible for past life experiences.
2) Nursing energetic interventions include meditation and journey work (i.e., a hypnotic technique in which the nurse guides a client in reaching the dimension of his or her self that can assist in healing).

c. Consciousness, overt and covert, is all dimensions of consciousness, such as those described by Assagioli. Nursing energetic interventions include counseling and cognitive therapy, journal writing, guided imagery, visualization, and other approaches that encourage recognition and synthesis of the content and dimensions of the psyche.

d. Body is the physical body to which Newtonian physics, biology, chemistry, and physics apply. Nursing energetic interventions include allopathic nursing care, nutrition, exercise, sensory influences, massage, acupressure, homeopathy, flower essences, and other approaches that affect the biologic/physiologic and electric/electromagnetic body.

e. The experiencing self (a level of being) is the aware self that corresponds to Assagioli's field of consciousness and personal self, I. Nursing interventions and results are experienced by the experiencing self.

6. A holistic energetic model of body-mind-spirit implies that energetic techniques directed to one level of the whole being can influence all types of experiences: physical, conscious, and transpersonal. Results may be reflected in the energy of the universe.

REFERENCES

1. K. Amdahl, *There Are No Electrons: Electronics for Earthlings* (Arvada, CO: Clearwater, 1991).

2. B.A. Brennan, *Light Emerging: The Journal of Personal Healing* (New York: Bantam Books, 1993).

3. R.O. Becker and G. Selden, *The Body Electric: Electromagnetism and the Foundation of Life* (New York: William Morrow, 1985).

4. Amdahl, *There Are No Electrons.*

5. V. Slater, Toward an Understanding of Energetic Healing, Part 1: Energetic Structures, *Journal of Holistic Nursing* 13, no. 3 (1995): 209–224.

6. F. Capra, *The Tao of Physics: An Exploration of the Parallels between Modern Physics and Eastern Mysticism*, 2nd ed. (New York: Bantam Books, 1984).

7. N. Herbert, *Quantum Reality; Beyond the New Physics. An Excursion into Metaphysics and the Meaning of Reality* (New York: Doubleday & Co., 1985).

8. R. Assagioli, *Psychosynthesis: A Collection of Basic Writings* (New York: Arkana, 1976).

9. C. Jung, *Alchemical Studies: Collected Works,* Vol. 13 (Princeton, NJ: Princeton University Press, 1960).

10. C. Jung, *The Structure and Dynamics of the Psyche: Collective Works,* Vol. 8 (Princeton, NJ: Princeton University Press, 1967).

Holistic Ethics

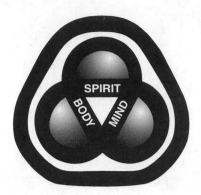

CHAPTER 8

Holistic Ethics

Lynn Keegan

KNOWLEDGE COMPETENCIES

- Review the classic principles of ethics.
- Synthesize the basic tenets of traditional ethical theorists.
- Explore the concept of holistic ethics.
- Relate ethical theory to clinical situations.
- Gain the knowledge necessary to serve on institutional ethics committees.
- Begin to see daily choices as opportunities to make a positive impact on the world.
- Clarify personal values and ideas.

DEFINITION

General Ethics: the study or discipline concerned with judgments of approval or disapproval, rightness or wrongness, goodness or badness, virtue or vice, and desirability or wisdom of actions, dispositions, ends, objects, or states of affairs; disciplined reflection on the moral choices that people make.

Holistic Ethics: the basic underlying concept of the unity and integral wholeness of all people and of all nature that is identified and pursued by finding unity and wholeness within the self and within humanity. In a framework of holistic ethics, an individual acts not for the sake of the law, precedent, or social norms, but rather from a desire to do good freely in order to witness, identify, and contribute to unity.

 Pause for a moment . . .

- ❑ *I am becoming more knowledgeable about the **AHNA Core Curriculum for Holistic Nursing** so that I can be a better holistic nurse.*
- ❑ *I am increasing my ability to articulate my holistic philosophy, mission, and work to my colleagues.*
- ❑ *I am becoming a wiser teacher with my clients.*

THEORIES AND RESEARCH

Ethics of Caring/Healing in Health Care Delivery[1]

1. The environment is best for healing when the intellect, will, emotions, and spirit of the healer are balanced and centered.
2. Holistic ethics provides guidelines for the development of spirit in the healer and spells out the steps needed to develop healing attitudes.
   a. Ethics assists the healer in tapping into the wisdom of the cosmos, teaching the individual strategies to release the self to become more participatory in the Greater Self.
   b. The participation in the Greater Self forms the linkages between the power of the cosmos, the healer, and the one to be healed.
3. Enlightened, ethical healers can focus and direct their caring energy to those in need of healing.

Role of Holistic Nursing in Health Care Reform

1. Holistic nurses deal with ethical questions that arise from all areas of life:
   a. Ramifications of the population explosion.
   b. Euthanasia.
   c. Genetic engineering.
   d. Allocation of health care resources.
2. Awareness of ethical issues is increasing because of several factors.[2]
   a. Advances in medical technology.
   b. Greater recognition of patients' rights.
   c. Malpractice cases and court-ordered treatment.
   d. Scarcity of resources.
3. Ethical dilemmas are usually characterized by the fact there is no right answer.[3]
4. Holistic nurses follow a code of ethics (Exhibit 8–1).

Nature of Ethical Problems, Morals, and Principles

1. There are three primary principles of ethical decision making.
   a. Respect for persons.
   b. Beneficence.
   c. Justice.
2. These principles represent obligations to respect the wishes of competent persons, obligations not to harm others, obligations to benefit others, obligations to produce a net balance of benefits over harm, obligations to distribute benefits and harms fairly, obligations to keep promises and contracts, obligations to be truthful, obligations to disclose information, and obligations to respect privacy and to protect confidential information.[4]

 Pause for a moment . . .

❏ *The study plan that I have developed includes*

_____ .

❏ *I am planning to take the holistic nursing certification (HNC) examination as soon as I can.*
❏ *My strengths are* _____ .
❏ *My weaknesses are* _____ .
❏ *I know where I need to start with my study plan.*

_____

Ethical Theories and Development of Holistic Ethics

1. A number of ethical theories have played a role in Western civilization and have laid the foundation for modern ethics.
2. Traditionally, there are two ways to view ethics.
   a. The deontologic approach assigns duty or obligation based on the intrinsic aspects of an act rather than its outcome.
   b. The teleologic approach finds an action morally defensible on the basis of the outcomes or consequences of the act.
3. Holistic ethics involves a basic underlying concept of the unity and integral wholeness of all people and of all nature that is identified and pursued by finding unity and wholeness within the self and within humanity.[5]

Holistic Ethics and Consciousness

1. The underlying principle of holistic ethics is being, and its corollary is consciousness. As each person develops an individual consciousness, people assess and direct the evolution of the consciousness of the species and contemplatively examine their relationship with the universal being.[6]
2. Each individual's personal will becomes the motivator for continued evolution. In the holistic concept of ethics, moral decisions affect both the spirit of humankind as a whole and each individual spirit.[7]
3. Holistic ethics is grounded in the conscious evolution of an enlightened individual who performs the act. Acts are judged by determining whether or not they promote wholeness and integration of either the collective whole or an individual.[8]

Ethical Dilemmas

1. Everyone daily confronts the need to make personal and professional ethical decisions.
2. In order to make appropriate decisions, it is necessary, first, to operate from a set of principles and, second, to have some sort of analytic method to help sort out and classify the elements of the problem.

Components of Ethical Case Analysis

1. Jonsen divides the ethical case analysis of a health care dilemma into four components:

Exhibit 8–1 American Holistic Nurses' Association Position Statement on Holistic Nursing Ethics

Code of Ethics for Holistic Nurses

We believe that the fundamental responsibilities of the nurse are to promote health, facilitate healing and alleviate suffering. The need for nursing is universal. Inherent in nursing is the respect for life, dignity and right of all persons. Nursing care is given in a context mindful of the holistic nature of humans, understanding the body-mind-spirit. Nursing care is unrestricted by considerations of nationality, race, creed, color, age, sex, sexual preference, politics or social status. Given that nurses practice in culturally diverse settings, professional nurses must have an understanding of the cultural background of clients in order to provide culturally appropriate interventions.

Nurses render services to clients who can be individuals, families, groups or communities. The client is an active participant in health care and should be included in all nursing care planning decisions.

In order to provide services to others, each nurse has a responsibility toward him/herself. In addition, nurses have defined responsibilities towards the client, co-workers, nursing practice, the profession of nursing, society and the environment.

Nurses and Self

The nurse has a responsibility to model health behaviors. Holistic nurses strive to achieve harmony in their own lives and assist others striving to do the same.

Nurses and the Client

The nurse's primary responsibility is to the client needing nursing care. The nurse strives to see the client as a whole, and provides care which is professionally appropriate and culturally consonant. The nurse holds in confidence all information obtained in professional practice, and uses professional judgment in disclosing such information. The nurse enters into a relationship with the client that is guided by mutual respect and a desire for growth and development.

Nurses and Co-Workers

The nurse maintains cooperative relationships with co-workers in nursing and other fields. Nurses have a responsibility to nurture each other, and to assist nurses to work as a team in the interest of client care. If a client's care is endangered by a co-worker, the nurse must take appropriate action on behalf of the client.

Nurses and Nursing Practice

The nurse carries personal responsibility for practice and for maintaining continued competence. Nurses have the right to utilize all appropriate nursing interventions, and have the obligation to determine the efficacy and safety of all nursing actions. Wherever applicable, nurses utilize research findings in directing practice.

Nurses and the Profession

The nurse plays a role in determining and implementing desirable standards of nursing practice and education. Holistic nurses may assume a leadership position to guide the profession toward holism. Nurses support nursing research and the development of holistically oriented nursing theories. The nurse participates in establishing and maintaining equitable social and economic working conditions in nursing.

Nurses and Society

The nurse, along with other citizens, has responsibility for initiating and supporting actions to meet the health and social needs of the public.

Nurses and the Environment

The nurse strives to manipulate the client's environment to become one of peace, harmony, and nurturance so that healing may take place. The nurse considers the health of the ecosystem in relation to the need for health, safety and peace of all persons.

Source: Reprinted with permission from *Position Statement on Holistic Nursing Ethics,* the American Holistic Nurses' Association, 4101 Lake Boone Trail, Raleigh, NC 27607, phone: (919) 787-5181; Fax: (919) 787-4916.

a. Medical indications.
b. Patient preferences.
c. Quality-of-life issues.
d. External socioeconomic factors.[9]
2. The holistic approach adds questions of relationships:
a. Who am I?
b. What is my relationship to others?
c. What other factors are contributing to my decisions?

d. Am I wise and courageous enough to perceive and respect others' differences and honor them as I would honor my own beliefs?

Advanced Medical Directives

1. The Patient Self-Determination Act of 1991 requires that all individuals receiving medical care also receive written information about their right to accept or refuse medical or surgi-

cal treatment and their right to initiate advance directives, such as living wills and durable power of attorney.[10]

2. There are two types of advance medical directives: treatment directives, often referred to as living wills, and appointment directives, often referred to as power of attorney or health proxies.

3. An advance directive applies only if a patient is incapacitated. It may not apply if, in the opinion of two physicians, the patient can make decisions.

4. Individuals may cancel advance directives at any time.

Nurses As Members of Institutional Ethics Committees

1. Many hospitals are developing ethics committees to participate in the decision-making processes when ethical dilemmas arise.

2. Ethically knowledgeable nurses who become active participants in ethics committees and decision-making discussions can begin to articulate a holistic approach that supports the essence of a comprehensive world ethical view.

Nurses As Political Activists

1. Nursing and ethics have been intertwined since the inception of nursing.
   a. Nurses have always concerned themselves with matters of public policy, such as urban slums and tenements, war and disaster, and special needs of the underserved.

b. Nurses are in the forefront of ethical decision making and public policy formation.
2. Many aspects of future health care delivery will be based on today's ethical decisions.
   a. Nurses who are politically active can gain knowledge about holistic ethics and intertwine the two philosophies into meaningful action.
   b. Many contemporary health care issues require the attention of politically active, enlightened nurses.

REFERENCES

1. B.M. Dossey et al., *Holistic Nursing: A Handbook for Practice,* 2nd ed. (Gaithersburg, MD: Aspen Publishers, 1995), 135–136.
2. F. Hendrickson and G.L. Deloughery, Ethical Influences on Nursing, in *Issues and Trends in Nursing,* ed. G.L. Deloughery (St. Louis: C.V. Mosby Co., 1991), 180.
3. M. Corley and D. Raines, An Ethical Practice Environment As a Caring Environment, *Nursing Administration Quarterly* 17, no. 2 (1993): 68–74.
4. R.M. Veatch, ed., *Medical Ethics* (Boston: Jones & Bartlett, 1989).
5. L. Keegan and G. Keegan, A Concept of Holistic Ethics for the Health Professional, *Journal of Holistic Nursing* 10, no. 3 (1992): 205–217.
6. L. Keegan and G. Keegan, Spirituality and the Technological Crisis, *Healing Currents* 11, no. 2 (1987): 26–28.
7. D. Singh, The Psychology of Consciousness, in *The Evolution of Consciousness,* ed. K. Gandi (New York: Paragon House, 1983), 68–86.
8. Keegan and Keegan, Concept of Holistic Ethics.
9. A.R. Jonsen, Case Analysis in Clinical Ethics, *Journal of Clinical Ethics* 1, no. 1 (1990): 63–65.
10. State of Texas, Patient Self-Determination Act of 1991.

Holistic Nursing Theories

CHAPTER 9

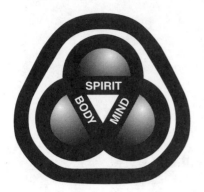

Nursing Theories

Noreen Cavan Frisch

KNOWLEDGE COMPETENCIES

- State similarities and differences among nursing theories.
- Describe the development of a theory over time.
- Describe the relationship of theory to research.
- Identify concepts basic to nursing theories, such as nursing's phenomena of concern (e.g., nursing, person, health, environment).
- Describe the ways in which selected nursing theories address nursing's phenomena of concern.
- Demonstrate the use of nursing theory in holistic nursing practice.
- Demonstrate the use of nursing theory with standard nursing diagnoses and classification systems.

DEFINITIONS

Nursing Theory: a framework from which professional nurses can think about their work. It deals with phenomena of concern to the discipline of nursing:[1] the practice of nursing, the person (or client), the nurse, health, and the environment. The use of nursing theory in practice gives a depth and richness to the nurse's work. Many persons define professional (as opposed to technical) nursing as being solidly grounded in theory-based practice. For example, a nurse adjusts the client's physical environment so that it becomes a calm, peaceful, quiet, and pleasing space to promote healing. A nursing theory would allow the nurse to look at nursing behaviors in light of controlling the environment to provide support of the client's innate healing process.

In another situation, if a nurse observes that a client's behavior is withdrawn, fearful, and socially isolating, the nurse will interpret such behavior differently, depending on the theory being used.

Theory: an abstraction of reality that serves some purpose;[2] a framework that provides a way of thinking about something. For example, most nurses understand the concepts of child developmental theory. When a nurse sees a toddler fearful of being separated from his or her mother, the nurse can interpret the observed behavior within the framework of child development and conclude that the child is exhibiting a normal and expected separation anxiety. In such a situation, the child development theory provides the framework and means of understanding what is observed.

 Pause for a moment . . .

❑ *I am studying small sections of content over a long period of time to increase my chance of success on the holistic nursing certification (HNC) examination.*
❑ *To avoid frustration and anxiety, I am learning carefully and will not cram.*

THEORIES AND RESEARCH

Similarities among Nursing Theories

1. Concepts basic to all nursing theories are nursing, person, health, and environment. These concepts are nursing's phenomena of concern.

2. Nursing theories suggest how all of these concepts are related to one another and explain how nursing care may affect the health of clients.
3. Nursing theories are testable through scientific research, which may be quantitative or qualitative.
4. Each nursing theory has a theory-specific language as a means of communicating information about nursing activities.

Differences among Nursing Theories

1. The levels of abstraction vary among theories. Some are global in nature, giving a nurse a means of thinking about the "big picture." Others are quite specific, providing direction on what to do in concrete practice settings.
2. Holistic nursing theories fall into two categories according to their definition of person.
   a. The person may be defined as a whole that is greater than the sum of its parts. These theories identify component parts that make up the whole (e.g., body-mind-spirit).
   b. The person may be defined as an irreducible whole, such that discussion or thought of component parts is inconsistent with the idea of "wholeness."
3. Some nursing theories have been subjected to several scientific investigations, while others have not.

Theory Development

1. Theories develop over time as concepts are introduced and relationships between concepts are suggested. By using concepts in practice and conducting research to validate the proposed relationships between concepts, nurses modify their theories.
2. As theories develop and mature, they serve increasingly complex purposes: description, explanation, prediction, and prescription.
   a. A theory that provides definitions of concepts and suggests a way of looking at the world gives the nurse a framework to describe the phenomena of nursing.
   b. A theory that suggests relationships between and among various concepts gives the nurse a means of explaining observed events.
   c. When research on a theory has established clear relationships between aspects of nursing, the nurse using that theory is able to

predict client outcomes based on certain activities.
   d. A very well developed theory permits a nurse to prescribe nursing activities, based on research, with confidence in the outcome.
3. Nursing theories are in the initial stages of development, so description and explanation based on theory are possible. Theorists and researchers are currently developing nursing theories to the point of prediction and prescription.
4. Research can validate any aspect of a theory. For example, if a theory states that a person is a human energy field, and suggests that there is an exchange of energy between two persons, research that indicates such an exchange exists serves to validate that theory.
5. Nurse researchers conduct studies over many years to validate current theories, and theories develop and change as new information emerges.

Specific Nursing Theories

1. Florence Nightingale. Known as the first "modern nurse," Nightingale in 1860 gave nurses the first published theory by which to reflect on nursing.[3]
   a. Nursing: Nursing is putting the patient in the best condition for nature to act upon him or her.
   b. Person: Nightingale does not define person, but describes person in relation to the environment.
   c. Health: Health is the "positive of which pathology is the negative"(p. 74). Furthermore, "nature alone cures" (p. 74).
   d. Environment: The theory stresses the healing properties of the physical environment, such as fresh air, light, warmth, and cleanliness.[4]
2. Callista Roy. Since she began her work in 1964, Roy has continued to develop her nursing theory. It is based on the idea of adapting to stressors and achieving health as a state of homeostasis, or balance.[5]
   a. Nursing: The role and activities of a nurse are to promote adaptive responses that support a client's health.
   b. Person: There is a constant exchange between the person and the environment, and a person must become an adaptive system, adapting to stimuli to maintain health.
   c. Health: Health is a state and process of being and becoming an integrated, whole person.

d. Environment: The environment includes any condition, circumstance, and/or influence that affects the development and behavior of persons and groups. Stimuli in the environment can be *focal* (the immediate situation), *contextual* (other current stimuli in the person's environment that provide the context for adapting to the current situation), or *residual* (all other internal factors).

3. Helen Erickson, Evelyn Tomlin, and Mary Ann Swain. Three individuals collaborated to develop and present the Modeling and Role-Modeling Theory in 1983.[6] The basis of this theory is to focus on the person receiving care and to individualize health care by creating a "model" of the client's subjective world.
   a. Nursing: Nursing is a process that requires an interpersonal and interactive relationship with the client. Facilitation, nurturance, and unconditional acceptance should characterize the nurse's caregiving.
   b. Person: A person is a holistic being with interacting subsystems (biological, psychological, social, and cognitive) and with inherent genetic bases and spiritual drives. The whole is greater than the sum of the parts.
   c. Health: Health is a dynamic equilibrium between subsystems.
   d. Environment: Perceived as both internal and external, the environment includes stressors as well as resources for adapting to stressors.

4. Madeleine Leininger. As a nurse-anthropologist, Leininger emphasized aspects of culture and cultural care for nursing. She called her theory Cultural Care.[7]
   a. Nursing: *Care* is the central focus of nursing and may occur without cure. Nurses perform activities to help others regain well-being or to cope with handicapping conditions or approaching death. All nursing care must be culturally congruent.
   b. Person: People are viewed as caring beings. Human care is seen in all cultures; caring is necessary, not only for health, but for survival.
   c. Health: Health is a culturally defined state of well-being. It reflects one's ability to perform culturally prescribed roles.
   d. Environment: Society, as the environment, is viewed from within the client's culture. Context is the totality of the situation.

5. Jean Watson. Watson first presented her work in the philosophy and science of caring in 1979.[8] Her theory emphasizes the humanistic aspects of nursing, combined with scientific knowledge.
   a. Nursing: Mediated by "professional, personal, scientific, esthetic, and ethical human care transactions,"[9] nursing is highly interpersonal and is grounded in human-to-human care.
   b. Person: A person is greater than, and different from, the sum of his or her parts. A person is a valued individual to be cared for and to be understood.
   c. Health: Health is a subjective state that has to do with unity and harmony. Illness can be understood as disharmony.
   d. Environment: Caring is achieved through societal and cultural interactions.

6. Martha Rogers. Rogers believed nursing is a "humanistic science dedicated to compassionate concern for maintaining and promoting health, preventing illness, and caring for and rehabilitating the sick and disabled."[10] Referring to her theory as an abstract system, Rogers established a new paradigm for nursing.
   a. Nursing: Nursing is the scientific study of human and environmental energy fields.
   b. Person: A person is a unified whole, defined as a human energy field. Human beings evolve irreversibly and unidirectionally in space and time.
   c. Health: Health is not defined as such within Rogers' theory. Health can be understood from within this framework in terms of cultural and subjective values.
   d. Environment: The environmental energy field is in constant interaction with the human energy field.

7. Margaret Newman. Newman included Rogers' concepts of energy patterns and unitary human beings in developing her own theory.[11]
   a. Nursing: Nursing is a profession, moving to an integrative role. Nursing is caring, and caring is a moral imperative for nursing.
   b. Person: A person is a dynamic field of energy that is continuous with a larger energy field. Human beings are identified by their field patterns.
   c. Health: Health is expanding consciousness; it includes an individual's total pattern. Pathologic conditions are manifestations of the individual's total pattern.

d. Environment: The environment is the wholeness of the universe; there are no boundaries.

8. Rosemarie Rizzo Parse. Since 1970, Parse has suggested the idea that there are two world views in nursing: a summative paradigm in which the person is viewed as a combination of component parts; and the simultaneity paradigm, in which a person can be viewed only as a unity.[12]

a. Nursing: Nursing is a scientific discipline, but the practice of nursing is an art in which nurses serve as guides to assist others in making choices that affect health.

b. Person: A person is viewed from within the simultaneity paradigm. The person is a unified, whole being.

c. Health: Health is a process of becoming; it is a personal commitment, an unfolding, a process related to a person's lived experiences.

d. Environment: The environment is the universe. According to Parse, the human–universe is inseparable and evolving together.

 Pause for a moment . . .

❑ *I have found my special place to be quiet, focused, and relaxed.*

❑ *I place healing objects around to remind me to be focused and relaxed while I study.*

Use of Nursing Theories in Holistic Practice

1. A theory provides the means of interpreting and organizing information. For example, observing a client situation from the perspective of the Theory of Cultural Care would lead the nurse to attend to differing assessment parameters than observing the same situation from the Theory of Human Becoming. However, using a theory gives the nurse a tool to ensure that nursing assessments are comprehensive and systematic, that nursing care is compassionate and meaningful.

2. Holistic nursing is "all nursing practice which has healing the whole person as its goal."[13] A nurse may use any nursing theory, as long as the nurse and the client perceive that the theory and the care are achieving the goal of holistic nursing.

3. Nursing theory provides language to communicate nursing assessment. A nurse may describe an energy pattern to another nurse (Theory of Human Becoming) or may describe aspects of the client's perceptions, needs, and wants (Modeling and Role-Modeling). Each nurse must understand which theoretical perspective is being used, however, so that the care delivered by a team of nurses can be consistent. A nurse who wishes to document care on the basis of a nursing theory may do so. In such a case the language of the theory will be used in assessment and outcome statements.

4. Diagnostic statements are atheoretical and serve to indicate the existence of a condition that requires a nursing response. In stating the etiology of the condition, however, the nurse may use the theoretical language to interpret the client's situation from within a particular framework (Exhibit 9–1).

5. Writing diagnostic statements in standard nursing vocabularies (e.g., nursing diagnoses and intervention statements) is increasingly important in the documentation of nursing outcomes.

6. Holistic nurses use all of these theories, and it is sometimes helpful to change from one perspective to another. The following are factors to consider when choosing a theory:

a. What theory is most comfortable for you, the nurse?

b. What theory is most comfortable for your client? Some clients have very strong feelings and opinions about what nursing is and what type of care they wish to receive.

Exhibit 9–1 Theoretical Interpretation of Nursing Diagnosis

A nurse is caring preoperatively for a 25-year-old woman who is about to undergo an appendectomy. Using Roy's adaptation theory, the nurse may assess that the client is fearful of surgery because of prior negative experiences with hospitals. This nurse may write a diagnostic statement such as "*fear* of surgery related to the contextual stimuli of past negative experiences in hospitals." Any nurse reading this diagnostic statement would understand the meaning of "contextual stimuli" and would further understand that care is being delivered from within the framework of Roy's theory.

Exhibit 9–2 Case Study: Fred

Fred is a 68-year-old white male, a retired engineer who was admitted to the hospital for a right carotid endarterectomy. His medical history includes coronary artery disease, severe; a myocardial infarction at age 43 years (he was told at age 43 years that he had the circulatory system of an 80-year-old); he has had two small strokes, leaving him with foot drop in the left foot and one calf muscle smaller than the other. He has a personal history of both drinking and smoking, although he quit drinking 5 years ago and smoking 4 years ago. He takes antihypertensive medications and aspirin daily. He lives with his wife. They have three grown children who live on their own in locations throughout the state in which Fred lives. His lifestyle is sedentary; he used to read extensively, but no longer reads much. He is 5'11" tall, weighs 135 pounds, and has a blood pressure of 140/90; hemoglobin/hematocrit and all other laboratory reports are within normal limits.

The morning of the scheduled surgery, Fred's blood urea nitrogen (BUN) and creatinine were elevated. Consultations with his physicians regarding the laboratory work delayed his surgery 6 hours. Fred's anxiety about the surgical procedure increased during the delay. He expressed ambivalence about the procedure, but gave consent for the operation.

On the operating table, his blood pressure rose to 280/140, and he had a massive, left-sided stroke. He was placed on a respirator for impaired breathing patterns. Nurses received him in the intensive care unit and identified his priorities as maintaining airway; monitoring blood pressure, urine output, and level of consciousness; and assessing for pain and fear. They proceeded to provide care as appropriate for these priorities.

Fred progressed physically and within 3 weeks was placed in a step-down unit; rehabilitation planning was initiated. Fred had had a left-sided stroke, leaving his right side impaired. He could stand only with assistance; he could not use his dominant hand; his visual field was diminished; and he had a right-sided sensory deficit. The nurses carrying out interventions for Fred's rehabilitation noted that he was angry and hostile, was "overly concerned" with his urine output, and wanted to urinate frequently. He was easily frustrated and did not communicate well with anyone at the hospital. His wife was at the end of her rope, and she expressed feeling guilty that he was such a difficult client. At this point, Fred's nursing care plan was developed and was aimed at keeping him active and involved. The initial nursing care plan is presented in Table 9–1. Nurses were consistent in carrying out the interventions. Fred did not improve; he only became more upset and hostile.

At this point, holistic nurse Myra entered the case. She evaluated Fred from the point of view of the Modeling and Role-Modeling Theory, understanding that the physical illness might well be a crisis for Fred and that his care needed to be individualized based on his world view.

The first consideration for Myra was the meaning of the experiences of illness, surgery, and the stroke to Fred. The second consideration was what Fred wanted in terms of recovery. Myra began by approaching Fred with an attitude of unconditional acceptance, a willingness to provide nurturance in whatever form Fred found acceptable. These actions are consistent with the five aims of intervention, starting from a place of building trust. Myra assessed Fred's adaptive potential and concluded that he was in arousal. He was frustrated and angry, with an escalating anxiety level. He was showing his state of arousal by being hostile and uncooperative. On one level, Fred was appealing to the nurses to notice him, to listen to him.

Myra assessed that the experience of illness was a crisis for Fred at this time. The experience of this illness was an encapsulating event. He was obsessed with urination in response to feeling completely out of control. Fred was responding to the crisis in the only way he could. His method of coping was to attempt to mobilize his resources. However, because of his debilitated state, the nursing staff were resources he had to use to accomplish anything. He wanted to direct his care, to feel independent, but he was not given the chance to do that. He wanted the nurses to know that he did not wish to be subjected to group therapy and social activities, nor did he wish to have his day so solidly structured with rehabilitation activities.

What did he want? Myra had to talk with him, spending time learning of his worries, needs, and wants. In time, he communicated with her, as he recognized that she wanted to help him begin to direct his own care. Fred had been an engineer; he was used to being in control of events. He liked having information to assist him in making his own decisions. He wanted someone to understand that he was tired, that his condition made him feel helpless, that he was experiencing the loss of his independence and his control over his life, and that he no longer liked his body.

Myra completely revised his nursing care plan. While not ignoring Fred's physiological needs (e.g., his needs for safety, nutrition, and elimination), Myra revised the nursing diagnoses so that they became fatigue, powerlessness, body image disturbance, and grieving. Table 9–2 presents Myra's care plan. With this new approach, all nursing care was directed to Fred's feelings, and the care helped Fred to regain control. With the new approach, Fred was permitted to explore his own feelings, to identify his resources, and to begin to direct his own rehabilitation.

Source: Adapted with permission from Wendy Woodward, PhD, RN, Humboldt State University, personal communication, 1993.

Table 9–1 Initial Nursing Care Plan for Fred

Nursing Diagnosis	Goal	Interventions
Activity intolerance r/t illness and debilitated state	Accomplish ADLs, controlled mobility	Gradual increase of activity; ambulate QID, utilization of aids (walker)
Social isolation r/t lack of contact with others	Return to premorbid level of socialization	Ward placement; therapy—personal/ group; reinforce social contact with family, especially wife
Sensory deficit r/t paralysis and visual field alteration	Positive adaptation to sensory losses	Training with ADLs, compensation with lipped plates, turning food tray, adaptive equipment; feed as needed
Altered elimination r/t atonic bladder	Patient will not be incontinent of urine	Offer urinal q 1 hour; assess for UTI
Nutrition: less than body requirements	Adequate nutrition; stable body weight	Offer supplements

Source: Adapted from Wendy Woodward, PhD, RN, Humboldt State University, personal communication, 1993. Used with permission.
Note: r/t, is related to; ADLs, activities of daily living; QID, four times a day; q, every; UTI, urinary tract infection.

Table 9–2 Revised Nursing Care Plan for Fred

Nursing Diagnosis	Goal	Interventions
Fatigue r/t illness and debilitated state	Provide balance between rest, sleep, and activities.	Permit Fred to set his own pace, allow him to set his daily schedule. Give uninterrupted time to sit quietly. Offer interventions to elicit the relaxation response (massage, guided relaxation, TT, healing touch techniques).
Powerlessness r/t loss of control over his life's events	Increase Fred's perception of control.	Allow Fred to set daily schedule. Provide Fred with control over daily events.
Body image disturbance r/t paralysis and debilitated state	Fred will accept his physical condition.	Emphasize strengths. Permit honest discussion of feelings.
Grieving r/t losses (health, mobility, independence, youth)	Fred will accept the loss of health and embark on a path toward rehabilitation.	Encourage Fred to describe the loss of health, youth, independence. Share grief with him.

Source: Adapted with permission from Wendy Woodward, PhD, RN, Humboldt State University, personal communication, 1993.

c. What theory is going to help you, as the nurse, communicate with others who may be providing care to the same client?

d. How will your nursing care be documented?

7. The use of theory really does change the nurse's perspective and may dramatically change the quality of care provided (Exhibit 9–2).

8. With a nursing theory to guide practice, patients such as Fred can be put in control, and the nurses can become resources for them (Exhibit 9–2). Any holistically based theory can help the nurse provide truly client-centered and compassionate care.

REFERENCES

1. P. Chinn and M. Jacobs, *Theory and Nursing: A Systematic Approach* (St. Louis: C.V. Mosby Co., 1983).

2. J. Fawcett, *Analysis and Evaluation of Conceptual Models of Nursing,* 2nd ed. (Philadelphia: F.A. Davis Co., 1989).

3. F. Nightingale, *Notes on Nursing* (London: Harrison, 1860). The First London edition of Florence Nightingale's *Notes on Nursing* was published the first week in January 1860 and became an overnight bestseller. It has been suggested that the first edition of *Notes on Nursing* was published in December 1859, but this first edition has yellow end papers with January 1860 advertisements. *Source:* Victor Skretkowicz, PhD, *Notes on Nursing Science,* Vol. 4, No. 2, 1991, p. 2.

4. L.C. Selanders, *Florence Nightingale: An Environmental Adaptation Theory* (Newbury Park, CA: Sage Publications, 1993).

5. C. Roy and H.A. Andrews, *The Roy Adaptation Model: The Definitive Statement* (Norwalk, CT: Appleton & Lange, 1991).

6. H. Erickson et al., *Modeling and Role-Modeling: A Theory and Paradigm for Nursing* (Lexington, SC: Pine Press, 1983).

7. M. Leininger, *Cultural Care Diversity and Universality: A Theory of Nursing* (New York: National League for Nursing, 1991).

8. J. Watson, *Nursing: Human Science and Human Care* (New York: National League for Nursing, 1988).

9. Ibid., 54.

10. M. Rogers, *The Theoretical Basis of Nursing* (Philadelphia: F.A. Davis Co., 1970), vii.

11. M. Newman, *Health As Expanding Consciousness,* 2nd ed. (New York: National League for Nursing, 1994).

12. R.R. Parse, Human Becoming: Parse's Theory of Nursing, *Nursing Science Quarterly* 5 (1992): 35–42.

13. Ibid.

Holistic Nursing and Related Research

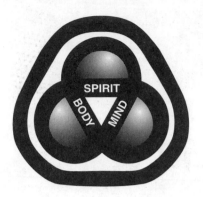

CHAPTER 10

Holistic Nursing and Related Research

Cathie E. Guzzetta

KNOWLEDGE COMPETENCIES

- Discuss ways in which the wellness model has redirected priorities in nursing research.
- Compare and contrast qualitative versus quantitative research methods.
- Discuss the advantages of qualitative research methods for evaluating holistic phenomena.
- Explore the implications of Heisenberg's Uncertainty Principle in conducting holistic nursing research.
- Discuss the ways in which the placebo response may be enhanced in nursing research and clinical practice.
- Examine the mission of the Office of Alternative Medicine in fostering the development of holistic alternative/complementary interventions.
- Outline various bio-psycho-social-spiritual variables that are affected by holistic interventions.

DEFINITIONS

Qualitative Research: a systematic, subjective form of research that is used to describe life experiences and give them meaning. Qualitative research focuses on understanding the whole, which is consistent with the holistic philosophy of nursing.

Quantitative Research: a formal, objective, systematic form of research in which numerical data are used to describe variables, examine relationships among variables, and determine cause-and-effect interactions between variables.[1]

Research: a diligent, systematic inquiry or investigation to validate and refine existing knowledge and generate new knowledge.[2]

Pause for a moment . . .

- ❑ *I highlight content in my own way with one or different colored markers as I study.*
- ❑ *I am proud of myself for choosing to prepare for the holistic nursing certification (HNC) examination.*

THEORIES AND RESEARCH

Wellness Model

1. The framework guiding client/patient research in nursing is shifting from an illness to a wellness model of health care.
2. The wellness model views people holistically as bio-psycho-social-spiritual individuals who assume responsibility for their own health.
   a. Each individual has the potential to use the healing power of his or her own body-mind-spirit.
   b. Accumulating research provides evidence of the devastating effects as well as the healing effects of consciousness on both health and illness.
   c. Research demonstrates that some holistic complementary/alternative therapies have the potential to change the clinical course and outcome of illness, prevent illness, and maintain high-level wellness.
   d. Such research has been instrumental in guiding the development of humanistic and holistic approaches to health care.

Quantitative Research Methods

1. In the seventeenth century, Descartes advanced medical research by using the scientific method used today.
2. Descartes' notion of reductionism in research—the idea of breaking down every question to its smallest possible parts—has been beneficial in isolating causative factors responsible for disease.
   a. The physiologic part of an individual can be divided into organs, cells, and biochemical substances; then into molecular, atomic, and subatomic levels.
   b. Such an approach is useful for identifying the etiology of disease (e.g., a virus causes AIDS) and offers direction for studying the cure of disease (e.g., antibodies are used to kill the bacteria associated with endocarditis).
3. This kind of research, called quantitative research, is the most commonly used method of scientific inquiry.
4. Quantitative research is classified into four categories.
   a. Descriptive research describes phenomena.
   b. Correlational research examines relationships among and between variables.
   c. Quasi-experimental research explains relationships, examines causal relationships, and clarifies the reasons that events happen.
   d. Experimental research examines cause-and-effect relationships.
5. The scientific or quantitative method was created for several reasons.
   a. Results in one study can be generalized to other similar patient populations.
   b. Results can be replicated in similar studies.
   c. Results can be used to predict and control outcomes.
6. Isolating parts for group comparisons and statistical analyses makes it possible to validate cause and effect.
7. The quantitative method, however, does not take into account:
   a. The response of the whole human being to variables.
   b. The characteristics of one individual's pathway to a particular problem.
   c. The unique patterns and interacting variables of one individual.
8. Bodymind researchers have challenged the biomedical paradigm.

a. The field of psychoneuroimmunology has generated research findings to support the interaction and connectedness of the mind and body.
b. There is conclusive evidence that thoughts and emotions affect the neurologic, endocrine, and immune systems at the cellular and subcellular levels.
c. Because quantitative methods seek to find answers to only parts of the whole, nurses have looked to alternate philosophies of science and research methods to investigate humanistic and holistic phenomena. Such methods have been termed qualitative research.

Holistic Qualitative Research Methods

1. Qualitative research is a systematic, subjective form of research that is used to describe an understanding of human experiences such as health, caring, loneliness, pain, and comfort.
   a. The context and meaning of observed patterns
   b. The whole which is consistent with the holistic philosophy of nursing
2. Qualitative research has been classified into six types.
   a. Phenomenologic research describes an experience as it is lived by the whole person (Exhibit 10–1).
   b. Grounded theory research uncovers the problems that exist in a social situation and the efforts of the persons involved to handle them.
   c. Ethnographic research studies a culture and the people within the culture.
   d. Philosophic inquiry analyzes meanings, identifies values and ethics, and studies the nature of knowledge.
   e. Historical research describes or analyzes the events that occurred in the past to understand the present situation better.
   f. Critical social theory explains how people communicate with one another and how symbolic meanings in society develop.
3. Although there are convincing data to refute the idea that the body is separate from the mind, many health care professionals remain tied to the biomedical model and view holistic principles and their corresponding qualitative research approaches as unscientific.
   a. The existence of a psychophysiologic link between the mind and body has been ques-

Exhibit 10–1 Use of the Phenomenologic Research Approach

Parse, Coyne, and Smith conducted a study to discover a definition of health as it is lived and experienced in everyday life. These researchers asked the question, "What are the common elements in experiencing a feeling of health among several different age groups?"* One hundred subjects between 20 and 45 years old were asked to write a description of their feelings, thoughts, and perceptions at a time when they felt healthy. The actual words used by the subjects were employed in reports of the findings. From the data collected, 30 descriptive expressions of health were identified (Table 10–1).

From these 30 descriptors, three central themes were recognized: spirited intensity, fulfilling inventiveness, and symphonic integrity. Based on these central themes, the researchers then formulated the following definition: "Health is symphonic integrity manifested in the spirited intensity of fulfilling inventiveness." Although some nurses may not understand this definition of health by itself, the fact that Table 10–1 provides such rich descriptors makes it possible to understand the lived experience of health. This understanding embodies a definition of health that is fuller and more holistic than the traditional biomedical view of health defined as the "absence of disease."

*R.R. Parse et al., The Lived Experience of Health: A Phenomenological Study, in *Nursing Research: Qualitative Methods,* eds. R.R. Parse et al. (Bowie, MD: Brady Communications Co., 1985), 27–31.

tioned because evidence to support the link has been provided in the form of anecdotes or personal testimonials.

b. "Hard core" researchers who embrace the quantitative method have not placed much value on the "softer" data obtained from qualitative studies.

c. Even when the results of quantitative research support the link, such studies are criticized because of their retrospective designs, methodologic problems, or lack of measurement tools with psychometric properties.

4. Before the mind–body link is universally accepted, additional research will have to be conducted. Nurses, by virtue of their day-to-day care of the client, are in a unique position to observe, document, analyze, and quantify the interactive relationship of the bodymind in health and illness.

5. The value of qualitative research methods will increase as important bodymind variables are discovered.

a. The respectability of qualitative research will make rapid gains also as the authors of nursing research texts dedicate more time to this content area, as research journal editors accept more qualitative studies for publication, and as more qualitative studies attract federal funding.[3]

b. The results of qualitative studies are supplying quantitative researchers with a plethora of potential research hypotheses.

Table 10–1 The Experience of Health—Descriptive Expressions from Participants in a Phenomenologic Study

Spirited Intensity	Fulfilling Inventiveness	Symphonic Integrity
1. Being enthusiastic	1. Finishing a project that takes up time	1. Being at ease
2. Catching a second wind	2. Accomplishment	2. Feeling of worth
3. Exercising and walking	3. Winning the game of life	3. Enjoying own space at that moment
4. Feel in peak condition	4. Trying some new endeavor	4. Peaceful feeling inside while bicycling
5. Positive outlook on life	5. Feeling something enriching my life	5. A "just right" feeling about everything
6. Feeling of refreshment	6. Doing what I struggled for	6. Drinking in the beauty of the day
7. Feeling full of energy	7. Pushing a little extra	7. Peaceful attitude
8. A glowing light of energy burning brightly in my eyes	8. Feel successful as a person	8. Rhythmical, easy, warm
9. A whip-the-world feeling	9. Ability to extend to limits of endurance	9. Glowing and good inside
10. A surge of energy	10. Accomplishing something	10. Feeling loved

Source: Reprinted with permission from R.R. Parse, A.B. Coyne, and M.J. Smith, *Nursing Research: Qualitative Methods,* p. 32, copyright © 1985, Appleton & Lange.

6. Both qualitative and quantitative methods are needed in holistic research.[4]
   a. Table 10–2 contrasts the characteristics of the quantitative and the qualitative approaches to research.
   b. Exhibit 10–2 illustrates the qualitative versus quantitative research method used to investigate an "apple." Clearly, each method is important in scientific investigation, and neither method is superior to the other.

Objectivity in Scientific Investigation

1. Most researchers believe that objectivity must govern scientific inquiry.
2. Werner Heisenberg, the Nobel Prize winner who studied information obtained from an electron, stated the principle, however, that one cannot look at a physical object without changing it.[5] Thus, objects and clients are changed when they are observed.
3. This principle, called Heisenberg's Uncertainty Principle, has various implications for the holistic researcher.
   a. The researcher does not stand apart from the research or research subject.
   b. The researcher is not an objective observer of the world, but rather a participant in that world.

Table 10–2 Quantitative and Qualitative Research Characteristics

Quantitative Research	Qualitative Research
Hard science	Soft science
Focus: concise and narrow	Focus: complex and broad
Reductionistic	Holistic
Objective	Subjective
Reasoning: logistic, deductive	Reasoning: dialectic, inductive
Basis of knowing: cause-and-effect relationships	Basis of knowing: meaning, discovery
Tests theory	Develops theory
Control	Shared interpretation
Instruments	Communication and observation
Basic element of analysis: numbers	Basic element of analysis: words
Statistical analysis	Individual interpretation
Generalization	Uniqueness

Source: Reprinted with permission from N. Burns and S.K. Grove, *The Practice of Nursing Research: Conduct, Critique and Utilization,* p. 27, © 1993, W.D. Saunders.

Exhibit 10–2 Investigating an Apple: A Qualitative versus a Quantitative Approach

A quantitative researcher might examine an apple using the following approach:
- Inspect the apple closely.
- Carefully weigh it.
- Cut into it.
- Separate the skin from the meat. For the skin and the meat,
  — Weigh each.
  — Analyze each for sugar, salt, water, fiber, calories, and vitamins and then statistically analyze the differences between the skin and the meat.
- Count the seeds, and examine the inside of the seeds.

A qualitative researcher might examine an apple using the following approach:
- Look at the apple from all sides, top, and bottom.
- Feel it.
- Smell it.
- Shine it.
- Roll it.
- Appreciate its wholeness.
- Bite into it, eat, and enjoy it, noting its
  — sound.
  — taste.
  — texture.
  — temperature.
- After finding its seeds, plant the seeds to determine what they might produce.

Courtesy of Dr. Elizabeth H. Winslow.

c. This participation, in turn, affects the results obtained through research.
d. Participation may be a word, an action, a touch, an observation, or simply presence.
e. The researcher becomes an integral part of the experiment and its outcomes.

4. Heisenberg also proposed that it is not possible to obtain a complete description of a physical object because, when we describe it, we change it.
   a. Because it is impossible to obtain all the data to describe an object, some information will always be unknown.
   b. Research effects are verified by observations. If it is impossible to obtain a complete description of a physical object, however, some outcomes will be unknown.

c. It is misleading to believe that research can always be validated in terms of testable or observational effects. The effects of a certain experiment, whether they are observable or not, will ultimately change the subject.

5. Certain phenomena related to holistic research may not be accessible to scientific investigation.
   a. Individuals may not be able to conceptualize or express certain experiences associated with alternative/complementary therapies or may be unable to translate or communicate their effects to another.
   b. Likewise, the researcher may be unable to interpret the effects because of a lack of experience with these feelings or because language is limited and inadequate for describing and communicating these phenomena.

 Pause for a moment . . .

❑ *I place my books and papers near to prepare to study.*
❑ *I gather other resources to assist me in studying.*

Evaluation of Holistic Interventions

1. Much research remains to be done in evaluating holistic interventions.
2. Many alternative/complementary therapies have been used to treat a variety of problems, but their appropriateness and adequacy in various populations and settings have not been assessed fully.
3. Outcome studies are needed to determine the comparative usefulness, indications, contraindications, and dangers of diverse alternative/complementary interventions. These interventions need to be evaluated for their potential to
   a. Change the clinical course and outcome of an illness.
   b. Promote high-level wellness.
   c. Prevent illness.
4. In 1992, the National Institutes of Health (NIH) created the Office of Alternative Medicine (OAM) to evaluate scientifically many alternative/complementary interventions.
   a. The OAM has funded 42 studies to evaluate such therapies as acupressure, massage therapy, electrochemical treatment, hypnosis, music therapy, guided imagery, biofeedback, prayer, and antioxidants.

b. The OAM recently has funded 10 Complementary and Alternative Medicine Research Centers.[6] Each center is responsible for researching a major health condition, such as cancer, pain, aging, women's health, stroke, low back pain, coronary artery disease, addictions, HIV/AIDS, asthma, allergy, and immunology.
   c. The results of these studies will provide the scientific basis for determining which alternative therapies are genuinely effective, safe, and relatively inexpensive when compared to conventional modalities in improving patient outcomes.[7]
   d. The ultimate goal of the OAM is not to supplant modern medicine with alternatives, but rather to integrate validated alternative/complementary approaches with the best of conventional health care practices.

The Placebo Response

1. Only recently have the power of the placebo effect and the mechanisms involved been understood.
   a. Placebo means "I will please."
   b. A placebo is a medically inert preparation or treatment that has no specific effects on the body and is intended to have no therapeutic benefit.
   c. This medically inert preparation or treatment can evoke a placebo response by relieving pain or dramatically affecting the client's symptoms or disease.
2. The placebo response has always been viewed as "getting in the way" of the research results.
   a. It is seen as a nuisance and an unreliable factor.
   b. It has been assumed to work only in illnesses that somehow were not real.
3. Recent evidence has shown that a placebo effect can activate the production of endorphins (i.e., peptide hormones produced and secreted by the brain with opiate properties that are exponentially more potent than morphine), which can modify or inhibit the transmission of pain stimuli throughout the central nervous system.[8]
   a. In an analysis of 15 double-blind studies, placebo medications were found to be effective in pain relief for one-third of patients with postoperative pain.[9]

b. An analysis of 11 more recent double-blind studies in which one-third of the patients received at least 50 percent pain relief from placebos confirmed these findings.[10]

c. The worse the pain or the more stressful the situation, the more effective the placebo.

4. The placebo effect may be even higher than the one-third rule of thumb governing placebo effectiveness. Approximately two-thirds of patients improved in preliminary trials of five new medical treatments (for asthma, ulcers, and herpes) that were considered promising,[11] but later proved useless. Thus, it appears that for more than one-third of patients, probably even more, the pharmacologically inert placebo is able to access and activate bodymind healing mechanisms.

5. The placebo response has been found to be present in all of the following conditions and therapeutic procedures:[12]

a. Hypertension, stress, cardiac pain, blood cell counts, headaches, pupillary dilation (suggesting the mind's ability to alter the autonomic nervous system).

b. Adrenal gland secretion, diabetes, ulcers, gastric secretion and motility, colitis, oral contraceptives, menstrual pain, thyrotoxicosis (suggesting the mind's ability to alter the endocrine system).

c. The common cold, fever, vaccines, asthma, multiple sclerosis, rheumatoid arthritis, warts, cancer (suggesting the mind's ability to alter the immune system).

d. Surgical treatments (e.g., for angina pectoris).

e. Biofeedback instrumentation and various medical devices.

f. Psychologic treatments such as conditioning (systematic desensitization) and perhaps all forms of psychotherapy.

6. The placebo response, also called the general healing response, occurs because of a communication link between the body and the mind that is probably present in all clinical situations and exists, more or less, in each one of us.

7. Many factors can affect the placebo response:[13]

a. The way in which a drug is given or a procedure performed.

b. The faith that the client has in the caregiver.

c. The client's expectation that the drug or therapy will work.

d. The faith that the caregiver conveys to the client regarding the drug or therapy.

e. The trust and rapport established between the client and caregiver.

8. Positive attitudes and emotions enhance the placebo response.

a. Many alternative/complementary therapies such as imagery, music therapy, relaxation, and exercise increase endorphin production.

b. When patients believe that they are doing something to enhance healing, endorphin levels can rise.

c. Patients, therefore, can influence the course of their own illnesses and their responses to therapy by using their own consciousness.

9. Because basic nursing interventions such as touching, giving back rubs, preoperative teaching, positioning, and distraction, all have the potential to enhance endorphin levels, nurses must learn to incorporate the powerful placebo as a part of nursing research and clinical nursing interventions.

Identification of Holistic Outcomes and Instruments

1. Although holistic interventions influence multiple bio-psycho-social-spiritual variables, there is a lack of holistic instruments or tools to measure the effects of such interventions.[14]

2. A variety of variables (e.g., heart rate, blood pressure, respiratory rate, temperature, cardiac output) and instruments make it possible to study the physiologic effects of holistic interventions.

a. Such variables need to be used in combination to develop a physiologic profile of observed outcomes.

b. Physiologic measurements tend to be used with more confidence than psychologic measurements, which are viewed as less reliable and less valid than their physiologic counterparts.

3. Many psychologic instruments are not sensitive indicators of the subtle yet significant psychologic outcomes associated with holistic interventions.

4. The finding that a psychologic variable is not significant in a research study does not necessarily disprove the existence of a significant psychologic effect.

a. The wrong variable may have been studied.

b. The psychologic instrument used may not have been sufficiently sensitive to measure the existence of a change.

5. Alternative/complementary interventions influence many psychophysiologic variables, but they do not necessarily influence the same variables in different individuals. Thus, researchers must use a number of psychophysiologic variables to evaluate the outcomes of these interventions.
   a. Physiologic and psychologic outcomes need to be used in combination and their effects correlated as a means of increasing the validity of the findings and discovering mind–body links.
   b. Psychologic and physiologic measurements need to be combined to develop various psychophysiologic tools.
   c. A rich, promising, and holistic source of data lies within the subjects' own estimates of their behavior and outcomes related to the effects of alternative/complementary interventions.
   d. Meaning and quality of life are essential tenets of the holistic model, and qualitative methods are well suited to tapping this subjective source of data.
6. Quantitative studies of subjective phenomena such as comfort, pain, and anxiety are appearing in the literature with more frequency.
   a. The outcome of comfort has been operationalized by total and subscale scores on a holistic instrument that measures the physical, psychologic, environmental, and social comfort of patients.[15]
   b. The Duke–University of North Carolina Health Profile has been used to assess the impact of medical interventions on daily functioning of clients in four areas: symptom experiences, physical function, emotional function, and social function.[16]
   c. A variety of visual analog scales, diaries, logs, and graphs also are being used with increased frequency as a method of capturing the holistic, longitudinal, and individualized perceptions of patient experiences.
7. A current research mandate is to develop psychophysiologic instruments that facilitate assessment, diagnosis, and selection of nursing interventions and measure the effectiveness of interventions designed to enhance body-mind-spirit outcomes.

REFERENCES

1. P. Flynn, *Holistic Health: The Art and Science of Care* (Bowie, MD: Brady Communications, 1980), 1–8.
2. N. Burns and S.K. Grove, *The Practice of Nursing Research: Conduct, Critique, and Utilization,* 2nd ed. (Philadelphia: W.B. Saunders, 1993), 3.
3. D.F. Bockmon and D.J. Riemen, Qualitative versus Quantitative Nursing Research, *Holistic Nursing Practice* 2, no. 1 (1987): 71–75.
4. L.C. Dzurec and I.L. Abraham, The Nature of Inquiry: Linking Quantitative and Qualitative Research, *Advances in Nursing Science* 16, no. 1 (1993): 73–79.
5. W. Heisenberg, *Physics and Philosophy* (New York: Harper & Row, 1978), 42.
6. W. Jonas, OAM Director outlines office mission and accomplishments. *Complementary and Alternative Medicine at the NIH, II* (1995): 1–8.
7. R. Cron, OAM Awards 30 Exploratory Grants in First Round, *Alternative Medicine Newsletter* 1, no. 2 (1993): 1.
8. A. West, Understanding Endorphins: Our Natural Pain Relief System, *Nurs 81* 2 (1981): 50.
9. H. Beecher, The Powerful Placebo, *Journal of the American Medical Association* 159 (1955): 1602.
10. F. Evans, Expectancy, Therapeutic Instructions, and the Placebo Response, in *Placebo: Theory, Research, and Mechanism,* ed. L. White et al. (New York: Guilford Press, 1985).
11. A. Roberts, Placebo Therapies Spark 'Improvement' for 7 of 10, *Brain Mind Bulletin* 18, no. 12 (1993): 1.
12. E. Rossi, *The Psychobiology of Mind-Body Healing* (New York: W.W. Norton & Co., 1993), 11–22.
13. L. Dossey, *Healing Words: The Power of Prayer and the Practice of Medicine* (San Francisco, CA: Harper, 1993), 134–135.
14. C.E. Guzzetta, Nursing Research and Its Holistic Application, in *Holistic Nursing: A Handbook for Practice,* 2nd ed., eds. B.M. Dossey et al. (Gaithersburg, MD: Aspen Publishers, 1995), 197–214.
15. K.Y. Kolcaba, Holistic Comfort: Operationalizing the Construct as a Nurse-Sensitive Outcome, *Advances in Nursing Science* 15, no. 1 (1992): 1–10.
16. G.R. Parkerson et al., The Duke-UNC Health Profile: An Adult Health Status Instrument for Primary Care, *Medical Care* 19, no. 8 (1981): 805–823.

CONCEPT VI

Holistic Nursing Process

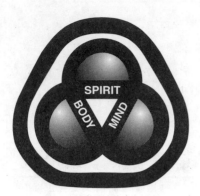

CHAPTER 11

Holistic Nursing Process

Pamela Potter Hughes

KNOWLEDGE COMPETENCIES

- Reflect on the origins of the nursing process and its applicability to holistic nursing.
- Discuss the application of the holistic nursing process within a theoretical framework. (See Chapter 9.)
- Describe the four patterns of knowing that guide the nursing process within the nurse–client interaction.
- Identify the interrelationships of the phases of the holistic nursing process.
- Describe the role of the nurse within the holistic nursing process.
- Identify the role of the client in the nursing process.
- Identify impediments to effective nursing process.
- Describe the six phases of the holistic nursing process.[1]
- Relate the AHNA Standards of Holistic Nursing Practice (see Appendix A) to the nursing process.

DEFINITIONS

Holistic Nursing Practice: the provision of nursing care in a way that "draws on nursing knowledge, theories, expertise, and intuition to guide nurses in becoming therapeutic partners with clients in strengthening the clients' responses to facilitate the healing process and achieve wholeness" (see Exhibit 1–1).

Holistic Nursing Process: a systematic framework for addressing and organizing information relevant to the nurse–unitary person interaction. It includes six steps: assessment, nursing diagnosis, client outcomes, care planning, implementation, and evaluation.

 Pause for a moment . . .

- ❏ *I use my time effectively.*
- ❏ *I know that there are no rules for how I actually study.*
- ❏ *I know my own personal style of studying.*

THEORIES AND RESEARCH

1. A systematic process for the practice of holistic nursing acts as a guiding structure for the novice and an internalized ballast for the experienced nurse; it "unifies, standardizes, and directs nursing practice."[2]
2. Originating as a problem-solving model based on the scientific method, the holistic nursing process expands to accommodate the human science paradigm.
   a. The holistic framework guides a client-centered process.
   b. This approach examines the clients' reality perceptions and life meanings for insight into their lived experiences of health and well-being.[3]
   c. The nurse collaborates with the client to identify and pursue goals for health enhancement.
   d. The whole person is considered in environmental context (e.g., family, culture, society, clinic, hospital).

Exhibit 11–1 Nine Human Response Patterns

1. Exchanging: mutual giving and receiving.
2. Relating: establishing bonds.
3. Valuing: assigning relative worth.
4. Choosing: selection of alternatives.
5. Moving: activity.
6. Perceiving: reception of information.
7. Feeling: subjective awareness of information.
8. Knowing: meaning associated with information.
9. Communicating: sending and receiving messages.

3. Information relevant to the client's care is gathered and processed according to a theoretical model. (See Chapter 9.)
   a. Nurses choose a theoretical practice model that is realistic, useful, and consistent with their professional values and philosophy.
   b. Client problems/strengths, probable outcomes, and appropriate nursing actions are identified through a synthesis of the theory base and client data.
   c. Client care is evaluated and documented in the language of the theory.
4. Insights derived from the four patterns of knowing identified by Carper[4] guide the nurse's process within the nurse–client interaction.
   a. Empirical or scientific knowledge is based on objective information measurable by the senses, including scientific instrumentation.
   b. Ethical knowledge flows from the "basic underlying concept of the unity and integral wholeness of all people and of all nature."[5]
   c. Esthetic knowledge draws on a sense of form and structure, beauty and creativity, for discerning pattern and change.
   d. Personal knowledge incorporates the nurse's self-awareness and knowledge, as well as the intuitive perception of meanings based on personal experiences, and is demonstrated by the therapeutic use of self.
5. Although the phases of the nursing process are described in a linear fashion, in practice they feed back to each other, are interrelated, often occur simultaneously, and rest in the nurse–client relationship.
6. Nurses focus on the care of the whole unique person.
   a. They respect and advocate for the client's rights and choices.
   b. They make decisions about client care based on a holistic assessment of relevant areas in collaboration with the client, other health care providers, and significant others.
7. Clients assume an active role in health care planning and decision making.
   a. They seek out the professional expertise of the nurse (via an office visit, hospitalization, or some other nurse–client interaction).
   b. They express health concerns and strengths.
   c. Participating as actively as possible, they take responsibility for their personal health and decisions for self-care.
8. Impediments to effective nursing process include the following:
   a. Excessive reliance on structure may decrease reliance on intuition and creativity.[6]
   b. Excessive reliance on objectivity may reduce the client to a mere object.

The Nursing Process in Theoretical Perspective

1. The conceptualization of nursing process as an orderly approach to the conduct of independent nursing activities was first formally identified as a nursing activity framework in 1957 by Kreuter.[7]
2. The nursing process incorporates the problem-solving component of natural science methodology, although it has been critiqued as potentially focused on "problems" rather than on the unique human individual.
3. The holistic nursing process is a synthesis of human and natural sciences.
   a. Awareness of an alternative approach to nursing knowledge has increased since 1970.
   b. Watson,[8] Leininger,[9] and others began to write about reemphasizing the unmeasurable human side of the traditional art of nursing.
   c. This paradigm is applied more and more often to nursing research, education, and practice.
   d. All nurse–client encounters are framed within the perspective of the unique wholeness of the unitary person.
4. The nursing process furthers outcomes research.
   a. Standardization of language about nurses' activities and responsibilities affords a unified structure for nursing research.
   b. The nursing process alone is not a substitute for nursing theory as the framework for nursing research.

Pause for a moment . . .

❑ *My family and friends are supporting me as I prepare for the holistic nursing certification (HNC) examination.*
❑ *I appreciate my peace and quiet without interruptions.*

HOLISTIC NURSING PROCESS

Assessment

Standard of Care:
Clients shall be assessed holistically and continually.

1. Assessment is the information-gathering phase in which the nurse and the client identify health patterns and prioritize the client's health concerns.
2. Its purpose is to identify and document the client's human response patterns (Exhibit 11–1) and willingness to participate in change.
   a. Assessment provides baseline data for evaluating changes that occur over time.
   b. The key to a holistic assessment is to discover the overall pattern of responses.
   c. A holistic assessment describes the client's total state of being.
3. The nurse gleans information about client patterns via interaction, observation, and measurement. Each pattern identification taps into the hologram of the person, contributing to the revelation of the whole.
   a. The nurse's interaction with the person reveals client perceptions, feelings, and thoughts.
   b. Nursing observation relies on information perceived by the five senses and intuition.
   c. Measurement is quantifiable information obtained from instruments.
4. The client is the primary source and interpreter of the meaning of information obtained by the assessment process. Family, significant others, other health care professionals, and measurable data provide supplemental information.
5. During assessment of the client's bio-psycho-social-spiritual patterns, the holistic nurse
   a. Looks for the overall pattern of interrelationships.
   b. Uses appropriate scientific and intuitive approaches.
   c. Assesses the state of the energy field.
   d. Identifies stages of change and readiness to learn.

e. Collects pertinent data from previous client records and other members of the health care team, if appropriate.
f. Incorporates new information into the holistic assessment.
g. Documents all pertinent data in the client's record (Holistic Nursing Assessment Tools, Appendixes 11–A and 11–B).
6. The holistic nurse sees the client as a whole and listen for the meaning of this current health situation to the person within the environment.
   a. The nurse reflects to the client patterns recognized from the assessment.
   b. The nurse acknowledges his or her personal patterns and their influence on the client.
7. Assessment and documentation are continuous within the nurse–client interaction.
   a. Changes in one response pattern always influence other dimensions.
   b. The client expresses the personal meaning of identified health patterns.
8. Impediments to holistic assessment include the following:
   a. Rigidity of the nurse's beliefs introduces a barrier to the flow of information.
   b. A nurse's lack of awareness of personal beliefs and patterns may influence the nurse–client interaction.
   c. There may be communication barriers between the nurse and client relative to culture, class, age, gender, education, or physical limitation.

Nursing Diagnoses

Standard of Care:
Client actual and high-risk problems/patterns/needs and opportunities to enhance health and well-being, and their priorities shall be identified based upon collected data.

1. A nursing diagnosis is a "clinical judgment about the individual, family, or community responses to actual or potential health problems/life processes"[10] and health-enhancing opportunities.
2. "Nursing diagnoses provide the basis for selection of nursing interventions to achieve outcomes for which the nurse is accountable."[11]
   a. The North American Nursing Diagnosis Association (NANDA) was formed for the purpose of standardizing the terminology used for nursing diagnosis.
   b. NANDA continues to define, explain, classify, and research summary health statements about health problems related to nursing.

c. Standardized labels facilitate communication and research validating the clinical outcomes of nursing interventions.

d. Nursing diagnoses are the basis for the remaining steps of the nursing process.

3. A systematic analysis of information, gleaned from the assessment and organized according to nine human response patterns (see Exhibit 11–1), makes it possible to formulate hypotheses as to the etiologic bases for each identified actual or high-risk problem/pattern/need and each opportunity to enhance health.

4. Nursing diagnoses are written as statements describing actual, risk, and wellness nursing diagnoses (Appendixes 11–A and 11–B).[12]

   a. An actual nursing diagnosis is a description of an individual's actual health problems in terms of a pattern of related cues (e.g., energy field disturbances related to slowing or blocking of energy flows secondary to surgical procedure[13]).

   b. A risk diagnosis is a description, supported by risk factors, of human responses to health conditions/life processes that may develop in a vulnerable individual, family, or community (e.g., risk for altered nutrition related to nausea, vomiting, fatigue, and activity intolerance associated with chemotherapy).

   c. A wellness nursing diagnosis[14] "describes human responses to levels of wellness in an individual, family, or community that have a potential for enhancement to a higher state"[15] (e.g., potential for enhanced spirituality).

5. The client's value system is the basis for holistic nursing decisions and diagnostic labeling.

   a. The nurse chooses diagnoses that most accurately reflect the client's perceptions.

   b. Preconceived notions about what would constitute health enhancement for the client are set aside.

6. The client collaborates with the nurse to prioritize nursing diagnoses.

7. Impediments to a holistic nursing diagnosis are neglecting to make the client the focus of the process; fitting the pattern of a dynamic, changing human being into an arbitrary diagnostic statement rather than reflecting the actual pattern of the person; and failing to have a continual focused awareness of the person as a whole.

Client Outcomes

Standard of Care:
Client's actual or high-risk problems/patterns/needs or opportunities to enhance health and well-being shall

have appropriate outcomes specified and revised as appropriate.

1. A client outcome is a direct statement of nurse–client identified goals to be achieved within a specified time frame; the client's significant others and other health care practitioners may participate in goal setting.

2. An outcome indicates the maximum level of wellness that is reasonably attainable for the person in view of objective circumstances and client perceptions.

3. Outcome criteria describe the specific tools, tests, observations, or patient statements that determine whether the client outcome has been achieved and include

   a. Changes that should or should not occur in the client's status.

   b. Level at which some change could occur.

   c. Client's verbalization about what the client knows, understands, or feels about the situation.

   d. Specific client behavior or signs and symptoms that are expected to occur as a result of intervention.

4. The holistic nurse selects interventions on the basis of desired client outcomes.

   a. The nurse discusses with the client possible ways for achieving desired outcomes.

   b. The client helps to establish observable milestones for knowing whether or not desired changes have occurred and makes a commitment to action in order to move toward those desired changes.

5. Assumptions made by the nurse concerning desired outcomes without client collaboration are impediments to client outcomes.

6. Neither the nurse nor the client should rigidly adhere to outcomes; rather, they should recognize the value of the journey (other paths/other possible outcomes).

Plan and Interventions

Standards of Care:
Clients shall have an appropriate plan of holistic nursing care formulated focusing on health promotion or health maintenance activities. Client's plan of holistic nursing care shall be implemented according to the priority of identified problems/patterns/needs, or opportunities to enhance health and well-being.

1. Identify interventions intended to achieve long- and short-term client outcomes.

2. Develop the plan in terms of "nursing prescriptions," which indicate the specific actions (in-

terventions) that the nurse will perform to help the client approach problems and accomplish outcomes.[16]

3. Develop appropriate client goals for each nursing diagnosis in collaboration with the client, the client's significant others, and other health care practitioners.

4. Determine nursing interventions for the diagnoses to enhance the health of the client and significant others.

   a. A nursing intervention has been defined as "any direct care treatment that a nurse performs on behalf of a client."[17]

   b. It may be nurse-initiated, based on nursing diagnoses, or physician-initiated, based on medical diagnoses.

   c. The Nursing Intervention Classification Code includes all direct care interventions that nurses perform for patients, both independent and collaborative (Exhibit 11–2).[18]

5. Organize the plan of care to reflect the priority of identified client opportunities to enhance health.

6. Establish priorities for intervention based upon assessment of the urgency of the threat to the client's life and safety.

7. Choose interventions based on utility, relationship to the nursing diagnosis, effectiveness, feasibility, acceptability to the client, and nursing competency.

8. Use interventions/holistic modalities that communicate acceptance of the client's and significant others' values, beliefs, culture, religion, and socioeconomic background.

9. Revise the plan of care to reflect the client's current status or ongoing changes.

10. Record the plan of care in the client record.

Evaluation

Standard of Care:
Client's results of holistic nursing care shall be continuously evaluated.

1. Evaluation is a planned review of the nurse–client interaction to identify factors facilitating or inhibiting expected outcomes.

Exhibit 11–2 Noninvasive Nursing Interventions*

Activity Therapy	Emotional Support	Limit Setting	Sexual Counseling
Acupressure*	Environmental (personal,	Massage (simple)	Shen Therapy*
Addictions Counseling*	community)*	Medication Management	Smoking Cessation
AMMA Therapy*	Exercise/Movement	Meditation	Spiritual Support
Animal Assisted Therapy	Family Integrity	Music Therapy	Spirituality
Anxiety Reduction	Promotion	Mutual Goal Setting	Counseling*
Aroma Therapy*	Family Involvement	Nutrition Counseling	Suicide Prevention
Art Therapy	Family Process	Pain Management	Support Groups
Assertiveness Training	Maintenance	Patient Rights Protection	Support System
Autogenic Training	Family Support	Play Therapy	Enhancement
Back Remedies*	Family Therapy	Polarity Therapy*	Sustenance Support
Behavior Modification	Foot Care	Presence	Teaching: Group
Bibliotherapy	Goal Setting/Contracts*	Progressive Muscle	Teaching: Individual
Biofeedback	Grief Work Facilitation	Relaxation	Therapeutic Touch
Biomagnetic Healing*	Hakoni Counseling*	Referral	Therapy Group
Body Image	Healing Touch*	Relationship Counseling*	Touch
Enhancement	Herbal Remedies*	Reminiscence Therapy	Values Clarification
Body Mechanics	Holistic Self-Assessments*	Role Enhancement	Violence Counseling*
Promotion	Humor/Laughter	Sacrocranial Therapy*	Weight Management
Calming Technique	Hypnosis	Self-Awareness	Wellness Counseling*
Caregiver Support	Imagery	Enhancement	
Cognitive Therapy	Journaling*	Self-Esteem	
Counseling	Lactation Management	Enhancement	
Crisis Intervention	Learning Facilitation	Self-Reflection*	
Deathing/Death/Grief	Learning Readiness	Sexual Abuse	
Counseling	Enhancement	Counseling*	

*Those marked are not yet recognized by Nursing Intervention Classification Code.
Source: Adapted from J.C. McCloskey and G.M. Bulechek, *Nursing Interventions Classification (NIC)* (St. Louis: Mosby–Year Book, 1996).

a. Data about the client's bio-psycho-social-spiritual status and responses are continuously collected and recorded throughout the nursing process.

b. The information is related to the nursing diagnoses, the outcome criteria, and the effect of the nursing intervention.

2. The goal of evaluation is to determine whether client outcomes have been achieved and, if so, to what extent.

a. Data are synthesized to identify successful repatterning behavior toward wellness.

b. Factors that contribute to deviations between the client's response and desired outcomes are identified.

3. After evaluating the effectiveness of nursing interventions to achieve client outcomes and opportunities to enhance health, the nurse and client may revise the plan of care.

4. Failure to recognize that all measurable outcomes may not be immediate, but are a process of becoming, is an impediment to evaluation.

REFERENCES

1. C.E. Guzzetta, Holistic Approach to the Nursing Process, in *Holistic Nursing: A Handbook for Practice*, 2nd ed., eds. B.M. Dossey et al. (Gaithersburg, MD: Aspen Publishers, 1995), 153–193.

2. J.W. Kenney, Relevance of Theory-Based Nursing Practice, in *Nursing Process: Applications of Conceptual Models*, eds. P.J. Christensen and J.W. Kenney (St. Louis: C.V. Mosby Co., 1995), 9.

3. P.J. Christensen and J.W. Kenney, eds., *Nursing Process: Application of Conceptual Models* (St. Louis: C.V. Mosby Co., 1995).

4. B.A. Carper, Fundamental Patterns of Knowing in Nursing, *Advances in Nursing Science* 1 (1978): 13.

5. American Holistic Nurses' Association, Code of Ethics for Holistic Nurses, in *Position Statement on Holistic Nursing*.

6. P. Benner, *From Novice to Expert* (Reading, MA: Addison-Wesley Publishing Co., 1982).

7. F.R. Kreuter, What Is Good Nursing Care? *Nursing Outlook* 5 (1957): 302–304.

8. J. Watson, *Nursing: The Philosophy and Science of Caring* (Boston: Little, Brown and Co., 1979).

9. M. Leininger, *Care: The Essence of Nursing and Health* (Thorofare, NJ: Charles B. Slack, 1984).

10. North American Nursing Diagnosis Association, *NANDA Nursing Diagnoses: Definitions and Classification, 1992–1993* (St. Louis: 1992), 5.

11. Ibid.

12. Ibid., 83–84.

13. L.J. Carpenito, *Handbook of Nursing Diagnosis*, 6th ed. (Philadelphia: J.B. Lippincott, 1995).

14. A.D. Houldin et al., *Nursing Diagnoses for Wellness: Supporting Strengths* (Philadelphia: J.B. Lippincott, 1987).

15. North American Nursing Diagnosis Association, 84.

16. C.E. Guzzetta and B.M. Dossey, Nursing Diagnoses, in *Cardiovascular Nursing: Holistic Practice*, eds. C.E. Guzzetta and B.M. Dossey (St. Louis: Mosby–Year Book, 1992).

17. J.C. McCloskey and G.M. Bulecheck, Classification of Nursing Interventions: Implications for Nursing Diagnoses, in *Classification of Nursing Diagnoses: Proceedings of the Tenth Conference*, eds. R.M. Caroll-Johnson and M. Paquette (Philadelphia: J.B. Lippincott, 1994), 114.

18. J.C. McCloskey and G.M. Bulechek, *Nursing Interventions Classification (NIC)* (St. Louis: Mosby–Year Book, 1996).

Appendix 11–A

Holistic Nursing Assessment Tool for Hospitalized Patients

Name: _____ Age: _____ Sex: _____
Address: _____ Telephone: _____
Significant other: _____ Telephone: _____
Date of admission: _____ Medical diagnosis: _____
Allergies: _____ Dyes: _____

Nursing Diagnosis
(Altered/High Risk for/
Potential for Enhanced)

Communicating—A pattern involving sending messages
Read, write, understand English (circle) _____   Communication
Other language _____   Verbal
Intubated _____ Speech impaired _____   [Nonverbal]
Alternate form of communication _____

"Valuing/Transcending"—A pattern involving spiritual growth
Religious preference _____   [Spiritual state]
Important religious practices _____   Spiritual
Cultural orientation _____   Well-being
Cultural practices _____   Spiritual distress
Meaning and purpose in life _____   Hopelessness
Inner strengths _____   Powerlessness
Interconnections (self, others, universe, higher power) _____

Relating—A pattern involving establishing bonds
[Alterations in role]
  Marital status _____   [Role performance]
  Age and health of significant other _____   Parenting
  _____   Sexuality patterns
  Number of children _____ Ages _____
  Responsibilities in home _____
  Financial support _____   Family processes
  Occupation _____
  Job satisfaction/concerns _____
  Physical/mental energy expenditures _____
  Sexual relationships (satisfactory/unsatisfactory) _____
  Physical difficulties related to sex _____

Source: Reprinted with permission from Cathie E. Guzzetta, Shelia D. Bunton, Linda A. Prinkey, Anita P. Sherer, and Patricia C. Seifert, *Clinical Assessment Tools for Use with Nursing Diagnoses,* pp. 15–22, © 1989, Mosby-Year Book.

[Alterations in socialization]

Quality of relationships with others _____

  Patient's description _____

  Significant other's description _____

  Staff observations _____

  Verbalizes feelings of being alone _____

  Attributed to _____

Impaired social interaction

Social isolation

Knowing—A pattern involving the meaning associated with information

Previous hospitalization/surgeries _____
_____

Educational level _____

History of the following diseases:

  Heart _____

  Lung _____

  Liver _____ Kidney _____

  Cerebrovascular _____ Rheumatic fever _____

  Thyroid _____

  Diabetes _____

Medication _____

Current health problems _____
_____

Current medications _____
_____

Knowledge deficit

Risk factors	Present	Knowledge of
1. Hypertension	_____	_____
2. Hyperlipidemia	_____	_____
3. Smoking	_____	_____
4. Obesity	_____	_____
5. Diabetes	_____	_____
6. Sedentary living	_____	_____
7. Stress	_____	_____
8. Alcohol use	_____	_____
9. Oral contraceptives	_____	_____
10. Family history	_____	_____

Knowledge of planned test/surgery _____
_____

Misconceptions _____

Readiness to learn _____

  Learning impeded by _____

[Learning]
Thought processes

Feeling—A pattern involving the subjective awareness of information

[Alterations in comfort]

Pain/discomfort

  Onset _____ Duration _____

  Location _____ Quality _____ Radiation _____

  Associated factors _____

  Aggravating factors _____

  Alleviating factors _____

[Alterations in emotional integrity]

  Recent stressful life events _____
_____

Pain
  Chronic
  [Acute]
[Discomfort]
  Chronic
  Acute
Anxiety

Nursing Diagnosis
(Altered/High Risk for/
Potential for Enhanced)

Verbalizes feelings of fear or anxiety _____

   Source _____ Fear

   Physical manifestations _____

_____

Moving—A pattern involving activity

[Alterations in activity]

  History of physical disability _____

_____

  Limitations in daily activities _____ Impaired physical

     mobility

_____ Activity intolerance

  Exercise habits _____

[Alterations in rest]

  Hours slept/night_____Difficulties _____

  Sleep aids (pillows, medications, food) _____ Sleep pattern disturbance

[Alterations in recreation]

  Leisure activities _____

  Social activities _____ Deficit in diversional

     activity

[Alterations in activities of daily living]

  Home maintenance management _____

  Size and arrangement of home (stairs, bathroom)_____ Impaired home

     maintenance

_____ management

_____

  Housekeeping responsibilities _____

  Shopping responsibilities _____

Health maintenance

  Health insurance _____

  Regular physical checkups _____ Health maintenance

[Alterations in self-care]

  Ability to perform ADL:

    Independent_____ Dependent _____ Self-care

     Feeding

  Specify deficits _____ Bathing

  Discharge planning needs _____ Dressing

     Toileting

Perceiving—A pattern involving the reception of information

[Alterations in self-concept]

  Patient's description of himself/herself _____

  Effects of illness/surgery on self-concept _____ Body image

_____ Self-esteem

[Sensory/perceptual alterations] Personal identity

  Vision impaired _____ Glasses_____

    Visual examination _____ Visual

  Auditory impaired _____ Hearing aid _____

    Auditory examination _____ Auditory

  Kinesthetics impaired_____ Romberg _____

  Gustatory impaired _____ Kinesthetic

  Tactile impaired_____ Examination _____ Gustatory

  Olfactory impaired_____ Examination _____ Tactile

  Reflexes: Biceps   R ___ L ___   Triceps   R ___ L ___ Olfactory

            Brachio- Reflexes

             radialis R ___ L ___   Knee   R ___ L ___

            Ankle   R ___ L ___   Plantar R ___ L ___

Nursing Diagnosis
(Altered/High Risk for/
Potential for Enhanced)

Choosing—A pattern involving the selection of alternatives
[Alterations in coping]
Patient's usual problem solving methods _____

_____

Family's usual problem solving methods _____

_____

Patient's method of dealing with stress _____

_____

Family's method of dealing with stress _____

_____

Patient's affect _____
Physical manifestations _____
[Alterations in participation]
Compliance with past/current health care regimen _____

_____

Willingness to comply with future health care regimen _____

_____

Ineffective individual
    coping
Ineffective family coping

Noncompliance
Ineffective management of
    therapeutic regimen

Exchanging—A pattern involving mutual giving and receiving
[Alterations in nutrition]
Teeth, gums, lesions _____
Dentures _____
Ideal body weight _____
Height_____Weight _____
Eating patterns
  Number of meals per day _____
  Special diet _____
  Where eaten _____
  Food preferences/intolerances _____
  Food allergies _____
  Caffeine intake (coffee, tea, soft drinks) _____
  Appetite changes _____
  Presence of nausea/vomiting_____
  Current therapy
    NPO _____ NG suction _____
    Tube feeding _____
    TPN _____
Laboratory results
  Na _____ K _____ Cl _____ Glucose _____
  Cholesterol_____ Triglycerides_____ Fasting _____
[Alterations in physical regulation]
  [Immune]
    Lymph nodes enlarged_____ Location _____
    WBC count _____ Differential _____
  Alteration in body temperature
    Temperature_____ Route _____
[Alterations in physical integrity]
  Skin integrity _____ Rashes _____ Lesions _____
    Petechiae_____ Surgical incision _____
    Bruising_____ Abrasions _____

Oral mucous membrane

More than body
    requirements

Less than body
    requirements

Infection
Hypothermia
Hyperthermia
Ineffective
    thermoregulation
Impaired skin integrity
Impaired tissue integrity

[Alterations in circulation]

Cerebral (circle appropriate response)

Pupils	Eye opening
L 2 3 4 5 6 mm	None (1)
R 2 3 4 5 6 mm	To pain (2)
Reaction: Brisk _____	To speech (3)
Sluggish _____	Spontaneous (4)
Nonreactive _____	

Cerebral tissue perfusion

Best verbal	Best motor
Intubated (0)	Flaccid (1)
Mute (1)	Extensor response (2)
Incomprehensible sound (2)	Flexor response (3)
Inappropriate words (3)	Semipurposeful (4)
Confused conversation (4)	Localized to pain (5)
Oriented (5)	Obeys commands (6)

Fluid volume
  Deficit
  Excess

  Glasgow coma scale total

_____

  Neurological changes/symptoms _____

Cardiac output

[Cardiac]

  Apical rate and
    rhythm _____
    PMI _____
  Heart sounds/murmurs _____
  Dysrhythmias _____
  Pacemaker _____

Cardiopulmonary tissue
  perfusion

BP: Sitting   Lying   Standing
    R ____ L ____   R ____ L ____   R ____ L ____

Fluid volume
  Deficit
  Excess

A-Line reading _____
Cardiac index _____ Cardiac output _____
CVP _____ PAP _____ PCWP _____
IV fluids _____
IV cardiac medications _____

_____
_____

Cardiac output

Serum enzymes _____

Peripheral

  Pulses: A = absent   B = bruits   D = Doppler
    + 3 = bounding + 2 = palpable + 1 = faintly palpable

Peripheral tissue perfusion
Peripheral neurovascular
  dysfunction

Carotid R ___ L ___	Popliteal	R ___ L ___
Brachial R ___ L ___	Posterior tibial	R ___ L ___
Radial R ___ L ___	Dorsalis pedis	R ___ L ___
Femoral R ___ L ___		

Fluid volume
  Deficit
  Excess

  Jugular venous distention   R ___ L ___
  Skin temperature _____ Color _____
  Edema _____ Capillary refill _____
  Clubbing _____ Claudication _____

Cardiac output

Gastrointestinal

  Liver: Enlarged _____ Ascites _____

Renal

GI tissue perfusion

  Urine output: 24 hour _____ Average hourly _____
  BUN _____ Creatinine _____ Specific gravity _____
  Urine studies _____

Renal tissue perfusion

Fluid volume
Cardiac output

Nursing Diagnosis
(Altered/High Risk for/
Potential for Enhanced)

[Alterations in oxygenation]
    Rate _____ Rhythm _____ Depth_____

    Labored/unlabored (circle) Chest expansion _____

    Use of accessory muscles _____

    Orthopnea _____

    Breath sounds _____

    Complaints of dyspnea _____ Precipitated by _____

    Cough: Productive/nonproductive _____

Sputum: Color _____ Amount _____ Consistency _____

    LOC _____ Splinting _____

    Arterial blood gases _____

    Oxygen percent and device _____

    Ventilator _____

[Alterations in elimination]
    Bowel

      Abdominal physical examination _____

      Usual bowel habits _____

      Alterations from normal _____

    Urinary

      Bladder distention _____

      Color _____ Catheter _____

      Usual urinary pattern _____

      Alteration from normal _____

Ineffective airway
  clearance
Ineffective breathing
  patterns
Ineffective gas exchange
Inability to sustain
  spontaneous ventilation

Dysfunctional ventilatory
  weaning response

Bowel Patterns
  Constipation
  Diarrhea
  Incontinence
Urinary Patterns
  Incontinence
  Retention

Energy Field Patterns

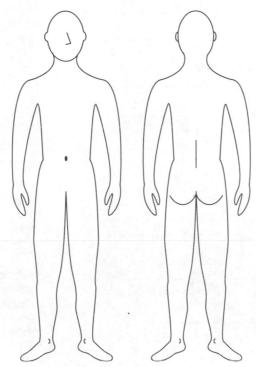

Energy Field Disturbance

ADL = activities of daily living; A-line = arterial line; BP = blood pressure; BUN = blood urea nitrogen; CVP = central venous pressure; GI = gastrointestinal; IV = intravenous; LOC = level of consciousness; NG = nasogastric; NPO = nothing by mouth; PAP = pulmonary artery pressure; PCWP = pulmonary capillary wedge pressure; PMI = point of maximal impulse; TPN = total parenteral nutrition

Appendix 11–B

Holistic Nursing Assessment Tool for Outpatients

Name _____ Date of Birth _____ Sex _____

Address _____ Telephone _____

Significant Other _____ Telephone _____

Date _____ Education _____ Employment _____

Medical Diagnosis _____

Reason for Seeking Holistic Nursing Care _____

_____

Height _____ Weight _____ B/P _____ T _____ P _____ R _____

Nursing Diagnosis
(Altered/High Risk for/
Potential for Enhanced)

Communicating—A pattern involving sending messages

Verbal: _____

Nonverbal: _____

[Communication, altered]
Verbal
Nonverbal

"Valuing/Transcending"—A pattern involving spiritual growth

Meaning and purpose in life: _____

Inner Strengths: _____

Interconnections (self, others, universe, higher power): _____

_____

[Spiritual State]
Spiritual well-being
Spiritual distress
Hopelessness
Powerlessness

Relating—A pattern involving establishing bonds

Role (marital status, children, parents): _____

_____

_____

_____

_____

_____

Role performance, altered
Parenting, altered
Parental role conflict
[Work]
Sexual dysfunction

Occupation: _____

Sexual Relationships: _____

Socialization: _____

_____

_____

_____

Family process, altered
Sexuality patterns, altered
[Socialization, altered]
Social interaction,
    impaired
Social isolation

Note: Holistic Nursing Assessment Tool: Developed by Pamela Potter Hughes and adapted by Barbara M. Dossey and Noreen Frish.
Source: Reprinted with permission from Cathie E. Guzzetta, Shelia D. Bunton, Linda A. Prinkey, Anita P. Sherer, and Patricia C. Seifert, *Clinical Assessment Tools for Use with Nursing Diagnoses,* copyright © 1989, Mosby–Year Book.

Nursing Diagnosis
(Altered/High Risk for/
Potential for Enhanced)

Knowing—A pattern involving the meaning associated with information
Orientation: _____
_____
_____
_____

Memory: _____
_____
_____
_____

Previous Illnesses/Hospitalizations/Surgeries: _____

Identified Health Problems (Present/History): _____

Current Medications (Medication Allergies): _____

Risk Factors (Smoking, Family History, etc.): _____
_____

Perception/Knowledge of Health/Illness: _____

Expectations of Holistic Health Intervention: _____
_____

Readiness to Learn (Ready, Willing, Able): _____
_____

Thought processes,
altered
[Orientation]
[Confusion]
[Memory]

Knowledge deficit
(Specify)

[Learning]

Feeling—A pattern involving the subjective awareness of information
Comfort: _____
_____
_____
_____
_____

Emotional Integrity States: _____
_____
_____
_____
_____
_____
_____
_____
_____
_____
_____

[Comfort, altered]
  Pain, chronic
  Pain, acute
  [Discomfort, chronic]
  [Discomfort, acute]
[Grieving]
  Anticipatory
  Dysfunctional
Anxiety
Fear
[Anger]
[Guilt]
[Shame]
[Sadness]
Post-Trauma Response

Moving—A pattern involving activity
Activity (Physical Mobility Limitations): _____
_____
_____
_____

Rest: _____
_____
_____
_____

[Activity, altered]
  Activity Intolerance
  Impaired physical
    mobility
  Fatigue
  Sleep Pattern
    disturbance
    [Hypersomnia]
    [Insomnia]
    [Nightmares]

Recreation: _____

_____

Environmental Maintenance: _____

_____

_____

_____

Health Maintenance: _____

_____

Self-Care: _____

_____

_____

_____

_____

_____

Perceiving—A pattern involving the reception of information

Sensory Perception: _____

_____

_____

_____

_____

_____

_____

_____

_____

_____

Self-Concept: _____

_____

_____

_____

_____

_____

_____

_____

_____

_____

Choosing—A pattern involving the selection of alternatives

Coping: _____

_____

Judgment/Decisions: _____

_____

Participation: _____

_____

Family Coping: _____

_____

_____

_____

Nursing Diagnosis
(Altered/High Risk for/
Potential for Enhanced)

Diversional activity
    deficit
Impaired home
    maintenance
    management
        [Safety Hazards]
Health maintenance,
    altered
Bathing/hygiene deficit
Dressing/grooming
    deficit
Feeding deficit
Toileting deficit

[Sensory Perception,
    altered]
    Visual
    Auditory
    Kinesthetic
    Gustatory
    Tactile
    Olfactory
    Unilateral Neglect
[Self-Concept, altered]
    Body image
        disturbance
    Personal identity
        disturbance
    Self-Esteem
        disturbance
        —Chronic low
        —Situational

Individual coping,
    ineffective
    Adjustment: impaired
    Conflict: decisional
    Coping: defensive
    Denial: impaired
    Noncompliance

[Family Coping,
    ineffective]
    Compromised
    Disabled

Nursing Diagnosis
(Altered/High Risk for/
Potential for Enhanced)

Exchanging—A pattern involving mutual giving and receiving

Nutrition: _____

_____

_____

_____

_____

_____

[Nutrition, altered]
  [Nutritional deficit]
  < or > Body
  Requirements
Oral mucus membranes,
  impaired

Elimination: _____

_____

_____

_____

_____

_____

[Bowel elimination,
  altered]
  Bowel incontinence
  Constipation: colonic
  Constipation:
    perceived
  Diarrhea
GI tissue perfusion

Renal/Urinary: _____

_____

_____

_____

_____

[Urinary elimination,
  altered]
  Incontinence (specify)
  Retention
  [Enuresis]
Renal tissue perfusion

Physical/Tissue Integrity: _____

_____

_____

_____

_____

_____

_____

_____

_____

[Tissue integrity,
    impaired]
  Impaired skin
    integrity
[Injury: Risk]
  Aspiration
  Disuse syndrome
  Poisoning
  Suffocation
  Trauma

Physical Regulation: _____

Immune: _____

_____

_____

_____

_____

_____

_____

[Physical regulation,
    altered]
  Infection: risk
  Altered protection
  Thermoregulation,
    ineffective
      —Hypothermia
      —Hyperthermia
Cardiac output,
  decreased

Circulation: _____

_____

_____

_____

_____

_____

_____

_____

_____

[Tissue perfusion, altered]
  Cardiopulmonary
  Cerebral
  Peripheral
[Fluid volume, altered]
  Deficit
  Deficit: risk
  Excess

Oxygenation: _____
_____
_____
_____
_____
_____

Hormonal/Metabolic Patterns: _____
_____
_____
_____
_____

Energy Field Patterns

Nursing Diagnosis
(Altered/High Risk for/
Potential for Enhanced)

[Respiration, altered]
   Airway clearance,
      ineffective
   Breathing pattern,
      ineffective
   Gas exchange, impaired
[Menstrual Patterns]
[Premenstrual syndrome]

Energy Field Disturbance

ADDITIONAL COMMENTS:
_____
_____
_____
_____
_____
_____
_____
_____
_____

Goals
1. _____
2. _____
3. _____
4. _____
5. _____

**Prioritized Nursing Diagnosis/Problem
List/Theory-Based Plan of Care**   **Date**

1. _____   _____
2. _____   _____
3. _____   _____
4. _____   _____
5. _____   _____

Signature _____ Date _____

Holistic Nursing Care Plan

Name: _____   Client Goals:
Date: _____   1. _____
                                            2. _____
                                            3. _____
                                            4. _____

Nursing Diagnosis and Related Factors	*Client/Patient Outcomes Outcome Criteria*	*Therapeutic Intervention*	*Evaluation*

Client Signature _____

Date _____

Caring and Healing of Clients and Significant Others

Meaning and Wholeness

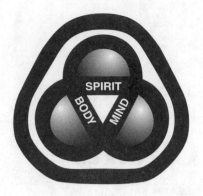

CHAPTER 12

Therapeutic Communication: The Art of Helping

Sharon Scandrett-Hibdon

KNOWLEDGE COMPETENCIES

- Delineate the skills of communication.
- Recognize barriers to communication.
- Describe the stages of effective helping.
- Determine which skills are used to deal with specific situations.
- Identify the influence of contextual, energetic, perceptual, and message-packaging factors on communicating effectively.
- Delineate criteria for effective communication.
- Evaluate effective communication.

DEFINITION

Therapeutic Communication: the purposive focusing of verbal and nonverbal interactions in such a way as to maximize the client's self-discovery, taking into account, and understanding. This builds positive regard or rapport between the communicator and the client in that the client feels heard and encouraged to express accurate states of experience or being. The main goal of therapeutic communication is the client's self-discovery, which places the client in position to make the clearest decisions and most desired changes.[1]

   Pause for a moment . . .

❑ *I can do _____ to improve my study skills just now.*
❑ *The AHNA Core Curriculum for Holistic Nursing is designed to help me learn and refine my knowledge and skills base.*
❑ *I congratulate myself for practicing good study skills.*

THEORIES AND RESEARCH

Basic Concepts for Communication

1. Communication is constant.
2. One cannot not communicate.
3. Communication is both verbal (i.e., content-oriented) and nonverbal (i.e., process-oriented).
4. Communication is nonlinear, multivariate, and simultaneous, and may have specific feedback loops. Communication occurs in many dimensions, including extrasensory realms such as intuitive knowing and energetic vibrations.
5. Communication may not necessarily change; rather, our understanding of it changes.
6. The effectiveness or occurrence of communication is determined by the client's ability to take into account, rather than by the sender's ability to send it.[2]
7. Communications that cut off or diminish what the client shares are considered detractive.
   a. Detractive communication leads to dissatisfaction within the helping relationship.
   b. Components of detractive communication include inaccurate empathy, interruption or cut-off, inattention, interpretation, attenuation of clients' responses, extensive self-disclosure, monopolization of discourse, and parrotting.
8. Accurately shared meanings produce feelings of being heard and understood, greater self-exploration, and maximum information from which the client can make the best decisions.
   a. Effective therapeutic communication can occur in a 5-minute interchange or can be extended to hours.

b. Effective therapeutic communication skills can be learned.

c. Core helping skills build positive regard between the person helping and the person being helped.[3]

d. The helper invests energy into the relationship by actively listening and selecting fresh words in which to convey meanings of what the helper understood.

9. Focused exploration is necessary if one is to see the underlying patterns that keep occurring in one's life. Understanding one's patterns does not guarantee change.

10. Further action through effective problem solving and initiating agreed-upon plans is necessary to promote life changes.

   a. Problem solving must be clearly based on the client's goals and must be broken down into steps manageable for success by the client.

   b. Mutual planning by the helper and the client is essential.

11. Outcomes of interchanges with others often depends upon the affective state the client experiences in the communications. Positive affective outcomes increase the likelihood that the client will continue future interchanges and comply with desired protocols.

12. Counseling is a supportive relationship in which clients are encouraged to see their patterns primarily through verbal means. With this support, a client can make desired changes with a coach, cheerleader, and troubleshooter.

   a. Counseling skills can be used in many situations to build rapport, invest in a relationship, and make changes in behavior. Such skills are used in psychotherapy.

13. Psychotherapy is a deeper therapeutic process in which the client learns much about himself/herself and can then make necessary changes in order to be more effective in one's life. Personality change often occurs. There are many theoretical and clinical approaches to psychotherapy. Like psychoanalysis, psychotherapy can take years, while brief therapy can occur successfully within 6 to 10 sessions. Corrective emotional experiences are especially important in psychotherapy.

14. Both counseling and psychotherapy have similar goals: to assist clients in understanding themselves clearly and to make the changes necessary to live more functionally. Counseling is often more problem oriented, while psychotherapy may focus on shifting the personality.

Therapeutic Communication Process

1. The process of therapeutic communication in a helping relationship occurs in stages. The initial stage is called building relationship. In this stage specific communication skills are used to enhance the helpee's feelings of being heard and understood. This understanding affords the client the opportunity to self explore.

2. Core helping skills are essential to build a positive relationship (Exhibit 12–1).[4,5]

Exhibit 12–1 Process of Therapeutic Communication: Operationalization of Therapeutic Helping Skills

Stage I:	Development of a Positive Relationship (Essential for helping relationship)
Empathy	Conveys meaning of what person is saying. Contains both an emotional and content component. Is foundational for establishing rapport and maintaining relationship.
	Helpful format: "You feel _____ because _____."
Respect	Conveyed with use of accurate empathy. Shows belief that client knows what is needed. Encourages self-determination by client. Highlights resources and strengths.
	Helpful approach: Use accurate empathy. Have client make own decisions. Reinforce client's strengths.
Genuineness	Acts as human being with feelings foremost. Shares parts of self that may impose on the relationship. Responds honestly, demonstrating freedom from role.
	Helpful approach: Be honest. Use self-disclosure when you have a strong feeling such as "We have been here before" (boredom) or "I am afraid" (when client threatening).

continues

Exhibit 12–1 continued

Concreteness	Clarifies any vagueness through use of descriptive questions except "why," which elicits the cause for the event. Uses summarization to clarify. *Helpful approach:* Ask how, what, when, where, under what circumstance.
Stage II:	**Focused Exploration (Essential for pattern recognition and goal identification)**
Additive empathy	Shows client bigger "picture" of one's behavior. Consists of three parts: a) underlying feelings, b) dysfunctional patterns, and c) ways dysfunctional patterns are set up and reinforced. Goal behavior is identified. Must have all parts to maximize information for client. *Helpful format:* "While you say you are feeling _____ (primary empathy), it sounds like you're also feeling _____ (underlying feeling), because _____ (cause of feeling). When faced with _____ (triggering event), you _____ (dysfunctional pattern) and it leaves you _____ (recurring consequence of pattern). You feel _____ (self-judgment) with yourself because you _____ (dysfunctional pattern) and you want _____ (desired response or pattern)." *Example:* While you say you're feeling sad, it sounds also like you're feeling ashamed because you feel responsible for the loss of a friend. When faced with a request to confront Jane's behavior, you are silent and it leaves you feeling dishonest and passive. You are distrustful of yourself because you are not open and honest with your friends and you want to be assertive and truthful with those you care about.
Self-disclosure	Purposeful sharing of poignant experiences and feelings of the helper designed to lead the client into deeper self-exploration. Must be short and take client back to own feelings. *Helpful format:* "When I _____ (event), I felt _____ (deeper feeling). I wonder if that's true for you." *Example:* When I went away to college, I was terrified that I might not make it on my own. I wonder if that fits for you.
Feedback	Mirrors what client is sending. Provides opportunities for client to receive information about own behavior. *Helpful format:* "May I share something with you? When I _____ (see, experience, hear, etc.) _____ (behavior), I feel _____ (specific feeling), I want to _____ (desired action), but instead I am _____ (actual action)." *Example:* When I hear you canceling our plans again, I feel frustrated and rejected. I want to stop inviting you to visit, but instead I'm letting you know.
Confrontation	Highlights discrepancies between what client says, feels, or does. Does not blame the client. *Helpful format:* "On one hand you _____ (feel, say, or do), but I also see you _____ (feel, say, or do)." *Example:* On one hand you say you really like your job, but I also hear you constantly criticizing your boss and co-workers.
Immediacy	Focuses upon what is occurring in the here and now between the helper and helpee. Poses the highest risk to the relationship in that it uncovers covert maneuvers between persons. *Helpful format:* "Right now I sense you want me to _____ (desired action or role)." *Example:* Right now I sense you want me to rescue you, but I will only listen to your plans.
Stage III:	**Problem Solving (Essential for change)**

1. Define the problem and goal: What specifically does the person want to change?

   Helpful approach: I intend to _____ (goal which is measurable) by _____ (time).

2. Brainstorming alternatives: What are some ways the goal could be achieved?

   Helpful approach: Both nurse and client list visually all possible alternatives as quickly as possible, even the most ridiculous. Remember you are breaking up old limitations by this act and it's a lot of fun.

continues

Exhibit 12–1 continued

3. Evaluating alternatives: use cost/gain analysis.

   Helpful approach: Have client list the three alternatives he or she is willing to begin first. Then do an analysis visually on each alternative of what it will cost the client to use this approach and what the gain will be. Have the client select which alternative to begin with in the actual planning, knowing the remaining alternatives are available for later use.

4. Plan for change: Make each step small enough so that the client can succeed.

   Helpful approach: Have the client visualize himself or herself successfully completing the goal and assess if he or she can support 100% having the goal actualize. If not, negotiate what needs to be changed. Have the client decide what can successfully be completed on the goal actualization before the next meeting with you. Ask the client how he or she will sabotage this goal; then plan an approach for client use if this begins to occur.

5. Troubleshoot: Figure out and plan to overcome rough spots in achieving goals.

   Helpful approach: What are the rewards for failing to change? Do goals need to be changed?

3. The second stage, focused exploration, deepens the communication experience so that information that is partially in and out of the client's awareness is brought into consciousness. Often this involves information shared through the helper's skills that focus on patterns and mirror the client's behavior. This stage is often deleted in helping, which leads to inaccurate goals.[6,7]

4. The third stage of the therapeutic communication process involves active problem solving. Use of strategies based on the client's goals ensures the client's success if he or she is willing to take the necessary risks in order to complete the growth-promoting tasks.[8,9]

 Pause for a moment . . .

❑ *I listen to my audio cassette tape with my own voice covering the most challenging core content (or all the core content).*

❑ *I listen to this important content over and over again at my own pace while in the car or while at home.*

Applications

1. Just as communication is necessary in life, it is necessary in all functions of nursing. In some ways, communication is the context as well as the tool for the fulfillment of nursing.

2. Those with any impairment in their ability to communicate—whether through sensory deficit, perceptual screens, or limits in expression—have a much harder time adapting to life.

3. The nursing diagnoses that are most directly considered by this intervention are
   a. Exchanging on all levels.
   b. Perceiving on all levels.
   c. Relating on all levels.
   d. Valuing.
   e. Choosing.
   f. Moving.
   g. Feeling.

Frequently Encountered Communication Problems

Perception

1. A person's ability to take into account, which is regulated by sensory (visual, auditory, kinesthetic, gustatory, and olfactory), intuitive or psychic, and energetic input.
   a. Limitations in any of these input channels alters the amount of information available to the person.
   b. Invisible screening filters out some information from a person's awareness (e.g., from belief systems, previous life experiences including traumas, self-esteem, meaning of the stimuli and unfulfilled needs).

2. Perceptions affect the thoughts and emotions that a person experiences, which, in turn, influence the person's reception of the next information input.

3. Perceptions are different for each person based on individual filters.

4. Assessment includes an examination of verbal and nonverbal abilities to take into account as well as the ability to express.

a. The examination for hearing, visual, kinesthetic, olfactory, or gustatory impairments addresses the possibility of misperception. Attention should be given to any toxicity or sensory altering stimuli.
b. It is also important to note any discrepancies in expression, such as between nonverbal and verbal content.

5. Guidelines for nursing interventions include the following:
   a. Validate with the client through use of accurate primary level empathy or questioning (e.g., "What did you hear me say?").
   b. Clarify any misperceptions.
   c. Encourage the client to check out any misperceptions by saying, "Let me make sure I understand what you said"; then repeat what was said.
   d. Match client's ability to communicate.

Self-Concept

1. All the beliefs that a person holds about one's self, including other's opinions and feelings, based upon past and current experiences, and body image.
   a. Self-esteem is based on the feelings that a person holds around his or her worth, which, in turn, is often based on goals, accomplishments, strengths, and limitations.
   b. Behavior is consistent with self-concept.
   c. Carefully listening to remarks made about oneself and observing the presentation of one's body reveals the self-concept.

2. Guidelines for nursing interventions include the following:
   a. Use good rapport-building skills, such as accurate empathy and clear honest communication.
   b. Do not overinflate feedback; rather, give data-based observations about strengths and resources.
   c. Explore self-depreciating comments and beliefs, challenge unrealistic opinions, reframe where possible, and encourage self-acceptance.
   d. Assist plan for desired changes.

Anxiety and Stressful Behavior

1. Unpleasant feelings experienced by perceived threats to the self may have physiologic symptoms, such as muscular tension, trembling, perspiration, dry mouth, increased heart rate, nausea, fatigue, insomnia or somnolence, repetitive body movements, or restlessness.
   a. A person can have a stress response to either nonthreatening (positive stress [eustress]) or threatening stimuli.
      1) Fear response usually results from a known threat.
      2) In anxiety response, threat may be unrecognized or unknown.
   b. Each stressor or threat is individually determined.
   c. Although people differ in their ability to cope with each threat or stress, most people attempt to find a way to deal with the stress to reduce the discomfort.
   d. Successfully facing the stressors preserves self-concept and enhances self-esteem.
   e. If a person feels inadequate to handle threats or stressors, anxiety may persist or defense mechanisms may be helpful in handling the discomfort.

2. Low levels of stressors can increase adaptation. As stress and anxiety escalate, however, the client needs greater energy to cope with stressors, often producing greater dysfunction.

3. Hypervigilance, hypovigilance, impaired decision making or problem solving, discomfort, feelings of inadequacy, increased tension, and helplessness decompensation are signs of a poor response to stress.

4. If possible, the nurse should ascertain with client the perceived stressors or threat.
   a. The nurse should determine the impact of the stressor.
   b. The nurse should investigate the possibility of distortions in perception and usual coping pattern with stressor.

5. Guidelines for nursing interventions include the following:
   a. Have client describe possible approaches to stressor.
   b. Use brainstorming to widen the client's usual frame of reference for possibilities.
   c. Help the client set a realistic plan of action through problem solving to alter handling of stressors or threats. Include tools to strengthen the client's ability to cope, such as relaxation or imagery.
   d. Reinforce strengths and resources displayed in previous coping.
   e. Highlight areas where the client displays self-control.

Pain

1. As a strong signal for location of a problem, pain can be physiologic in origin; it also has a

heavy psychologic component involving unpleasant perceptions.

   a. Often, the person feels vulnerable or unprotected.

   b. Pain is usually compounded by previous experience.

2. Pain involves the individual's beliefs and values and is unique for each person.

   a. Emotional pain is often triggered when past conflicts or traumas remain unresolved.

   b. Pain may emerge especially when energy or body work is being completed or when change is being resisted.

3. It is essential to determine the intensity, duration, quality, location, history, meaning, dysfunction from pain, and what relieves it.

4. Guidelines for nursing interventions include the following:

   a. Provide support during the exploration and working through of pain; know that pain is real to the client.

   b. Promote immediate comfort through use of medications, energetic, touch, hypnotic, or relaxation procedures.

   c. Focus on the origins and meaning of the pain (e.g., using imagery or active imagination to dialogue with pain).

   d. Determine what is needed to resolve the conflict or issue behind the pain (e.g., necessitating some psychotherapy work on traumas).

     1) Tools such as journaling, art therapy, or letter writing may help the client work on the painful issues.

     2) Referral may be made to other professionals for psychotherapy or emotional release work if needed.

Crisis

1. Crisis (a state of feeling overwhelmed and unsuccessful in coping with the stimuli) is a chaotic state in which the usual structure of responses and coping is weakened or disintegrated. This shifting of structure affords an opportunity to learn new, more adaptive ways to handle one's life.

2. Individuals determine what they feel is a crisis. Life events that require major changes and developmental tasks often produce crisis.

3. Phases of crisis include

   a. shock, in which the person feels overwhelmed,

   b. defensive maintenance of usual coping responses,

   c. recognition that usual responses are ineffective,

   d. adaptation.

4. Individuals can fail to adapt, maintain themselves the same, or develop a new sense of strength and confidence to handle life in new, more adaptive ways.

5. Assessment focuses on signs of emotional upset; nature of crisis, including duration and intensity; functionality of client; coping patterns; and support system.

   a. Short, directive communications may be helpful during the disorganization or shock phase.

   b. It is important to explore the meaning of this crisis with the client.

6. Guidelines for nursing interventions include the following:

   a. Offer the client support and validation.

   b. Help clarify the problem and correct distortions.

   c. Help the client identify effective coping mechanisms and alternative approaches.

   d. With the client, plan successful constructive steps to accomplish needed changes.

Interpersonal Communication

1. Often, problems occur in one's ability to communicate with others (see Chapter 14).

2. Therapeutic communication and basic counseling approaches can address many specific problems.

3. Helping skills like active listening or primary level empathy can greatly facilitate communication for the client.

4. Learning to use second-stage skills can empower the client to give constructive feedback and increase assertive behaviors.

REFERENCES

1. A. Turok, *Interpersonal Skills Laboratory Experience* (Iowa City, IA: University of Iowa, Mental Health Authority, 1979).

2. L. Thayer, *Communication and Communication Systems* (Homewood, IL: Richard D. Irwin, 1968).

3. G. Egan, *The Skilled Helper: A Problem Management to Helping*, 5th ed. (Pacific Grove, CA: Brooks/Cole Publishing Co., 1994).

4. Ibid.

5. R.R. Carkhuff, *The Art of Helping IV*, 4th ed. (Amherst, MA: Amherst Resource Development Press, 1980).

6. G. Egan, *The Skilled Helper*.

7. A. Turok, *Interpersonal Skills Laboratory Experience*.

8. G. Egan, *The Skilled Helper*.

9. A. Turok, *Interpersonal Skills Laboratory Experience*.

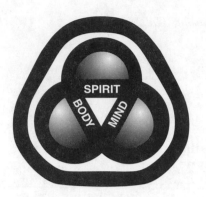

CHAPTER 13

Cultural Diversity and Care

Joan Engebretson

KNOWLEDGE COMPETENCIES

- Discuss components of cultural competence.
- Discuss the principles necessary for building cultural competence.
- Compare common value orientations associated with cultures.
- Analyze components of cultural diversity.
- Describe barriers to cultural competence.
- Discuss cultural influences on beliefs and explanatory systems related to health and illness.
- Discuss the role of culture in the interaction between provider and client/patient.
- Apply theoretical knowledge of cultural diversity to the nursing process.
- Analyze the components of a transcultural assessment.
- Identify appropriate nursing diagnosis in the cultural domain.
- Explore appropriate interventions that reflect cultural competence.
- Discuss an appropriate approach for evaluation of nursing actions in relation to cultural competence.

DEFINITIONS

Cultural Competence for Nurses: the ability to deliver health care with knowledge of and sensitivity to cultural factors that influence the health/illness behavior of an individual client/patient or family.

Culture: "the complex whole including knowledge, beliefs, art, morals, laws, customs and any other capabilities and habits acquired by one as a member of society."[1(p10)] Culture is learned through language and socialization and is shared by members of the same cultural group. All cultures are inherently dynamic and changing, and are adapting to the environment, historical context, technology, and availability of resources.

 Pause for a moment . . .

❏ *My good study skills enable me to organize, acquire, remember, and use the information I need to pass the holistic nursing certification (HNC) examination.*
❏ *I will accomplish this important endeavor.*

THEORIES AND RESEARCH

Five Components of Cultural Competence[2]

1. Awareness and acceptance of cultural differences require an open-minded attitude about other world views.
2. An awareness of one's own biases and attitudes that create barriers to direct interaction with a group or groups makes it possible to overcome them.
3. It is essential to understand dynamic differences and to recognize basic differences among cultures without promoting the superiority of one culture over another.
4. Basic knowledge about a client/patient's culture permits the development and sharing of

knowledge and skills in a straightforward manner. Knowledge may be gained through literature, observation, participation, interaction, and communication with people from diverse cultures.

5. Adaptation skills include being receptive to different cultures, actively seeking advice and consultation from individuals of that culture, and incorporating those ideas into one's practice. Skills also include the ability to articulate an issue from another's perspective, recognizing and reducing resistance and defensiveness, and the ability to admit errors and perceive that making errors may be better than playing it safe.[3]

Considerations in Developing Cultural Competence[4]

1. The process of sharing information in a straightforward manner demystifies other cultures and makes it possible both to find common ground and to understand the context of differences.

2. Consensus has not been reached on terminology. Many individuals consider some ethnic/racial terms inappropriate and possibly offensive. Individuals working together in provider–client/patient interaction, as well as collaborators and scholars, need to ascertain that terminology is mutually understood and acceptable.

3. The heterogeneity of ethnic groups is often underestimated. The variations within an ethnic group may be as great or greater than those among ethnic groups. For example, the Hispanic culture includes persons of Puerto Rican, Cuban, Spanish, and South and Central American origins. This grouping includes those from many different socioeconomic backgrounds and represents the Caucasian, Mongoloid, and Negroid racial groups.

4. In a culturally pluralistic society such as the United States, it is important to understand the historical context of the immigration of groups and individuals. Many African-Americans arrived involuntarily and endured a lengthy history of slavery; Hispanics may be immigrants seeking economic opportunity (voluntary), refugees from political upheavals, or descendants of people living in the Southwest before it became part of the United States.

5. Immigration status affects cultural practices and has health implications. For example, many Asian immigrants find it necessary to take a job with lower status than they had in their country of origin. This creates cultural and economic hardship for the family. Health issues may also arise due to low income and lowered self-esteem.

6. Acculturation is the process of the adaptation, assimilation, or accommodation of an individual immigrant or immigrant group to a new culture. The theory of orthogonal cultural identification proposes that this process is not along a single continuum but has numerous dimensions that operate independently from each other.
   a. Intergenerational gaps with the traditional culture may occur as youth become more quickly acculturated to the dominant society, threatening the more traditional values, beliefs, and customs of their parents.
   b. This difference has implications for the integrity and lines of respect in the family, and roles within the family (e.g., the role of women).
   c. Conflicts can lead to the alienation of young people from both the ethnic culture and the general dominant culture.

7. It is necessary to distinguish between cultural identification and socioeconomic status. For example, the experience of being poor in our society is different from that of being Hispanic and must be further distinguished from being both poor and Hispanic.

8. Culture has a variety of medical implications.
   a. Strictly biologic differences between groups of people may lead to disease. For example, genetic predisposition for sickle cell disease affects people of African and Mediterranean descent; predisposition for Tay-Sachs disease affects Askenazi Jews.
   b. The higher prevalence of certain diseases among some groups may be attributed to a *combination* of genetic predisposition and lifestyle, including nutrition patterns (e.g., diabetes in Native Americans and Hispanics).
   c. Certain social behaviors connected to health risks, such as substance abuse, may have a cultural component. There is also an association between the prevalence of specific types of substances used and various ethnic groups.

9. People of biracial heritage have unique concerns in the recognition of their bicultural heritage.

Value Orientations and Beliefs Associated with Culture

Cultural Values

1. All cultures hold certain values in high regard and worthy of emulation. These values can be either implicit or explicit.
2. Values influence an individual's perception of others; direct individuals' responses to each other; reflect a person's identity and are the basis for self-reflection; serve as the foundation for positions on personal, professional, social, political, and philosophic issues; motivate behavior and direct goals; and give meaning to life.[5]
3. Variants of value orientations reflect cultural solutions to universal problems of human nature.
   a. Innate human nature. Cultures' dominant views of human nature range from seeing human beings as basically *evil* or perfectable only with discipline and effort to seeing human beings as *good* and being unalterable or incorruptible. A third category sees human nature as *mixed*, a combination of good and evil, but with the capacity for self-control.
   b. Relationship to nature.
      1) Various cultures are *fatalistic*, seeing human beings as subjugated to nature in their destiny.
      2) *Mastery* over nature is the perspective that natural forces are to be overcome and put to humanity's use.
      3) Another variant views human beings and nature existing together in *harmony*.
   c. Relationship to time. Some cultures focus on the past, emphasizing tradition and ancestors, while others focus on the present. Future-oriented cultures focus on progress and change.
      1) In the United States, most middle-class citizens tend to be *future-oriented* with a very structured time schedule. They often delay gratification to pursue education or career, and they set high future goals. They plan their actions to save time, as time is money. They value punctuality and efficiency. Future-oriented people may alter their lifestyle to ensure better health in the future. Emphasis is on youth and new ideas.
      2) *Present-oriented* people live in the moment. They may often be late for appointments, as they are involved in the activity of the moment rather than thinking about future events.
      3) *Past-oriented* people have great respect for the wisdom of the past and reverence for ancestors and elders. They value tradition and are suspicious of change.
   d. Purpose of being.
      1) In cultures oriented toward *being*, impulses and desires are expressed spontaneously and the focus is not on development.
      2) *Being-in-becoming* cultures are oriented to self-development and self-realization wherein the self is contained and controlled within, and this detachment from the outer world brings enlightenment.
      3) In *doing* cultures, people actively strive to meet goals, and their accomplishments are evaluated competitively against externally applied standards of achievement.
   e. Relationship to other persons.
      1) Expressed in heredity, kinship ties, and orderly succession, *lineal* relationships have continuity through time.
      2) The welfare of society, group goals, and family orientation are the hallmarks of the *collateral* value.
      3) *Individual* orientations, where personal autonomy and independence are primary, subject group goals to individual goals.
4. Values in the United States are generally perceived as having a strong moral orientation and an emphasis on active instrumental mastery over the world according to external standards.
   a. Individual and peer relationships rather than hierarchical relationships are stressed.
   b. The focus is on progress and change with a rationalistic rather than traditional approach.
   c. Orderliness and attention to structure and form are also important.[6]

Cultural Beliefs

1. Beliefs are tenets with a shared meaning in a group. Held by the group to be true, beliefs are a set of metaphorical explanations used to explain the phenomena of nature. They form a world view, or a paradigm.
2. Beliefs and values derived from the basic world view determine the explanatory models of health and healing. Three major cultural paradigms operate: magicoreligious, holistic, and sci-

entific. Although aspects of all three are found in most cultures, one usually predominates.[7]

a. Magicoreligious health paradigm. The fate of the world depends on God, gods, or supernatural forces. Events possibly responsible for illness include sorcery, breach of taboo, intrusion of a disease object, intrusion of a disease-causing spirit, or loss of soul. These systems relate to a psychic or metaphysical need of humanity for integration and harmony.

b. Holistic health paradigm. The forces of nature must be kept in harmony according to natural laws and the larger universe. The Chinese concept of balance through the forces of yin and yang is a good metaphor for health. In Western culture, the humoral theories are exemplified by the concepts of balancing hot and cold held by Hispanic, Arab, African, and Caribbean societies.

c. Scientific or biomedical paradigm. The scientific paradigm is characterized by

  1) Determinism. A cause-and-effect relationship exists for all natural phenomena.

  2) Mechanism. The relationship of life to structure and function of machines suggests the possibility of control through mechanical or engineered interventions.

  3) Reductionism. The division of all life into isolated smaller parts, such as the dualism of mind and body, as a method to better study the whole.

  4) Objective materialism. That which is real can be observed and measured.

3. Religious systems are the institutionalization of a belief set. They are the source of many of the assumptions that people have about creation, reality, behavior, and rituals.

a. The Western belief in monotheism and the separateness of the Creator contrasts with the Eastern views of essential unity, or the belief in the divine in all.

b. Many indigenous or agricultural traditions have a belief in pantheism, believing that several aspects of the divine are found in objects, places, and other living things.[8]

Communication Patterns

1. In literate Western society, technology determines not only the medium by which knowledge and information are communicated, but also the information and epistemology.

2. Many forms of communication may co-exist in a culture.

a. Traditionally, knowledge was passed on by oral means in stories, parables, and poetry. Essential knowledge (e.g., pieces of cultural wisdom) was distilled through a process of discourse and discussion over time. The tone, rhythm, rhetoric, and sound of the words were important.

b. Written culture allows for "frozen speech" that can be referred to across time and space.

  1) The written word can be scrutinized for accuracy and precision in a way that oral speech cannot.

  2) It facilitates lengthy discussions of logic and rational argument, as the reader can reread complex thoughts and arguments.

  3) This medium is the heart of academe and rational discourse. The demand for precision and verification is congruent with the development of scientific methods and quantification in modern scholarship.

c. Today, there is an electronic culture, dependent upon telephones, radio, television, and computers to communicate.[9] This medium is focused on image. Lengthy scholarly discourses have been replaced by short messages meant to capture the attention of the viewer and convey a message in a short period of time, but with no context and, as a result, often little relevance or coherence for the viewer.

3. Individuals from many cultures show overt respect to people representing authority and prestige. In their interaction with medical practitioners, for example, Asians, Hispanics, Native Americans, and African-Americans often demonstrate modesty, deference, and respect that is sometimes misinterpreted as shyness, inexpressiveness, or even sullenness, hostility, and noncommunicativeness.

4. Members of other cultures are often high-context communicators in that they rely less on the verbal content of the message than on the accompanying verbal style and nonverbal cues.[10]

Cultural Diversity

1. Cultural grouping can be attributed to multiple factors that determine values, beliefs, and behaviors.

a. Ethnicity. Values, perceptions, feelings, assumptions, and physical characteristics are associated with ethnicity, the most common cultural demarcation. Frequently, ethnicity refers to nationality, a group sharing a common social and cultural heritage. In contrast, race is typically a reference to a biologic, genetically transmitted set of distinguishable physical characteristics. Race is a loose and largely misused term.

b. Religion. All religions have experiential, ritualistic, ideologic, intellectual, and consequential dimensions. Religion refers to an organized system of beliefs and should be differentiated from spirituality, which is born out of each person's unique life experience and efforts to find meaning and purpose in life.[11]

c. Socioeconomic status/education. One's standing in society may be determined by social status, occupation, education or economic status, or a combination of these. Socioeconomic status has been shown to be highly associated with measures of health of groups.

d. Social or professional orientation. Often, professional orientations constitute a type of subculture. For example, the biomedical orientation of many hospitals constitutes an unfamiliar, alien culture for many lay people.

e. Region. Local or regional manifestations of the larger culture may vary.

f. Age. Because value systems are tied to historical events that were shared in childhood, each generation develops a unique value system. Persons born in the United States prior to the 1940s generally maintain "traditional values," for example, while those born in the 1940s and 1950s often consciously try to reject those values.

g. Common belief/idealogy. Perspectives and practices can unite a group and differentiate that group from the larger culture. These value systems may be related to religion (e.g., the Amish), lifestyle (e.g., communal groups), sexual orientation (e.g., gay and lesbian groups), or political ideologies (e.g., feminist separatist groups).

2. It is important to be aware of common myths and errors about cultural diversity in the development of cultural capacity.

a. Stereotyping. Those who define the world by strict categories of race or ethnicity may presume that all members of another culture conform to a common pattern without regard to individual characteristics or the variety within one categorization.

b. Ethnocentrism. Some people have an unconscious tendency to look at others through the lens of their own cultural norms and customs and take for granted that their own values are the only objective reality. This is a restrictive view of the world in which differences are often seen as inferior.

c. Cultural imposition. The view that successful adaptation means a change to the cultural views of the dominant group, regardless of one's personal beliefs, assumes that the dominant culture is inherently superior.

d. Xenophobia and cultural conflict. An inherent fear of cultural differences often leads people to bolster their security in their own values by ridiculing the beliefs and traditions of others.

e. Cultural blindness. Often disguised as treating everyone equally. Proceeding as if there are no cultural differences ignores real diversity and the importance of other perspectives.

f. Melting pot. The view that in the process of acculturation and assimilation, everyone takes on significant aspects of the dominant culture is being challenged by concepts of heritage consistency, which is the degree to which one maintains practices and beliefs that reflect one's own heritage.[12]

Impact of Culture on Health Care

1. Health care systems of all cultures have certain sectors in common.

a. In the United States, the orthodox or professional, biomedical sector of health care has held a legal/political monopoly for most of this century. Nurses are part of this sector.

b. The popular sector includes all the personal and social networks that lay people use to organize their health. Individuals, family, and social networks determine whom to consult and when, what treatments to follow, when to switch, and how to determine efficacy and satisfaction with treatment.

c. All secular and sacred healers that are generally outside the professional sector make up the folk sector. This also includes healing devices and practices to promote health and treat illness.

2. Concepts of health and healing are rooted in culture and influence health behaviors.

   a. The definitions of health, healing, illness, and disease are culturally determined; they include the interpretation of symptoms and treatment possibilities.

   b. Some cultural determinants influence an individual's behavior to promote, maintain, and restore his or her health or to cope with illness or dying.

   c. Explanatory models are interpretations of the culture's world view as it pertains to health and healing. They provide an understanding of disease and direct treatment.

3. Interactions between the provider and client/patient are based on the communication between the two and reflect their respective cultures (Figure 13–1). This interaction affects the transfer of information, decision making, adherence to treatment, and the healing outcomes.

   a. Personal beliefs, values, and ethnic background influence the perspective from which providers view the world and subsequent interventions and behaviors.

      1) All health care providers of the professional sector have acculturated to the biomedical model and accompanying science technology and teaching by virtue of their education and the sociology of the health care institutions.

      2) Healers often approach health from a holistic perspective and attend to the psychologic and spiritual domains, as well as to the physical domain.

   b. Beliefs, values, and explanatory models reflect the personal cultural background of the client/patient.

      1) Cultural rituals and practices related to health may have both pragmatic and symbolic meaning.

      2) Barriers to health care can be physical (access to care), ideologic (explanatory models), or related to communication (language, both verbal and nonverbal).

   c. Communication between the provider and client/patient generally involves individuals of nonequal positions, often is nonvoluntary, concerns vitally important issues, and is emotionally laden.

      1) The purposes of communication are to create an interpersonal relationship, exchange information, and allow for decision making.

      2) Communication behavior may be instrumental (i.e., task-focused, cure-oriented, and often intended to give the client/patient information) or affective (i.e., socioemotional, care-oriented, and nonverbal, such as voice tone, eye contact, and body positioning).

   d. Roles in the relationship can be seen as a spectrum of control ranging from paternalist to mutualist.

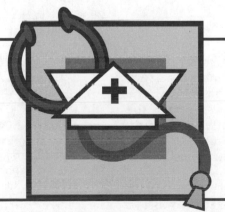

Patient/Client Cultural Background	Provider Cultural Background
Individual personality	Biomedical and cultural explanatory models
Experience and situation	Institutional culture
Explanatory models	Medical language
Everyday language	

Figure 13–1 An understanding of the cultural world of the patient/client and the cultural world of the health care system enables the nurse to facilitate communication and deliver culturally appropriate care. In developing cultural competence, the nurse must also be aware of his or her own cultural beliefs and values.

1) In a paternalistic (provider-centered) relationship, the provider has the control, directs care, makes decisions about treatment, and is authoritative.

2) A mutual (client/patient–centered) relationship involves shared decision making and is egalitarian.

Nursing Implications

1. Nurses need to approach cultural competency through knowledge of self and knowledge of other cultures.
2. In order to develop the ability to interact with clients/patients appropriately, nurses also need to
   a. Clarify their personal values.
   b. Recognize the health care system as a culture.
   c. Learn about the specific culture of each client.
   d. Interact and intervene in a culturally consistent manner.
   e. Elicit feedback from the client/patient.

Pause for a moment . . .

❑ *I study to learn, not to memorize.*
❑ *I frequently ask myself:*
   — *How can I apply this information in my clinical practice, education, or specific practice environment?*
   — *How can I apply this information to more deeply understand myself as an instrument of healing?*

HOLISTIC NURSING PROCESS

Assessment

1. The integration of knowledge about cultural diversity into nursing care requires an assessment of several parameters (Exhibit 13–1).
2. Because cultural traditions are passed on by the community through the family, frequently through the women, it is helpful to ask what practices or beliefs the client's mother or grandmother had.
3. During the assessment, it is essential to obtain specific details for interventions such as diet or healing modalities to develop a culturally acceptable plan.
4. Six cultural phenomena that are evidenced in all cultural groups have variations relevant to providing culturally competent nursing assessment and care.[13] These six areas have been

identified as important components of a transcultural assessment whereby an individual or a group can be systematically assessed. An example of the variation among four ethnic groups according to these six categories is provided in Table 13–1.

a. Communication. There are cultural variations in expression of feelings, use of touch, body contact, gestures, and verbal and nonverbal communication.

1) Verbal communication. Language shapes experiences and influences perceptions and actions. Areas for assessment include names and the process of naming children; speech pattern structure that links a person with a region, social class, or particular group (jargon); voice quality and intonation; and use of silence.

2) Nonverbal communication. The meanings of touch, facial expression, eye movement or eye contact, and body posture vary among cultural groups.

3) Combined verbal and nonverbal elements. Warmth and humor are interpreted differently through various cultures.

b. Personal space. Spatial behavior refers to the comfort level related to personal space, the area that surrounds a person's body. Spatial behavior/territoriality is the need to have and to control personal space.

1) Proximity to others. Western culture has three zones that differ from those in other cultures: intimate zone (<18 inches), per-

---

Exhibit 13–1 Cultural Areas Critical to a Nursing Assessment

- Nutritional patterns
- Exercise and physical activities
- Decision making: how made, who is involved, and why
- Health and healing practices
- Family organization, structure, and role differentiation and child care practices
- Social support networks and relationships
- Spiritual beliefs, rituals, and practices
- Cognitive attributive style and personal/family coping approaches
- Demographics and socioeconomic status, employment patterns
- Immigration and cultural history
- Communication style and relationship toward authority

Table 13–1 Cultural Variation in Human-Environmental Responses (Four Examples)

Response Variants	Asian American (Hmong)	Native American	Black American	Hispanic
Communication	Oral tradition. Gender- and age-specific patterns. Group learning. Spiritual link. Taboos guiding topics. Conversation focus to promote harmony. Language barrier—interpreter.	Oral tradition. Storytelling. Group learning. Spiritual foundation of life. Only able to speak for self, nonaggressive. Role of elder.	Black English. Specific dialect. Significance of names/terms. Nonverbal: talk-look at, listening-look away, prolonged eye contact, frequent touch, emotional sharing. Group learning.	Language barrier—interpreter. Verbal: privacy, avoid conflict, emotionally expressive. Nonverbal: touch, handshake, avoid prolonged eye contact. Group learning.
Space	Avoid eye contact. Sacred parts of body. Avoid public display of affection and extreme emotions.	Avoid eye contact, limit touch. Negative significance rt handshake.	Often space much closer than "Anglos."	Familial closeness—demonstrative.
Time	Cyclical, present-oriented, holistic, fatalistic. Social time vs clock time.	Circular, holistic, present-oriented, fatalistic.	Wide variation. Social time vs clock time.	Present-oriented, "Latin Time," Polychronic.
Social Organization	Clan structure. Decision-maker: elder male, clan leader. Family—patrilineal. Male dominant in affairs extending beyond the home. Female more active role within the home. Clearly defined roles/responsibilities—age and gender. Children indulged until the age of five then more strict discipline—"communal focus."	Clan/family/tribes. Role of elder. Role definition. Social relations—wheel of life. Core values: thanks, harmony, sharing, and hospitality.	Disruptive influence of slavery and discrimination on the family structure. Today variance, a link with social economic status (SES). Lower SES: matrifocused—present focused. Mid/Upper SES: egalitarian. Children—socialized to be in control, independent at earlier age. Importance of extended kinship.	"Lafamilia": patrilineal, extended, gender significance. Machismo: decision maker, protector. Marianismo: nurturer, mediator. Respect elders. Children a priority, dependency. Family value: respect, pride, responsibility, spirituality (Catholic).
Environmental Control	Explanatory Model of Health/Illness (H/I): H: Mandate for life, predetermination, maintain harmony. I: Supernatural, soul loss, spiritual, disharmony, imbalance, sins of ancestors, self in relation to others. Curers: Herbalist, Shaman. Tx: foods, maintain harmony with the forces, spiritual divination, massage, herbs, foods, coining, pinching, cupping. Special Tx for certain conditions, e.g., childbirth.	Explanatory Model of Health/Illness (H/I): H: Beliefs—balance with mother nature, predetermination—Creator. I: lack of harmony, failure to live according to code of life, evil spirits, fear and jealousy of other nations. Curers: Shaman/faithkeeper, Midwiwln, False Face Society, Herb specialist. Tx: herbs, ceremonies, e.g., sweat and medicine lodge, vision quest, talking circle, etc. Significant elements.	Explanatory Model of Health/Illness (H/I): I: an inability to function due to a hex, sins, disharmony, natural or supernatural. Curers: family first, "Old lady" or "Granny," voodoo priest, spiritualist, root doctor. Tx: includes use of teas, cod liver oils, dietary choices, laxatives for purging, wearing of garlic, amulets, copper or silver bracelets. Folk practices include: silver dollar to navel, oil—baby's bath, cradle cap, prayer cloth to diaper, PICA.	Explanatory Model of Health/Illness (H/I): I: Severity rt pain or blood, unable to perform roles/ADLs. Illness: mild or severe, lg of time. Causes: sins, will of God, "evil eye," "nerves," "bad blood"—loss of respect, imbalance of humors or hot and cold. Direct re between certain illnesses—supernatural intervention. Many folk illnesses. Curers: family, curandero herbalist, spiritualist. Tx: prayer, massage, ceremonies rt specific illnesses.

continues

Table 13–1 Continued

Response Variants	Asian American (Hmong)	Native American	Black American	Hispanic
Biological	Small stature, small bone structure, Mongolian spots, eye. Disease susceptibility: Hepatitis, TB, lactase deficiency, hemoglobinopathies, altered drug metabolism.	Taller, bigger, heavier bone structure. Cheek bones, dark eyes. Disease susceptibility: Diabetes mellitus, ETOH abuse, TB, SIDS, AIDS. Health Risks: Pneumonia, malnutrition, adolescent suicide, MVA, homicide.	Skin variance: Mongolian spots, keloids, vitiligo, nigra. Heavier/denser bones, shorter trunk, longer legs. Body fat link to economics. Disease susceptibility: TB, Hypertension/CV, sickle cell anemia, enzyme disorders, diabetes. Health Risks: Obesity, ETOH abuse, infant mortality, homicide, AIDS.	Skin color. Susceptibility to disease: Diabetes, TB, AIDS. Health risks: Obesity, alcoholism, adolescent pregnancy.

Source: Used with permission from Kathleen McGlynn Shadick, RN, MSN, "A Practice Model for Promoting Cultural Diversity," American Nephrology Nurses Association Annual Conference, Dallas, Texas, 1994.

sonal zone (18 inches to 3 feet) and social zone (3 feet to 6 feet).[14] In many cultures, people are more comfortable with closer proximity.

  2) Objects in the environment. Cultural background often influences orderliness, cleanliness, color and appearance of the environment, and the structural boundaries of architecture and furniture.

c. Time. Cultures vary in their orientation to time.

  1) Social time vs. clock time. Social time refers to patterns and orientations related to the ordering of social life, while clock time represents an objective, ordered approach of viewing time in a linear fashion that infers causality. Cyclic approaches attach time to natural events that repeat (i.e., seasons or migration patterns). In mystical thought, magic or ritual may negate the temporal order of causality and reverse a bad event.

  2) Temporal orientations. All cultures combine the three orientations of future, present, and past, with one being dominant.

d. Social organization. Significant social structures include the family, religious organizations, and kinship and special interest groups.

  1) Families vary by structure, dynamics, roles, and organizational patterns. Kinship structures and relative geographic location of family members may have cultural implications.

  2) Religious organizations provide not only social connections, but also a context in which to understand one's relationship to the world and the cosmos.

e. Environmental control. Those in different cultures have different views of the ability of an individual or person to plan activities that control nature, the environment, and relationships.

  1) The locus of control may be perceived as external (i.e., an event contingent on luck or fate), internal (i.e., the event is contingent on one's own behavior or characteristics), or outside (i.e., the event is in harmony with nature, as in some Asian cultures).

  2) Natural events have to do with the world as God intended according to laws of nature. Illness is related to environmental hazards such as cold, impurities, etc. Health is being in harmony in the interconnectedness of nature.

  3) Unnatural events upset the harmony of nature and are outside of world of nature. Illness is related to divine punishment for wrongdoing or witchcraft.[15]

f. Biologic variations. In a pluralistic culture, it is important to determine those factors that are strictly biologic (genetic), ethnic adaptations related to a particular environment (e.g., availability of certain types of food) or related to other social conditions (e.g., socioeconomic status or lifestyle). Among the factors to be considered are the following:

1) Body size and structure, including variation in teeth and facial structure.
2) Skin color and variations, such as formation of keloids.
3) Enzymatic and genetic variations, including group tendencies for variations in metabolism and enzyme production that result in drug reactions, interactions, and sensitivities.
4) Susceptibility to disease (e.g., hypertension, diabetes, sickle cell anemia).
5) Nutritional issues, including food preferences, habits and patterns, and lactose intolerance and other nutritional issues.

Nursing Diagnoses

1. Nursing diagnoses that focus on the cultural domain, primarily on biophysical and psychologic disturbances, alteration, impairments, and distresses, are derived from the conceptual ideas of normalcy based in North American culture and are heavily influenced by biomedicine.
2. The following diagnoses are related to the common human response patterns associated with communication:
   a. Communicating: Altered or impaired communication related to language differences or communication style.
   b. Relating: Altered or impaired social interaction related to sociocultural dissonance.
   c. Valuing: Altered adherence to traditional beliefs.
   d. Choosing: Noncompliance related to noncoherent value systems between provider and client/patient.
   e. Feeling: Anxiety related to culturally unusual expectations for behavior and treatment; fear related to unknown environment or customs.

Client Outcomes

1. The desired outcomes are established prior to the implementation of the plan and interventions.
2. The client will actively participate in care as appropriate.

Plan and Interventions

1. Incorporate into the plan of care knowledge and acceptance of the client's right to alternative solutions and modalities so that the plan is mutually designed.
2. Discuss the explanatory models and meaning of illness.
3. Present and negotiate interventions in a manner that makes them culturally acceptable.
4. Focus on the concept of *engagement,* not compliance, in recommended health behaviors,[16] because the concept of compliance implies an authoritative relationship in which the provider is active and in control while the client/patient is in a passive, accepting role.
5. Incorporate cultural healing practices into the client's care if they are not contraindicated.
   a. It is essential to convey respect for the practices; to acquire appropriate foods, people, and artifacts; and to secure the necessary space and time to practice.
   b. Three modes of intervention involve clinical decision making and nursing actions that incorporate the client's cultural practices.[17,18]
      1) Cultural preservation and/or maintenance refers to professional actions that retain relevant care values in health promotion, restoration, or management of handicaps and/or death.
      2) Cultural accommodation and/or negotiation refers to professional actions to bridge the gap between the client's culture and biomedicine for beneficial health outcomes.
      3) Cultural repatterning and/or restructuring refers to professional actions that help a client improve his or her life pattern while respecting cultural values and beliefs.
   c. Incorporate a variety of healing modalities.
      1) Touch as communication has culturally specific meaning. In some Arab and Hispanic cultures, male providers may be prohibited from examining or touching parts of the female body. Some Asians believe strength lies in the head, and touching the head is a sign of disrespect or threat. Gentle touch is often seen as a caring gesture.
      2) Many cultures have traditions of healing touch or laying-on-of-hands. Touch can be instrumental, but healing touch should be viewed from an energetic or spiritual framework. Clients in Western biomedical cultures are usually unfamiliar with these techniques for healing, so it is very important to give an explanation and receive permission prior to use.

3) Herbs or foods may be used for many different purposes:
   a) To balance the body. The use of hot/cold foods or other preparations may remedy an imbalance.
   b) To purify the body. Many preparations, such as emetics, purgatives, and colonic irrigations, are commonly used for cleansing toxins from the body. Other oils or preparations are applied for the purification.
   c) To treat specific maladies. Many herbs used in traditional healing have antiseptic and other therapeutic functions.
   d) To protect health. For example, many ethnic groups eat raw garlic to prevent illness.
   e) To enhance and facilitate body processes. Chamomile and mint teas are used to aid digestion, and barley water is used to promote lactation.
4) Many cultures approach healing from a spiritual perspective:
   a) Rituals and practices to protect one from evil, disease, or danger. These may include the use of amulets, talismans, ritualistic behavior, and the avoidance of taboos.
   b) Purification or cleansing rituals.
   c) Rituals for life transitions, birth, initiations to adulthood, marriage, death, entrance into a social group.
   d) Rituals and practices related to spiritual growth, redemption, and initiation into higher spiritual levels.
   e) Healing rituals. Often viewed as having a divine gift, healers are able to negotiate with the spirit world through prayer, meditation, blessings, chants, and other primal religious experiences, many incorporating altered states of consciousness. Healing rituals include exorcizing bad spirits and protecting others from evil forces. Individuals may also seek healing by sacrifice, penance, and pilgrimages.

6. Since many nursing interventions involve teaching, use the acronym LEARN—listen, explain, acknowledge, recommend, and negotiate—when caring for culturally diverse client/patient populations.[19]

7. Discuss referrals with the client/patient to establish their acceptability. Follow up to determine if referral sources have been a good match culturally.

Evaluation

1. All evaluation should be a collaborative effort between the nurse, the client/patient, and any member of the extended family or social group whom the client feels is significant.
2. Each component of the health care plan and each nursing intervention should be carefully examined to ensure that it is understandable and acceptable to the client, effective, and appropriately revised, when necessary.
3. Cultural modifications can be made based on a careful evaluation.

REFERENCES

1. M.M. Andrews and J.S. Boyle, *Transcultural Concepts in Nursing Care* (Philadelphia: J.B. Lippincott Co., 1995).
2. P.D. Barry, *Psychosocial Nursing: Care of Physically Ill Patients and Their Families* (Philadelphia: J.B. Lippincott Co., 1996).
3. K.H. Kavanaugh and P.H. Kennedy, *Promoting Cultural Diversity: Strategies for Health Care Professionals* (Newbury Park, CA: Sage Publications, 1992).
4. M.A. Orlandi, ed., *Cultural Competence for Evaluators* (Rockville, MD: U.S. Department of Health and Human Services, 1992).
5. Andrews and Boyle, *Transcultural Concepts in Nursing Care*.
6. Ibid.
7. Ibid.
8. J. Engebretson, "Considerations in Diagnosing in the Spiritual Domain," in *Nursing Diagnosis* 7: 100–107.
9. N. Postman, *Technopoly* (New York: Vintage Books, 1993).
10. D. Sue and D.W. Sue, *Counseling the Culturally Different: Theory and Practice*, 2nd ed. (New York: John Wiley & Sons, 1990).
11. Andrews and Boyle, *Transcultural Concepts in Nursing Care*.
12. R.E. Spector, *Cultural Diversity in Health and Illness* (Norwalk, CT: Appleton & Lange, 1996).
13. J.N. Giger and R.E. Davidhizar, *Transcultural Nursing: Assessment and Intervention* (St. Louis: Mosby–Year Book, 1991).
14. Ibid.
15. Ibid.
16. B.M. Dossey et al., *Holistic Nursing: A Handbook for Practice*, 2nd ed. (Gaithersburg, MD: Aspen Publishers, 1995).
17. Andrews and Boyle, *Transcultural Concepts in Nursing Care*.
18. Kavanaugh and Kennedy, *Promoting Cultural Diversity*.
19. E. Arnold and K.U. Boggs, *Interpersonal Relationships: Professional Communication Skills for Nurses*, 2nd ed. (Philadelphia: W.B. Saunders Co., 1995).

CHAPTER 14

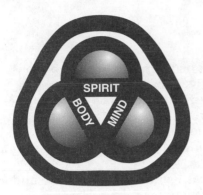

Relationships

Dorothea Hover-Kramer

KNOWLEDGE COMPETENCIES

- Name three areas in which nurses must develop effective relationships.
- List eight characteristics of effective communication that builds relationships.
- Name one way that Jung expanded our understanding of the human psyche.
- Name two contributions of Maslow to holistic thinking.
- Describe Berne's concept of the three major ego states.
- Distinguish a complementary transaction from a distorted, crossed, or game-like interaction.
- Name the ego state that is most often triggered in nurses when they are interacting with persons seen to be in authority.
- Name the four archetypes of human relatedness that address physical, emotional, mental, and spiritual domains.
- Explain how nurses can enhance effectiveness in relationships by activating the four relationship archetypes.
- Name two ways that nurses can move out of the Adaptive Child ego state for conflict resolution.
- Give two elements of effective negotiating.
- Describe the importance of reframing in conflict resolution.

 Pause for a moment . . .

- ❑ *My study skills are working.*
- ❑ *I may need to study in a study group.*

- ❑ *My goal of holistic nursing certification (HNC) is a wonderful endeavor.*
- ❑ *I hold the vision of myself as a certified holistic nurse.*

THEORIES AND RESEARCH

1. Nursing effectiveness requires interactions in three arenas of relationships:
   a. Day-to-day aware and insightful interaction with clients; those *for* whom nurses accept responsibility because of their diminished self-care capacity.
   b. Daily interactions with colleagues, peers, co-workers; those *with* whom nurses work as ethical, caring professionals.
   c. Interactions with persons in leadership, including supervisors, managers, administrators, insurance companies and their representatives, physicians, and the public; those *to* whom we are accountable.
2. Because they encompass all of the nursing experience, the communication skills required to establish and maintain effective relationships in the three arenas are different from the specific skills for listening to and counseling clients (see Chapter 12).
3. Effective communication characteristics that facilitate and reinforce all three types of relationships include the following:
   a. Self-esteem, confidence, sense of self-worth, positive outlook.
   b. Flexibility, but no yielding or overcompliance.

c. Goal orientation, directness, maintenance of a sense of purpose.
d. Motivation to be understood, ability to find common ground.
e. Caring without appeasement or overeagerness to please.
f. Honesty, respect for self and others.

Specific Theorists

Carl Gustav Jung[1]

1. In the early twentieth century, Jung expanded the idea of individual personality beyond Sigmund Freud's notion of mind as conscious and unconscious domains.
2. Jung included the vast realms of the subconscious (e.g., personal creativity, intuition, a sense of interconnectedness between all humans) in what he called the Collective Unconscious. Thus, he believed that we are all aligned through our shared human experience.
3. Specific patterns of the collective awareness, called archetypes, became symbolic representations of human potentials, such as the healer archetype, the visionary, and the warrior.

Abraham Maslow[2]

1. Abraham Maslow moved the study of psychology from a focus on pathology to an understanding of healthy individual functioning and relationships.
2. He explored the realm of interpersonal relationships in view of each person's hierarchy of needs as follows:
a. Safety.
b. Belonging.
c. Status.
d. Meaning.
e. Self-actualization.
f. Emerging transpersonal spirituality.
3. He focused on health as ever expanding human potential for self-actualization. His ideas brought about the birth of the "human potential movement" and with it the founding of the Association of Humanistic Psychology and the Association of Transpersonal Psychology.
4. His work prepared the way for holistic philosophies in the past two decades.

Eric Berne[3]

1. Eric Berne, a psychiatrist, in the early 1970s began popularizing Transactional Analysis, an approach to human relatedness in which relationships are viewed as a series of understand-

able transactions between two or more persons who each have five powerful ego states.
a. The Parent ego state is characterized by accumulated knowledge, including rules of behavior, values, and ethics.
1) The Nurturing Parent is accepting and supportive.
2) The Critical Parent is judgmental and discriminating.
b. The Adult ego state is associated with thinking clearly, making decisions, moving purposefully toward a stated goal, assessing problems and finding solutions, and asserting oneself effectively. The nursing process comes from the Adult ego state but receives input from the other ego states.
c. The Child ego state relates to the capacity for feeling, playfulness, creativity, spontaneity, and capacity for fun. It can be manifest as follows:
1) The Free Child is lively, creative, and playful.
2) The Adaptive Child is compliant, deferring, shamed, withdrawn, frustrated, codependent, fearful, or angry.
2. Human transactions are actually the complex interaction of these five related states of awareness in varying combinations.[4]
a. Complementary transactions are those in which the ego states match each other.
1) A Parent-to-Parent communication may include agreement about mutual criticism such as "kids are getting worse each year."
2) An Adult-to-Adult communication may be a mutual exploration of ways to get things done and make agreements.
3) A Child-to-Child communication is about mutual playfulness and creativity—"Let's just have fun." On the more adaptive side, interchild communications focus on how bad both people are feeling about a work situation.
b. Uncomplementary transactions are those in which ego states cross each other, mutual agreement is lacking, the outcome is unexpected, or a less than desirable pattern results in a "game" (Exhibit 14–1).

Angeles Arrien[5]

1. An anthropologist and transpersonal psychologist, Angeles Arrien advanced the concept of four guiding principles, or archetypes, that are manifest in all cultures.

Exhibit 14–1 The "Psychological Game"

Eric Berne coined the term *psychological game* to refer to repeated, uncomplementary transactions resulting in an emotional payoff or a sense of being "had." For example, an insurance representative (Parent ego state) tells nurses via the supervisory staff (Parent ego state) that, for better patient care, they must limit client home visits to 10 minutes and plan 5 minutes of charting per patient on their own time. The nurses agree, because they (Child ego state) are afraid of supervisor disapproval. Later, after this pattern is well established in the agency, someone questions it (Adult ego state) and is roundly chastised (parent-to-child transaction) for questioning authority. The nurses become frustrated, experience "burn-out," and consider other careers (all Child behaviors) rather than unionizing or exploring other options (Adult capacities). Overall, the game may be called "Gotcha!" or "Dehumanizing the Caring Profession."

2. These archetypes provide a helpful framework in the physical, emotional, mental, and spiritual dimensions for understanding and enhancing nurses' relationships with the many influences that surround the profession. Healthy individuals use all four principles as needed rather than limiting themselves to one or two of the archetypes.
   a. The Warrior archetype corresponds to the physical dimension of the relationship.
      1) Stands firm and is well-grounded.
      2) Knows facts and statistics.
      3) Has worldly knowledge and uses it effectively.
      4) Works with courage to modify behavior in self and others.
      5) Translates ideas into action and honors professional code of ethics.
   b. The Healer archetype relates to the feeling dimension of relationships:
      1) Addresses others with love and compassion.
      2) Is highly motivated to bring about emotional release so others can become whole.
      3) Brings caring quality into all interactions.
      4) Values self and others.
   c. The Teacher archetype is associated with the mental dimension of relatedness:
      1) Brings wisdom and knowledge to others.
      2) Assists others in developing perceptions and insight.

Exhibit 14–2 Self-Awareness Exercise

- Note how you feel at the end of the day. What happened that pleased you? What happened that distressed you? What do you wish you had done differently?
- Note an unpleasant interaction. Who was the critical parent, the adapted child, the adult? What would be the choices available to all participants?
- Diagram the transaction that keeps happening to you when you feel cheated or diminished. What is it that you say or do (or do not say or do) that maintains the pattern?
- Name the game for the fun of it and decide how you will do things differently the next time. Practice the new responses with a friend or co-worker to make sure you know exactly what you will do.

      3) Enjoys sharing accumulated wisdom and is always willing to learn.
   d. The Visionary archetype relates to the spiritual aspect of relationships.
      1) Uses qualities of clarity and perception to discern conflicts and assist resolution.
      2) Is a fair and nonjudgmental witness.
      3) Senses intuitively and brings others to an awareness of the highest good for all concerned.

Exhibit 14–3 Example for Using a Different Ego State

- *Example:* Day shift nurse to tired night nurse: "You probably did not turn your patients again. It's always the same with you people." Night nurse feels cowed, helpless, or angry.
- *Diagram:* Critical Parent to Adaptive Child transaction. No Adult in sight. New possibilities for transactions:
   Admit the feelings, acknowledge the Child: "I feel bad when you say that. We both have strong feelings about this problem; when can we take 10 minutes to sort this out?" (Adult invitation to have a Child share feelings.)
   — Counter with nurturing Parent: "I'm so glad you have this concern, and I support you fully in finding solutions. Maybe we could all learn from your caring."
   — Go to Adult: "You're right. This is a problem. We could work out some compromise that is good for both shifts. Let's sit down and explore the options."

Exhibit 14-4 Example for Employing Different Archetypes

Nurse N. is a sweet and gentle person who evokes predominantly the Healer archetype. She becomes totally flustered and tongue-tied when a patient refuses to take his bath, eat his breakfast, or go for treatments. Her new choices include the following:

- As a Warrior, with courage and inner conviction, ask, "What is going on within you? Please tell me your concerns. My intent is to help you as best I can at this time."
- As a Teacher, with wisdom and knowledge, say, for example, "Hospital schedules are designed to accomplish the most for the greatest number of people. There are some areas of choice and some that cannot be redesigned. It is helpful to know your goals in being here, and then perhaps we can figure out a schedule that will work for you."
- As a Visionary, who brings fair witness, consciousness, and intuition through centered presence, allow a moment for breathing together with the patient. Ask what the bigger picture is in this situation and how illusions or projections can be diminished.

Communication for Building Relationships

1. Nurses are generally effective in nurse–patient and nurse–peer interactions but may find it difficult to communicate with the people in power and leadership (of which there are many).
2. Establishing and maintaining effective relationships with administrative personnel, third-party payers, medical organizations, and the greater public require specific skills and valuing of oneself.
3. Every interaction either builds or detracts from a relationship. As nurses seek to communicate effectively who they are to the larger society and the value of their profession, they must develop skills at identifying detracting communications and countering discounts with effective assertiveness.
   a. Analyze confusing, uncomplementary, or crossed communications to find out what keeps happening (Exhibit 14–2).
   b. Move in consciousness to change ego states and with that the whole character of interactions (Exhibit 14–3).
4. In determining their own unique relation to each of the four cross-cultural archetypes, nurses can learn the areas that they need to develop further in order to become holistic, balanced practitioners.
   a. Nurses seem to be very strong in the Healer archetype.
   b. Some nurses have difficulty manifesting the Warrior or the Teacher archetypes, which require standing firm, being clear, and willingly teaching others to widen their view of the importance of caregiving skills (Exhibit 14–4).
5. Negotiation is a special form of relatedness in which both parties find mutually accepted, common ground.
   a. Negotiating requires enough flexibility to understand all one's own ego states and to comprehend the dynamic of any discounting transaction:
      1) Revisiting all situations that are unsatisfactory.
      2) Coming to clear adult agreements—the best outcome of good negotiations.[6]
   b. When there is agreement about the commonality of purpose, specific agreements can be made.
   c. Agreements need to be clearly defined, realistic, and pertinent to the issue.
   d. All agreements must include means of monitoring to ensure that they are honored, not just given lip service (Exhibit 14–5).
6. Reframing is a specific way of maintaining positive intent in all relationships and resolving conflicts by finding the mutually accepted objectives and common ground.
   a. Although specific behaviors and attitudes may vary, the positive intent behind the activity is maintained. "Hard on the issues, soft on the people" may be the slogan of reframing.
   b. Mutual respect as a basis for all relatedness includes a willingness to honor and value ourselves as well as others (Exhibit 14–6).

 Pause for a moment . . .

- ❑ *I formulate my own questions and give rationale for my answers while I study.*
- ❑ *I can do _____ to motivate myself to study more.*
- ❑ *My study group helps as each participant adds questions during the discussion process and discusses his or her rationale.*
- ❑ *My studying is worth it!*

Exhibit 14–5 Example To Show Negotiation Principles

Nurses in a large health maintenance organization (HMO) are told that costs must be cut, and they have a choice to reduce staff or reduce their salaries by 10%. The nurses vote to reduce salaries by 10%, but 3 months later, half of them are laid off. They cry "foul!" and feel totally discounted.

The basic steps of negotiation were not honored. If the nurses had been able to demonstrate the cost-effectiveness of their services to the HMO, it might have been possible to reach an agreement about finances as a common ground. If the agreement about the pay cut had clearly stated that no one would be laid off for a specific period of time, the nurses could seek legal relief. Better yet, they should have built a provision for legal monitoring into the pay cut agreement from the start.

Unfortunately, these kinds of dilemmas are all too common. Nurses sometimes jump too quickly to preserve jobs without looking at the bigger picture and ways of ensuring effective negotiations.

HOLISTIC NURSING PROCESS

Assessment

1. Assessment of a relationship interaction requires discernment and awareness.
2. Transactional analysis gives nurses a quick tool for assessing the dynamic of an interaction.
3. The communicator's intent must be clear and the desired outcome identified. For example, "I am going for a job interview. I could feel intimidated, like a child, in this awesome task. I want to stay in my Adult ego state by thinking this through, practicing it, trying it out with my friends. My intent is to learn all I can, be clear in my communication, and feel good about myself when I leave the interview."
4. Among the factors that should be addressed in a transaction with a client are the following:
   a. the client's reason for seeking help at this time and the duration of the problem.
   b. the client's perception of the problem/situation with a person or specific relationship, including who is doing what (that presents a problem), to whom, and how the behavior constitutes a problem.
   c. the client's perception of all the people involved in the situation. If appropriate, the nurse may ask to meet the people involved.
   d. the client's current approach to the problem.
   e. the client's position in the relationship/current problem.
   f. the client's body and verbal language as the situation is being described.
   g. the client's minimal goals in regard to the perceived problem.

Nursing Diagnoses

1. The following nursing diagnoses compatible with relationship interventions and related to the nine human response patterns are as follows:
   a. Communicating: Altered communication
   b. Relating: Altered parenting
      Altered sexual dysfunction
   c. Valuing: Spiritual distress
   d. Choosing: Coping, ineffective individual or family
      Altered family process
   e. Moving: Self-care deficit
      Self-care dysfunction
   f. Feeling: Anxiety
      Grieving
      Violence
      Fear
      Rape-trauma
2. Nurses can use the diagnostic categories in self-assessments to look at their own strengths and weaknesses, as well as those of others in any transaction. For example, the nurse who predominantly invokes the Healer archetype may begin to activate the Teacher or Warrior arche-

Exhibit 14–6 Example of Reframing

A reframe of the situation in which the HMO laid off the employees is to suggest that management is responding in the only way it has considered. Life in the twenty-first century is going to require different skills from everyone. The HMO could become the first corporation to explore new options, design a new concept that emphasizes human values. There are, in fact, other values than the dollar, and genuinely wise corporations pay attention to their own hierarchy of needs.

Another reframe is for nurses to look at the need for more than one way of operating within themselves. Nurses must develop a wide variety of skills as effective communicators while keeping the ethic of caring alive in a changing and stressful work environment.

type as a way of increasing his or her own sense of wholeness and balance. Centering before each interaction is a powerful way to bring in the visionary archetype.

Client Outcomes

1. In working on relationships, there are a great many desirable client outcomes.
   a. The client will recognize family and relationship systems patterns.
   b. The client will demonstrate awareness of the effect of human dialogue on the body-mind-spirit.
   c. The client will learn new strategies to improve the quality of relationships.
2. As nurses plan for identifiable outcomes in transactions, they begin to actualize them.
3. A healthy sense of "I'm okay, you're okay" creates an expectation of mutual respect.[7]
4. It is possible for everyone to come out winning in some way, even though compromises may be necessary.

Plan and Interventions

1. Acknowledge feelings (Child ego state).
2. Consider values and beliefs (Parent ego state).
3. Propose options (Adult ego state).
4. A limitation to only one solution is clear evidence that adult thinking is missing.
5. Facilitate relationships through effective communication skills.
   a. Throughout any communication, the nurse builds and maintains rapport. This includes attention to matching the language, as well as the nonverbal communication, of the client.
   b. The positive intent of the communication is maintained, even though the exact content may be questioned.
   c. Whenever possible, negative ideas are reframed to include positive, growthful aspects.
   d. It is wise to make "I " statements when speaking about one's inner state rather than accusing another person. For example, "I feel uncomfortable when you criticize my co-workers, and the result is diminished trust in you" is preferable to "You are always on someone's case about something; I wish you would just go away!"

6. Use the following guidelines for interaction:
   a. Before beginning any transaction, plan the intent and focus, allowing yourself to center and align with your sense of purpose. This may be accomplished through
      1) Taking several deep breaths.
      2) Rehearsing a new pattern mentally.
      3) Imaging the successful outcome.
      4) Acknowledging your positive intent.
   b. During the transaction, note the ego states that are in evidence and specifically the feelings that are triggered in yourself.
   c. Consider options for interventions that get back to the subject and address the goal of the communication.
   d. Set limits that maintain boundaries such as time frames, selection of settings, and topics for discussion.
   e. After the interaction, evaluate your communication skills and the specific archetype that you activated in yourself. Honor yourself and others in the ongoing process of learning to become more effective in relationships. Consider ways that make trying out new behaviors safe and enjoyable.

Evaluation

1. Evaluation of relationships is an ongoing process.
2. Daily review is helpful to take stock of what is effective and what needs further development.
3. Relatedness is an open-ended process of changing, trying out the new, and re-evaluating.
4. Rogers held in the concept of helicy that "our patterns are continually changing, innovative and creative."[8]

REFERENCES

1. C.G. Jung, *Man and His Symbols* (London: Aldus Books, 1964).
2. A. Maslow, *The Farther Reaches of Human Nature* (New York: Penguin Books, 1971).
3. E. Berne, *Transactional Analysis in Psychotherapy* (New York: Grove Press, 1961).
4. E. Berne, *Games People Play* (New York: Grove Press, 1964).
5. A. Arrien, *The Four-Fold Way* (San Francisco: HarperCollins Publishers, 1993).
6. R. Fisher and W. Ury, *Getting to Yes* (New York: Penguin Books, 1981).

7. T.A. Harris, *I'm OK—You're OK* (New York: Avon Books, 1969).

8. M. Rogers, *Portraits of Excellence,* Video (Oakland, CA: Studio 3, Helene Fuld Trust Fund, 1987).

SUGGESTED READING

D. Hover-Kramer et al., *Healing Touch: A Resource for Health Care Professionals* (Albany, NY: Delmar Publishers, 1996).

M. James and D. Jongeward, *Born To Win* (Reading, MA: Addison-Wesley Publishing Co., 1971).

C.G. Jung, *The Portable Jung,* ed. J. Campbell (New York: Penguin Books, 1971).

L. Laskow, *Healing with Love* (San Francisco: HarperCollins, Publishers, 1992).

G.I. Nierenberg, *The Art of Negotiating* (New York: Simon & Schuster, 1981).

F. Vaughan, *Shadows of the Sacred* (Wheaton, IL: Quest Books, 1995).

CHAPTER 15

Death and Grief

Melodie Olson

KNOWLEDGE COMPETENCIES

- Discuss the characteristics of a "peaceful death."
- Explain how theories of family, grief, pain, and transcendence guide the care of dying people.
- Analyze the comfort needs of individual patients who are dying and their families.
- Plan care strategies to assist dying patients and their families with pre-death planning and anticipatory grief.
- Plan care strategies to help dying people achieve comfort and a peaceful death.
- Recognize, value, and use the multiple talents of all members of the health care team who can help the dying patient to achieve end-of-life goals.
- Identify legal requirements related to dying (e.g., those related to home death, violent death, death by infectious process).
- Discuss ethical issues related to death and dying.
- Use strategies for self-care to manage one's own grief when caring for people who are dying.

DEFINITIONS

Comfort: a multidimensional concept experienced by an individual in the present moment, resulting in the elimination or reduction of discomfort and an improved ability to live in a more satisfying way until death occurs.

Conscious Dying: an active mental process of awareness and preparation for one's own death.

Death: cessation of physiologic processes that sustain life; a passing or parting; letting go of this life, or loss of life. It has also been defined as a "moment in time."[1]

Dying: the dynamic and individualized process of death.

Grief: a pervasive, individualized, and dynamic process that may result in physical, emotional, or spiritual distress because of the loss (through death) of a loved one. Described by some as normative, it may be acute (intense) or chronic.

Pain: a subjective experience, defined by an individual as something that hurts and involves the whole person. More than a physical sensation, pain has meaning to people.

Palliative Care: "the active total care of patients whose disease is not responsive to curative treatment. . . . The goal of palliative care is achievement of the best quality of life for dying people and their families."[2]

 Pause for a moment . . .

- ❏ *I use my relaxation and imagery strategies.*
- ❏ *My positive affirmations help me study to successfully pass the holistic nursing certification (HNC) examination.*
- ❏ *My positive feedback right now is _____.*
- ❏ *I reward myself in my own special way while I study to follow my concentrated study session.*

THEORIES AND RESEARCH

Family Theory

1. Families include not only traditional family members, but also those who have a close association with the person who is dying.

2. According to developmental theory, families have a life cycle and need to achieve certain tasks at each stage of life.
   a. Each family member may have a different role to fulfill at each stage.
   b. Care of the dying requires the caregiver to identify tasks that the dying client or family wants or needs to complete to achieve peace at the end of life.
3. Structural/functional family theory assigns five functions of role to a family: personality maintenance for the individuals, socialization, reproduction, economics, and health care.[3]
   a. The role fulfilled by the dying person must be reassigned.
   b. Plans for that role shift must be made in order for the family to fulfill its functions and go on during and after the death.
4. In family systems theory, families are self-regulating social systems. Disruption of the social system, as in the case of death, requires new channels of communication (feedback) and the creation of new ways of relating to each other (adaptation).
   a. Families that have open communications and are free to find new ways of relating are able to seek support, express feelings, and find appropriate emotional outlets.
   b. Families that are not open may need help to do those things.[4]

Grief Theory

1. People go through defined stages of grief, from shock and denial (protest) through feelings of anger, despair, bargaining, detachment, depression, acceptance, or resolution.
   a. Not all people go through each stage.
   b. Grief is personal, and each person goes back and forth between the stages, sometimes spending more time in one stage, almost skipping another stage.
   c. The stages of grief are transient.
   d. They may also be defined by the time that elapses between the identification of a terminal diagnosis (acute crisis), through a stage of living–dying, to the terminal stage.[5]
2. Grief is pervasive, dynamic, and normative.
   a. Pervasive grief affects all areas of one's life; it is acute. Some may have physical symptoms, including a sense of being unable to swallow, palpitations of the heart, and hyperventilation. Others may not be able to concentrate, make choices, or take action.
   b. The dynamic nature of grief is seen in the fact that people move from one stage of grief to another, have grief rekindled by a birthday or anniversary years after a death, or remember previous times of grieving.
   c. Normative grief is a value that society or a cultural group puts on certain grief practices, deeming them normal, atypical, or pathologic. The concept of normality is useful only in the assessment of dysfunctional grieving, that is, grieving that keeps the griever from functioning to achieve life's goals.
3. The consequences of those who successfully complete the grieving process are the development of a new reality and a new identity.
   a. The new reality is that life is different, that the family and other close associates must relate in new ways and fulfill new roles because of the death of a family member.
   b. Each person in the extended relationships has a new identity that includes memories, but not the presence, of someone. New skills must be learned.
   c. Dysfunctional grief can result in poor communications, social isolation, depression, physical signs of stress, and lack of achievement or progress toward life's goals.
4. Grief of the person who is dying extends from the time one realizes that the diagnosis has a fatal outcome, to the death itself.
   a. The person first copes with an unstable period of multiple small losses, physical and otherwise, and cycles of hope and denial. This person needs to integrate care, like treatments and examinations and the like, into an already full schedule of work and family.
   b. Increasingly, as energy and time wane, the client must give up some aspects of control and care to others. The preservation of energy for accomplishing end-of-life goals is important. Relationships are a priority, focusing on leave taking, resolving old arguments or conflicts, and sharing hopes for the family's future.
   c. The turning inward of self to work toward peace during the death process is the final goal.

Pain Theory

1. The perception of pain requires two sets of events: the transmission of pain stimuli from the pain receptors to the brain and the interpretation of those signals in the brain.

2. Advocates of the gate control theory of pain propose the following path of transmission of pain:
   a. Nocioceptors (cells that respond to injury or pain, located on the ends of neurons) release chemical substances that, in turn, stimulate peripheral sensory neurons.
   b. Peripheral nerve fibers conduct sensory impulses of various sizes to the dorsal horn of the spinal cord.
   c. Neurotransmitters (e.g., acetylcholine) carry the impulse over the synapses, and the impulse travels to the opposite side of the spinal cord, then along the spinal-thalamic tract to various centers in the brain, including the thalamus, hypothalamus, brain stem, and cortex.
3. "Closing the gate," or interrupting the transmission of pain, by avoiding the stimuli; filling up the transmission pathways with other sensations, such as touch or cold; or using chemicals that interrupt the conduction of pain within the central nervous system (e.g., endorphins) can lessen pain.
4. Interpretation of pain transmission signals occurs within centers of memory, emotion, and learning. Therefore, previous experiences, culture, pain education, and emotions all contribute to the way in which any individual feels pain.
5. A variety of cognitive and educational techniques, including imagery, relaxation, hypnosis, breathing, and focusing techniques may alter the perception of pain.
   a. Education about near-death experiences, therapeutic touch, and appropriate counseling (including standard techniques such as listening and allowing ventilation, verbalizing problems) may decrease anxiety.
   b. Pharmacologic control of pain may affect either the transmission of pain or the perception of pain.

Transcendence

1. Transcendence implies a sense of connectedness between self and a greater reality or the environment. It integrates self with past and future, giving meaning to life. It is a set of introspective activities that reflect concern for others or for meaning.
2. Positive outcomes for the self-transcendent person, even when approaching death, include less depression, self-neglect, and hopelessness; greater sense of well-being and ability to cope with grief; and the ability to live and find meaning in the present. This sense of meaning is often spiritual, an ability to connect with God (or Deity).

Awareness of Impending Death

1. People become aware of their own impending death in stages, and this awareness leads to conscious dying.
   a. One marker of the beginning of the process is the diagnosis of a terminal illness, but some people seem to know before they learn of the diagnosis that they will die. Others deny the impending death for a time.
   b. The best markers are actual statements of awareness.
2. The goals of becoming aware of impending death, or conscious dying, are to live fully until death comes and to direct or participate in the death process until one is comfortable with accepting the ministrations of others.
3. In addition to participating in treatment decisions and determinations about the kinds of care, the dying client should plan to say goodbye to friends and family members, finish things he or she has wanted to do (e.g., take a special vacation, go fishing, learn to speak another language), make final disposition of property, and clarify his or her wishes concerning organ and tissue donation.
4. Emotional and spiritual tasks with which the nurse may assist the client are learning to forgive self and others; experiencing a sense of continuity (e.g., "life has mattered and the world is different because I was here"), and recognizing and accepting love as one changes in the dying process.
5. Awareness of death, conscious dying, allows the client to rehearse the dying process and learn to reduce fear of death and to "let go of this life" when it is time to do so. Rehearsals are a special form of imagery, carefully scripted (see Chapter 24) to demonstrate the release of grief and pain, the creation of comfort and peace, and the achievement of closure. Hypnosis, relaxation skills, meditation and prayer, and rituals all help in this process.

Rituals, Prayer, and Meditation

1. Rituals are timeless. They help individuals maintain connectedness with something beyond self:

other people, a sense of the Eternal, or universal truths.[6] They provide comfort to the dying person and the grieving family. Some rituals are religious in nature: sharing sacraments, fasting at holidays like Yom Kippur or Ramadan, or Native American drumming. Providing time, place, and resources, as well as support for rituals, is a nursing responsibility.

2. Death bed rituals can be created. They are meant to provide for connectedness with a loving group of people throughout the dying process.
   a. The family decides what they want to occur, within the constraints of the dying process. One group of people may hold hands and pray, forming a prayer circle. Another group may chant. Another may sit quietly and put hands on the dying person.
   b. There may come a moment in which it is appropriate to let the dying person know that it may be time to "let go," as when the person relaxes, acts as if he or she feels or sees other worldly beings, and is becoming peaceful in that knowledge. This requires sensitivity, as doing it too early can leave a person feeling abandoned.
   c. The one dying may also determine it is time to go and say good-bye. Music may ease the transition.
3. Prayer is a conversation or a personal connection with God. The person may communicate feelings, concerns, and a sense of awe or worship, and God communicates a sense of presence and peace back to the person.[7] Prayer is a form of nonlocal healing.[8]
   a. Chants may be a kind of prayer, a timeless song creating connection, sometimes with the past.
   b. Prayers may be ritualistic, as in the case of a child who learns to say one prayer every night before bed.
4. Meditation is a clearing of the mind by an inner focusing of attention to reach a relatively pure experience of self.
   a. An experienced meditator brings this experience of self to the dying process, achieving calm and often a knowledge of purpose.
   b. Time, privacy, and support for a particular physical position may be necessary for the client's practice of meditation.
   c. The nurse who prays or meditates can bring a personal sense of peace to the caring of the dying patient and share the experience with those who also practice.

Near-Death Experiences

1. People who report near-death experiences have generally had an intense episode involving a trauma or life-threatening event.
   a. The cluster of perceptions most often reported includes a feeling of being outside of the physical body (perhaps floating above one's body); feelings of peace and calmness, or well-being; absence of pain; absence of fear; panoramic memory (i.e., a review of all the events in one's life occurring at the same moment); ineffability (difficulty in relating the experience accurately); and, sometimes, an "otherworldliness" (e.g., seeing religious figures or family members who are dead).
   b. These experiences are each unique, not always dramatic, and sometimes leave lasting effects.
2. The lasting effects of near-death experiences are usually positive and may include absence or lessened fear of death, a sense of purpose in life, a belief that relationships are the most important thing in life, and greater altruism. Sometimes, there is a greater interest in spiritual things.
3. In caring for the person who has had such an experience, the nurse should listen without judgment and help the person to share the story with the family.
4. Referrals to clergy or spiritual guides may be helpful if the client's life is disrupted or changed by the experience; it may be beneficial to introduce the client to others who have had a near-death experience.
5. The family may not understand the changes in their loved one after the near-death experience. The nurse can help them to value that experience for its ability to decrease fear and anxiety, to talk about it with the client, to deal with the change, and not to give an inappropriate meaning to the event. For example, the experience can be helpful in resolving end-of-life issues, but it is not proof of life after death. That concept is a matter of faith, not of proof.

HOLISTIC NURSING PROCESS

Assessment

1. The goals of the client and family for the time that remains, and for the kind of death desired (e.g., to fight to the end, to be at peace, to avoid disfigurement, to resolve conflict) must be a primary focus of assessment.

2. The nurse also assesses comfort needs, including physical needs such as sleep, movement (or function), and relief of pain; psychospiritual needs, including one's sense of meaning in life; environment, including light, noise, odor, and temperature; and social needs, especially relationships.
3. The degree of fear and/or anxiety related to end-of-life issues merits assessment.
4. Final tasks, including legal issues such as making a will, establishing advanced directives, and providing organ donation instructions, must be accomplished.
5. Resources needed by both client and family, including referrals to social workers and other professionals who can bring intellectual, physical, fiscal, or support services to the care of the dying person, should be assessed.
6. Caregivers need to carry out a self-assessment to ensure that they maintain good health, focus on client needs, and render excellent care without "burnout."

Nursing Diagnoses

1. The following nursing diagnoses compatible with and commonly associated with the care of dying patients are related to the human response patterns:

   a. Exchanging: Altered circulation
                         Altered oxygenation
                         Altered body systems
   b. Communicating: Altered communication
                         Ineffective
                            communication
   c. Valuing: Spiritual distress
   d. Choosing: Ineffective individual/
                            family coping
   e. Moving: Self-care deficit
   f. Perceiving: Body image disturbance
                         Powerlessness
                         Hopelessness
   g. Feeling: Pain
                         Anxiety
                         Grieving
                         Fear

Client Outcomes

1. The client will experience the kind of death desired, generally having reached life's goals; having said good-bye to important others; having found meaning in life and a sense of peace and/or wisdom; feeling comfort in the minis-

trations of others; feeling little pain or discomfort; and having sufficient time, but not too much, in the dying process.
2. The family will say good-bye to the one who dies, value the memories they share with that person, resolve grief in a healthy way, and work to attain their own life goals.

Plan and Interventions

1. Prioritize interventions based on the client's/family's goals.
2. Continually reassess the client's condition for changes and effectiveness of interventions.
3. Encourage the verbalization of emotions, fears, worries, changes in condition (including pain assessment), and current goals (to resolve unfinished business). Offer reassurance as appropriate.
4. Allow and encourage the client to spend time with family and others who can give support and hope. Include family lawyers, clergy, and the physician. Assess the effect of these interactions on the client's status.
5. Provide for comfort needs.
6. Focus on the client's strengths.
7. Provide privacy as needed, but stay with the client when death is imminent.
8. Provide opportunities for death bed rituals, such as prayer circles, appropriate sacraments, and music (as determined by family and client).
9. Use referrals to bring care to the client who is beyond the scope of nursing practice or requires special skills, such as physical therapy, massage therapy, or music therapy.
10. Know and obey laws related to the care of the dying, including notification of appropriate authorities when one dies at home, of infection, or from violence.
11. Use a variety of specific nursing interventions in the care of the dying and their families.

Planning an Ideal Death[9]

1. Prepare yourself to care for this person.
   a. Center; be focused and in a caring state of being.
   b. Plan to take breaks from intense situations, and practice good health habits for yourself (e.g., good nutrition, exercise, relaxation).
   c. Be fully present in each moment that you are with the dying person.
   d. Collaborate with team members who are supportive and caring; accept the situation as it is.

2. Consider the environment. For example, where does the client want to die? What are the relative benefits of each possible setting, when there is a choice?
   a. Provide a quiet, calm environment with access to familiar things and people.
   b. Determine relative costs if the setting is changed and who will be responsible for them.
   c. Consider the need and availability of respite care.
3. Determine the care needed.
   a. Prepare for the medications, technology, and equipment that will be needed.
   b. If the client's goals include medical and nonmedical therapies that are believed to be complementary, prepare for those additional therapies with knowledge and referrals, as required.
4. Incorporate all senses (e.g., touch, smell, hearing, seeing, and tasting) in care and rituals.
5. Help the family prepare for the moment of death by giving information about the changes in the body during the death process.
6. Be prepared to care for someone who is restless, whose state of consciousness is changing, and who will later become unresponsive. Help the family know what to do as these changes occur.
7. At the moment of death, continue to talk with the dying one, and/or encourage the family to do so. Relate to the client as it seems right, using touch, hand holding, prayer, or encouraging words; it may be helpful to give permission to "let go." If the family has planned rituals for this moment, participate if you are invited and it seems right.
8. Be sure to plan follow-up visits with the family to give support and encouragement as they resolve grief.

Relieving Pain

1. Interview the client to find out the intensity of pain, its location, the interventions that help, the duration, and the patterns of pain.
   a. Regular, consistent recording of pain data by means of rating scales helps all caregivers manage pain consistently. Scales can be used to determine the efficacy of the treatments being used, to decide when treatments need to be upgraded or changed, and to identify and validate pain patterns.
   b. Special assessment techniques used to measure a child's pain are dependent on the child's age. Scales that use frown to smile faces may be more useful than numbers that adults use. Children's pain can be managed, and the child involved should take an active part in the description of "hurt" and what helps make it better.
2. When appropriate, provide pain relief through pharmacologic treatment.
   a. There is no reason to withhold needed medication because of unfounded fears of addiction or potential side effects or a belief that the pain is not treatable. Pain is manageable for at least 90% of clients.
   b. A variety of administration methods may be used for pharmacologic pain control, depending on the symptoms and the way that the medication is best absorbed:
      1) Oral.
      2) Rectal.
      3) Sublingual.
      4) Transdermal patch.
      5) Intravenous, by infusion pump.
      6) Patient-controlled analgesia (PCA).
      7) Spinal anesthesia.
      8) Nerve block.
   c. A change in the route of administration may mandate an adjustment in the dosage.
3. When appropriate, use nonpharmacologic treatments for pain.
   a. Methods that "close the pain gate" by stimulating large nerve fibers include the following:
      1) Massage (e.g., back rubs, hand and foot massage, some shiatsu, reflexology).
      2) Temperature changes, such as alternating heat and cold.
      3) Transcutaneous nerve stimulation (TENS). A portable device delivers mild electrical stimulation through electrodes placed on the skin near the site of pain. The client can control the intensity, rate, and duration of the stimulation. Good skin care of the electrode site and reduction of the intensity of the TENS unit if muscle contraction occurs is a part of care. Continuous use can reduce the effectiveness of the unit.
   b. Behavioral and cognitive interventions for pain include those that use distraction or change perception of pain.
      1) Visualization, relaxation, and imagery are effective in pain control. With severe pain, these techniques should be used in conjunction with pharmacologic methods to achieve maximum control.

2) Creative arts are useful, in part because of distraction. Similarly, humor, pets, and art and music therapy are useful.

Reminiscence and Life Review

1. Encourage the dying person to reminisce.
   a. Reminiscence is a naturally occurring process in which the experiencer remembers life events in no apparent order and with no predetermined goal. It occurs in all people as they age or approach the end of life.
   b. Reminiscence groups are efficient ways to encourage this kind of verbalization, although individual interviews are also effective.
2. There are generally six to eight sessions in a structured life review. Systematically ask questions designed to help the client remember events at each stage of life.
   a. Begin by asking open-ended questions about childhood, earliest memories; then listen. All memories have relevance, whether happy or sad. Support the client when remembering sad events.
   b. Proceed through the next sessions with open-ended questions through adolescence, family and home, adulthood, and later life.
   c. Have a summary session to ask questions such as "On the whole, what kind of life do you think you have had?" and "What would you do over again?"
   d. Be prepared to handle any kind of responses to these questions. If you have never done a life review, use a printed format, such as Haight's Life Review and Experiencing form.[10]
3. The goal of life review is integration of self, the sense that this life was personal and unique. There is some sadness in this process, but achievement is also evident. The process helps an individual to see meaning in his or her own life.

Managing Grief

1. Be sensitive to the needs that arise during the period of anticipatory grief.
2. Give knowledge as it is needed—about the dying process, about legal requirements, about treatments and options available.
3. Support and encourage connections and sharing between family and the dying client.
   a. The planning of shared time, such as vacations, weekends, evenings, and, when death is close, time in the room together, promotes a sense of connectedness.

   b. The client and family can use multiple means of communication, including touching; leaving notes for others with pleasant or meaningful messages; reading together (e.g., poems, scriptures, letters, stories); and planning future events, such as a child's graduation, even if it is likely to occur after the death.
   c. Taping cassettes for future use can be helpful.
   d. Developing spiritual awareness through prayer and other means is also helpful.
4. Provide a safe place to express emotions. Support groups that include a dying client and members of the family allow expression of anger, guilt, and secrets to be shared. The love generated in the group becomes a great source of comfort when families meet after the death to celebrate the life and remember the individual.
5. Encourage family and loved ones to be present in an atmosphere of forgiveness and peace.
6. Create an environment that is familiar because all present have planned for the death. If the client has rehearsed what will happen and has practiced relaxation, breathing, and imagery exercises, the nurse or family member becomes a coach for the process.
7. Use touch, music, co-meditation (i.e., meditate, chant, or pray together), and preplanned rituals like a prayer circle. Talk quietly to each other, including the client, sharing life until it is released.
8. Continue comfort measures and regular nursing care as required. Allow the family to share that care.
9. Have clergy or other invited guests present to meet the family's needs and provide frequent breaks for meals or just to leave the room. Having decisions made in advance about legal issues (e.g., organ donation) is helpful. Most important, the family should know that they can talk with their loved one, share anything as yet left unsaid, and when it is time, let the person dying know that they will be all right.
10. After death, encourage the family to join or continue their participation in a support group.
    a. Remembering anniversaries, maintaining other rituals (e.g., setting a place at the holiday table for the one not present for the first year), or celebrating a birthday may be useful.

b. Unsaid messages can be written in a letter, and the letter burned so that the message goes into the universe.

c. Visits to the burial site or planting a special tree in memory of the individual help bring a sense of closure while not forgetting the person.

11. Help family members move forward.

a. The survivors must make plans for the future that do not include the deceased family member.

b. Grief may last for a long time; however, healing memories will gently push away pain, and a new level of awareness will be present.

Evaluation

1. The client was able to experience the kind of death desired, generally having reached life's goals; having said good-bye to important others; having found meaning in life and a sense of peace and/or wisdom; having felt comfort in the ministrations of others; was without pain or discomfort; and, with sufficient time, but not too much, in the dying process.

2. The client's family was able to say good-bye to their loved one, valued the memories that they share with their loved one, and is resolving grief in a healthy way and working toward attainment of life goals.

REFERENCES

1. B.M. Dossey et al., *Holistic Nursing: A Handbook for Practice,* 2nd ed. (Gaithersburg, MD: Aspen Publishers, 1995), 429.

2. D. Doyle et al., *Oxford Textbook of Palliative Medicine* (London: Oxford University Press, 1993), 3.

3. M.M. Friedman, *Family Nursing: Theory and Assessment,* 2nd ed. (Norwalk, CT: Appleton-Century-Crofts, 1986).

4. M. Olson, *Healing the Dying* (Albany, NY: Delmar Publishers, 1997).

5. P. Hess, Loss, Grief and Dying, in *Principles and Practice of Adult Health Nursing,* ed. P. Beare and J.L. Myers (St. Louis: C.V. Mosby Co., 1990), 431–433.

6. J. Achterberg et al., *Rituals of Healing* (New York: Bantam Books, 1994), 1–33.

7. V. Carson, *Spiritual Dimensions of Nursing Practice* (Philadelphia: W.B. Saunders, 1989).

8. L. Dossey, *Healing Words: The Power of Prayer and the Practice of Medicine* (San Francisco: HarperCollins Publishers, 1993).

9. Dossey et al., *Holistic Nursing: A Handbook for Practice,* 429.

10. B. Haight, Psychological Illness in Aging, in *Perspectives on Gerontological Nursing,* ed. E.M. Baines (Newbury Park, CA: Sage Publications, 1991), 316.

CONCEPT VIII

Client Self-Care

CHAPTER 16

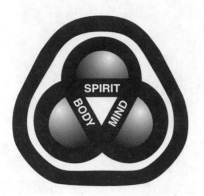

Self-Assessments

Anneke Young

KNOWLEDGE COMPETENCIES

- Discuss 10 areas of self-assessment.
- Describe four tools of self-assessment.
- Discuss the idea of self-responsibility and its relationship to obtaining maximum wellness.
- Explore self-assessments and the nursing process.
- Describe guidelines for holistic self-assessment.
  —Energy system or field assessment.
  —Physical self-assessment.
  —Mental/intellectual self-assessment.
  —Emotional self-assessment.
  —Social self-assessment.
  —Spiritual self-assessment.
- Describe ways to facilitate and interpret self-assessment tools.
- Describe ways to develop one's own healing awareness.

DEFINITION

Holistic Self-Assessment: the multidimensional process of assessing one's own physical, emotional, mental/intellectual, social, energetic, and spiritual well-being for the purpose of making necessary adjustments in order to maximize one's level of health/wellness. The process requires an awareness of the whole being greater than and different from the sum of its parts.

 Pause for a moment . . .

❏ *I have much to contribute to the dynamic changes that are occurring in holistic nursing and in health care.*

❏ *These changes provide me with a great opportunity to integrate caring and healing in my work and life.*

THEORIES AND RESEARCH

Physical Self-Assessment

1. Poor nutrition is a common source of illness.
   a. A diet consisting of fresh organic vegetables, fruits and meats, whole grains and adequate water intake is preferred over a diet filled with salt, fats, refined sugars, and preservatives.
   b. Foods laden with preservatives, pesticides, colorings, hormones, antibiotics, saturated fats, salt, simple sugars, dairy products, no-cal sweeteners, and other nonfood substances negatively affect the bodymind.
2. Constitution is related to the overall health of the parents, particularly their health at the moment conception takes place.[1]
   a. When the mother takes care of her health during pregnancy, the fetus is more likely to be healthy.
   b. If the mother smokes, drinks, takes drugs (including medications), or suffers severe emotional stress during pregnancy, the health of the fetus may be compromised—not only at birth, but also later in life.
3. Exposure to environmental stressors (e.g., pesticides, air and water pollution, noise pollution, ongoing stressful living and/or working conditions) challenges the bodymind complex.
4. When the bodymind is in a state of homeodynamic balance, it tends to tolerate the pres-

ence of viral, bacterial, fungal, or parasitic organisms in the system. When a person is in a compromised state of health, however, such microorganisms will proliferate in the body and cause infection.

5. The proper quantity and quality of exercise is associated with good health.
   a. Proper exercise also implies proper rest.
   b. General lack of exercise results in weakness and atrophy of muscles, skeletal misalignment, poor circulation of blood and energy, and poor metabolism.

6. Any damage or trauma to the body can disrupt the physiologic system.

7. Damage or trauma may also include psychologic trauma; a serious shock to the bodymind, such as the death of a loved one; divorce; or a change in careers.

8. Proper posture can augment health as it allows for the free flow of energy or Q^i.[2] Poor posture, skeletal misalignment, or muscular tension can block the free flow of energy in the system and can result in various health problems.

9. Indications of sleep deprivation include a decrease in attention span, irritability, slowed reaction time, an inability to perform tasks that require fine motor skills, reduction in the production of red blood cells, and altered body chemistries.

Other Types of Self-Assessment

1. Emotions have been described as etiologic factors of disease when they extend over a long period of time, when they are intense, and when they are not expressed but repressed. Because the body, mind, and emotions form a gestalt within the human being, emotions can also result from illness. Health and disease are multifactorial.
   a. Self-esteem has a great influence on all other aspects of well-being.
   b. Psychoneuroimmunologists have discovered connections between emotional states and the immune system, demonstrating that stress is associated with immunosuppression.
   c. According to Selye, there is eustress (positive stimulus) and distress (negative stimulus). The fact that eustress results in much less damage than distress suggests that it is how one perceives the stressor that makes the difference.[3]

   d. A significant body of research has linked emotional stress with cardiovascular and respiratory problems, which is easily understood in terms of the fight-or-flight mechanism in animal physiology.[4]

2. Mental/intellectual well-being can involve the ability to direct one's attention and perceive the world accurately.
   a. The intellect needs continual stimulation to optimize functioning.
   b. With interventions such as the relaxation response and meditation, individuals learn to participate with active attention to thought processes and to be present in the moment.

3. Social well-being is associated with open and honest communication.
   a. Different individuals satisfy different social needs.
   b. Social well-being involves both the ability to give to others in need and the ability to receive when in need oneself.

4. Spiritual well-being requires an awareness that human beings are part of the cosmos and that they do not exist in a vacuum.
   a. The spiritual dimension of our lives guides us in finding answers to questions about the meaning of life and death.
   b. Spirituality encompasses a belief in a more powerful being.

Self-Responsibility and Its Relationship to Optimizing Wellness

1. Self-confidence, assertiveness, decision-making ability, and openness to active participation in change make up self-responsibility.

2. The ability to assume self-responsibility must evolve as the personality develops.

3. Accepting personal accountability for the activation of one's inner resources can lead to optimal wellness.

4. The client and the practitioner are both assuming responsibility for the client's health/wellness.

5. Self-responsibility includes the capacity to make sound decisions and follow through with them.

6. Power is defined as the capacity to participate knowingly in the nature of human and environmental change, freedom to act intentionally, and involvement in creating change.[5]

Pause for a moment . . .

❏ *I find satisfaction in the art and science of holistic nursing.*
❏ *I find joy in assisting others toward the wholeness inherent within them.*
❏ *I love the broad and eclectic academic background of holistic nursing, which integrates artistic, scientific, analytic, and intuitive skills.*

HOLISTIC NURSING PROCESS

Assessment

1. The nurse evaluates the client's mental, physical, and emotional ability to do self-assessment.
2. The client makes a commitment to do self-assessment.

Nursing Diagnoses

1. Nursing diagnoses compatible with self-assessment interventions and related to the human response patterns of unitary person are as follows:
   a. Knowing: Knowledge deficit
               Altered thought process
   b. Feeling: Ineffective coping
               Self-esteem deficit
   c. Valuing: Powerlessness
               Spiritual distress
   d. Moving: Self-care deficit
               Sleep pattern disturbance
               Altered health maintenance
   e. Relating: Social isolation
               Altered role performance
               Impaired social interactions

Client Outcomes

1. Before the session, the nurse and the client establish desired outcomes.
2. The client will carry out self-assessments.

Plan and Interventions

1. Explain the positive effects on wellness by doing regular self-assessment; understanding the positive effects will promote active participation.
2. Demonstrate the self-assessment tools.

   a. Have the client explain the purpose of the self-assessment tools.
   b. Have the client give a return demonstration of the self-assessment tools.
3. Positively reinforce the client's compliance.

Physical Assessment Guidelines

1. Identify the client's current knowledge of holistic physical self-assessment (see Exhibits 16–1 and 16–6).
2. Provide the client with specific nutritional guidelines to assist in a self-assessment of nutritional status. A food intake inventory form may be helpful.
3. Teach the client about potential risk factors and ways to identify them:
   a. Hereditary illnesses within the client's family that can potentially weaken the constitution.
   b. Smoking history.
   c. Environmental risk factors, such as the exposure to radiation, pesticides, chemical-laden foods, and water, air, and noise pollution.
   d. Use of over-the-counter or prescription drugs, alcohol, and caffeine.
4. Provide the client with information on hygiene, principles of cleanliness, microorganisms, and the infectious process.
5. Educate the client on the benefits of daily exercise, including Yoga, and T'ai Chi, along with moderate aerobic exercise, such as walking or bicycling.
6. Discuss with the client for the purpose of self-assessment the following potential effects of the lack of exercise:
   a. Weak muscle tone and atrophied muscles.
   b. Increased blood sugar levels.
   c. Increased blood cholesterol levels.
   d. Decreased endurance for physical activities.
   e. Decreased cardiovascular tone.
   f. Decreased sense of well-being.
   g. Decreased ability to control weight.
7. Teach the client to assess his or her home and work environment for safety hazards.
8. Evaluate the client's ability to assess his or her own skills in emergency and first aid care, and provide necessary information.
9. Provide guidelines for the client to assess proper quality and quantity of sleep and rest; teach relaxation, imagery, and breathing exercises that the client can use to encourage restful sleep and clarity of thought.

Exhibit 16–1 Physical Self-Assessment

I	Most of the Time	Often	Sometimes	Seldom
Have a good level of energy	3	2	1	0
Exercise daily	3	2	1	0
Do not smoke	3	2	1	0
Drink alcohol in moderation	3	2	1	0
Consume limited amounts of saturated fats and refined sugars	3	2	1	0
Consume no artificial sweeteners	3	2	1	0
Have regular physical and dental checkups	3	2	1	0
Practice safe sex	3	2	1	0
Am aware of the potential negative effects of my prescription and over-the-counter drugs, as well as illegal drugs	3	2	1	0
Feel rested after a night's sleep	3	2	1	0

Physical Score _____

Source: Adapted from *Self-Care: A Program To Improve Your Life.* Lynn Keegan and Barbara Dossey with permission of Bodymind Systems, © 1987.

10. Explain how to use a physical self-assessment form, if available (Exhibits 16–1 and 16–6).

Mental Assessment Guidelines

1. Evaluate the client's ability to assess himself or herself mentally.
2. Explain that it is not possible to assess mental health in isolation from physical and emotional health. Health is inclusive of body, mind, and spirit. Good physical health can positively influence mental health and vice versa.
3. Discuss and explain the following specific areas of mental self-assessment:
   a. Problem solving.
   b. Cognitive ability, thought processes.
   c. Coping strategies.
   d. Perceptions of feelings/emotions.
   e. Developmental tasks.
   f. Role performance.
   g. Situational stressors.
4. Identify the role of poor nutrition, drugs, caffeine, and alcohol on mental state, as well as

Exhibit 16–2 Mental Self-Assessment

I	Most of the Time	Often	Sometimes	Seldom
Am open to new ideas	3	2	1	0
Have broad interest in many subjects	3	2	1	0
Set reasonable and challenging goals	3	2	1	0
Anticipate stress and am prepared to cope with it	3	2	1	0
Stay up-to-date on current events	3	2	1	0
Have a good attention span	3	2	1	0
Take care of my role responsibility	3	2	1	0

Mental Score _____

Source: Adapted from *Self-Care: A Program To Improve Your Life.* Lynn Keegan and Barbara Dossey with permission of Bodymind Systems, © 1987.

Exhibit 16–3 Social Self-Assessment

I	Most of the Time	Often	Sometimes	Seldom
Have a good support system	3	2	1	0
Make friends easily	3	2	1	0
Am assertive	3	2	1	0
Participate in activities that help meet the needs of others	3	2	1	0
Feel that I am a productive part of society	3	2	1	0
Participate in social activities with family and friends	3	2	1	0
Trust others easily	3	2	1	0
Am open and honest in my relationships with others	3	2	1	0

Social Score _____

Source: Adapted from *Self-Care: A Program To Improve Your Life.* Lynn Keegan and Barbara Dossey with permission of Bodymind Systems, © 1987.

ways to assess their negative effects on one's own mental functioning.

5. Explain how to use a mental self-assessment form, if available (Exhibits 16–2 and 16–6).

Social Assessment Guidelines

1. Evaluate the client's ability to assess himself or herself socially.
2. Discuss and explain the following areas of social self-assessment:

a. Social support (e.g., significant others who give one a subjective feeling of belonging).
b. Adequate means for communication with others.
c. Relationships with others.
d. Self-actualization (i.e., fulfilling one's potential).
e. Social, cultural, and ethnic identity (i.e., links with the past or present that give a sense of belonging).

Exhibit 16–4 Emotional Self-Assessment

I	Most of the Time	Often	Sometimes	Seldom
Have a high level of self-esteem	3	2	1	0
Acknowledge and accept my feelings	3	2	1	0
Accept others' feelings without judgment	3	2	1	0
Am able to express my feelings appropriately	3	2	1	0
Have an adequate means for self-expression	3	2	1	0
Know that not expressing emotions can lead to illness	3	2	1	0
Seek help when I am not dealing effectively with my emotions	3	2	1	0
Feel a sense of contentment with my life	3	2	1	0

Emotional Score _____

Source: Adapted from *Self-Care: A Program To Improve Your Life.* Lynn Keegan and Barbara Dossey with permission of Bodymind Systems, © 1987.

Exhibit 16–5 Spiritual Self-Assessment

I	*Most of the Time*	*Often*	*Sometimes*	*Seldom*
Center, pray, or meditate daily	3	2	1	0
Have a relationship with a higher power	3	2	1	0
Attend regular religious services	3	2	1	0
Live in accordance with my spiritual values	3	2	1	0
Am tolerant of others' spiritual beliefs	3	2	1	0
Have faith in other human beings	3	2	1	0
Believe that the universe has meaning	3	2	1	0

Spiritual Score _____

Source: Adapted from *Self-Care: A Program To Improve Your Life.* Lynn Keegan and Barbara Dossey with permission of Bodymind Systems, © 1987.

---

f. Contribution to others, society and generative behaviors.

3. Explain how to use a social self-assessment form, if available (Exhibit 16–3).

Emotional Assessment Guidelines

1. Evaluate the client's ability to assess himself or herself emotionally (see Exhibits 16–4 and 16–6).
2. Explain the connection between the emotions and illness.
3. Discuss and explain the following areas of emotional self-assessment:
   a. Acknowledgment and acceptance of one's feelings.
   b. Acknowledgment and acceptance of others' feelings.
   c. Ability to express feelings appropriately.
   d. Available means for self-expression.
   e. Healthful self-concept, level of self-esteem, self-understanding.
   f. Healthful acceptance of body and physical appearance.
4. Help the client to understand the role of emotional self-assessment and to seek outside help for emotional difficulties when needed.
5. Explain how to use an emotional self-assessment form, if available (Exhibit 16–4).

Spiritual Assessment Guidelines

1. Evaluate the client's ability to assess himself or herself spiritually (Exhibits 16–5 and 16–6).
2. Discuss and explain the following areas of spiritual self-assessment:

a. Centering daily through prayer, meditation, or some other activity that produces inner awareness.

b. Identification of a higher power in his or her life to clarify the meaning and purpose of existence.

Exhibit 16–6 Self-Assessment Scores

Total Scores of 91–120

Your score demonstrates a high potential for achieving and maintaining optimum wellness. You are setting a good example for your family and friends by assuming responsibility for your health and well-being.

Total Scores of 60–90

Your health patterns are good in this area but you need to improve in some aspects of this category. Examine the "Seldom and Sometimes" answers to see how you can improve your score.

Total Scores of 30–59

Your score shows that you are lacking knowledge to maintain a sufficient level of health.

Total Scores of 0–29

You are not practicing healthy lifestyle patterns. If you make the appropriate changes now, you will be able to avoid potential illness.

Source: Adapted from *Self-Care: A Program To Improve Your Life.* Lynn Keegan and Barbara Dossey with permission of Bodymind Systems, © 1987.

    c. Regular attendance at religious services, if personally satisfying.

    d. Living and acting from one's spiritual values and beliefs.

    e. View of death and the acceptance of it.

3. Explain how to use a spiritual self-assessment form, if available (Exhibit 16–5).

Evaluation

1. It is essential to determine if client outcomes were achieved.

2. The client's skill of self-assessment and the regularity of the client's self-assessment must be evaluated (Exhibit 16–6).

REFERENCES

1. G. Maciocia, *The Foundations of Chinese Medicine* (New York: Churchill Livingstone, 1989), 135.

2. T. Sohn, *A Complete Textbook of Oriental Bodywork and Medical Principles* (Rochester, VT: Healing Arts Press, 1996).

3. M. Oermann, *Professional Nursing Practice* (Philadelphia: J.B. Lippincott Co., 1991), 59–62.

4. D. Ornish, *Reversing Heart Disease* (New York: Ballantine Books, 1990), 139–142.

5. E. Barret, *Visions of Rogers' Science-Based Nursing* (New York: National League for Nursing, 1990), 105–108.

CHAPTER 17

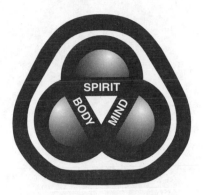

Cognitive Therapy

Eileen M. Stuart and Carol L. Wells-Federman

KNOWLEDGE COMPETENCIES

- Discuss the physiologic effects of cognitions.
- Identify the potential biopsychosocial responses to stress and their effects on health and illness.
- Identify four major contributors to the development of cognitive theory.
- Discuss the major diagnoses and health problems that respond favorably to cognitive therapy.
- Identify the three main principles of cognitive therapy.
- Discuss the roles of contracting and goal setting in cognitive restructuring.
- Describe ways to facilitate cognitive restructuring.
- Identify stress warning signals.
- Describe and identify automatic thoughts.
- Describe and identify cognitive distortions and irrational beliefs.
- Describe a simple model for cognitive restructuring.
- Discuss guidelines for organizing a session.
- Describe different practice settings in which cognitive restructuring can be used.
- Evaluate client progress toward goals by assessing both short-term and long-term goals of therapy.

DEFINITIONS[1,2]

Cognition: the act or process of knowing; perception, including both awareness and judgment.
Cognitive: of, relating to, or being conscious; intellectual activities (as thinking, reasoning, imagining).
Cognitive Distortions: inaccurate, defective thinking; irrational thoughts.

Cognitive Restructuring: examining and reframing one's interpretation of the meaning of an event.
Cognitive Therapy: a therapeutic approach that addresses the relationships among thoughts, feelings, beliefs, behaviors, and physiology. Cognitive therapy was first used as a short-term treatment for depression and anxiety, but it has been successfully applied in reducing health-risking behaviors, physical symptoms, and the emotional sequelae of a variety of medical illnesses.

Pause for a moment . . .

- ❏ *I believe that health and disease are part of the human experience.*
- ❏ *My holistic nursing knowledge helps me to understand that health involves the harmonious balance of body, mind, and spirit in an ever changing environment.*

THEORIES AND RESEARCH

Effects of Cognitions on Health and Illness

1. The major theorists responsible for developing cognitive therapy include Aaron Beck,[3] Albert Ellis,[4] Donald Meichenbaum,[5] and David Burns.[6]
2. Psychologic stress (the perception of a threat) can stimulate a cascade of significant biochemical events initiated by the central nervous system[7] (Figure 17-1).

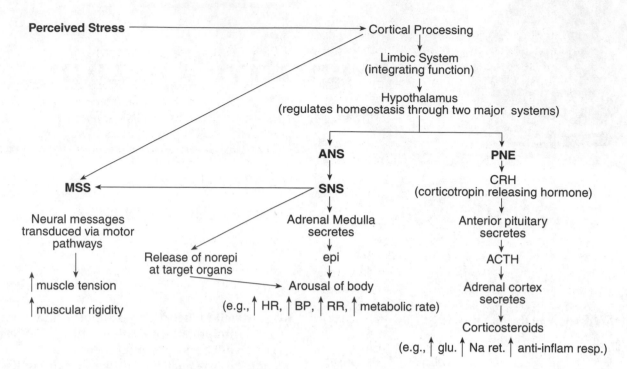

Figure 17–1 Stress Response. *Source:* Reprinted with permission from C.L. Wells-Federman, et al., *Clinical Nurse Specialist,* Vol. 9, No. 1, p. 60, © 1995, Williams & Wilkins.

a. Termed the fight-or-flight response by Walter B. Cannon and the stress response by Hans Selye, this heightened state of sympathetic arousal affects the skeletal musculature, the autonomic nervous system, and the neuroendocrine system.

b. Acute and chronic responses to stress differ, both in etiology and psychophysiologic response.

c. Prolonged negative mood states such as depression, anxiety, hostility, and anger have been correlated with increased morbidity and mortality in certain diseases.

d. The influence of stress on the etiology and exacerbations of a wide variety of illnesses is documented in extensive experimental and clinical literature.[8]

3. Behavior patterns, such as how and what individuals eat, drink, smoke, and exercise, as well as how they take prescribed or illegal drugs, have important ramifications on the incidence and progression of disease.

a. Stressful events can increase unhealthy behaviors, such as overeating or excessive drinking of alcohol. The inability to control health-risking behaviors in the presence of increased stress is called the "stress-disinhibition effect."

b. Social isolation, which may be influenced by stress and negative thinking patterns, has been shown to be associated with higher morbidity and mortality in the first year after myocardial infarction.[9]

c. Stress hardiness has been shown to correlate with decreased incidence of illness.[10] Individuals who were classified as stress hardy engaged in social support, exercised, and viewed life with a sense of commitment (as opposed to alienation), challenge (as opposed to threat), and control (as opposed to helplessness/hopelessness).

d. An optimistic explanatory style has been associated with better health.[11]

e. A study demonstrating lifestyle change across biopsychosocial domains showed a regression of coronary atherosclerosis.[12]

4. In a 30-year retrospective, Beck gave a comprehensive overview of several outcome studies.[13]

a. A meta-analysis of 27 studies has demonstrated the efficacy of cognitive therapy in unipolar depression and its superiority to other treatments, including the administration of antidepressant drugs.

b. Five published studies have indicated that cognitive therapy has a greater effect on maintaining gains and preventing relapses than does antidepressant medication.

c. An almost complete reduction of panic attacks after 12 to 16 weeks of treatment has been reported.

d. The successful application of cognitive therapy to generalized anxiety disorder, eating disorders, heroin addiction, and inpatient depression has been reported.

5. Emmelkamp and van Oppen published an overview of the contribution of cognitive approaches to a reduction in physical symptoms and emotional sequelae in hypertension, bulimia, chronic pain, tension headache, AIDS, cancer, and asthma.[14]

6. Other authors have reported its effective use for insomnia,[15] infertility,[16] and medically unexplained physical symptoms.[17]

7. Cognitive therapy, as integrated into behavioral medicine and clinical health psychology, has been shown to be cost-effective.[18]

Cognitive Restructuring

1. The basic principles of cognitive therapy are as follows:[19,20]

a. Our thoughts, not external events, create our moods.

b. The thoughts that cause stress are usually unrealistic, distorted, and negative.

c. Distorted, illogical thoughts and self-defeating beliefs lead to painful feelings, such as depression, anxiety, and anger.

d. By changing maladaptive, unrealistic, distorted thoughts, we can change how we feel.

2. The basic goals of cognitive therapy include training clients to accomplish the following:[21]

a. Pinpoint the negative automatic thoughts and silent assumptions that trigger and perpetuate their emotional upsets.

b. Identify the distortions, irrational beliefs, or "cognitive errors."

c. Substitute more realistic, self-enhancing thoughts, which will reduce the stress, symptoms, and/or painful feelings.

d. Replace self-defeating "silent assumptions" with more reasonable belief systems.

e. Improve social skills, as well as coping, communication, and empathic skills.

Pause for a moment . . .

❑ *I view disease and distress as opportunities for increased awareness of the interconnectedness of body, mind, and spirit.*

❑ *The teaching–learning process enables me to assist clients to assume personal responsibility for their own health.*

HOLISTIC NURSING PROCESS

Assessment

1. Before using cognitive therapy interventions, the nurse assesses the following parameters:

a. The client's ability to monitor/appraise inner dialogue and communicate.

b. The client's ability to identify stress warning signals.

c. The client's perception of the problem.

d. The client's readiness/openness to changing thoughts or behaviors.

2. The client's level of experience with each of the interventions to be used is also important.

Nursing Diagnoses

1. The following nursing diagnoses compatible with cognitive therapy are related to the human response patterns:[20]

a. Communicating:	Altered verbal/nonverbal communications
b. Relating:	Altered, actual or potential Impaired social interaction Social isolation Parenting
c. Choosing:	Coping, ineffective individual and family
d. Perceiving:	Altered self-concept Disturbance in self-esteem, body image, role performance, personal identity
e. Knowing:	Altered thought processes
f. Feeling:	Anxiety, fear

Client Outcomes

1. Long-term goals (outcomes) are established prior to therapy, and short-term goals are set prior to each session.

2. Goals are set with the client and must be mutually acceptable.
3. A general list of optimal cognitive therapy outcomes is that the client will be able to accomplish the following:
   a. Recognize connections among cognitions, emotions, behaviors, and physiology.
   b. Identify physical, psychologic, and behavioral stress warning signals.
   c. Demonstrate the ability to recognize cognitive distortions, and examine the evidence for and against key beliefs.
   d. Change the way that he or she thinks (views situations), and try out alternative conceptualizations or more rational responses independently.
   e. Report a decrease in arousal, anxiety, fear, depression, or somatic complaints and an elevation in well-being after correcting cognitive distortions.

Plan and Interventions

1. Establish a therapeutic relationship.
2. Create a space in which both you and the client feel physically and emotionally comfortable.
3. Provide materials for recording cognitive distortions and alternative rational thoughts and statements (e.g., paper and pen, blackboard, pre-printed forms).
4. Center yourself; clear your mind of personal or professional issues in order to be fully present and nonjudging.
5. Establish the long-term goals (outcome) of therapy with the client.
6. Assess the client's level of anxiety, discomfort, or relaxation.
7. Review homework from the previous session, if appropriate. Have the client describe any changes that have occurred since the previous session.
8. Determine, with the client, which issues need to be addressed, and set short-term goals for the session.
9. Listen and guide with focused intention. Provide appropriate feedback, clarification, support, or interpretation.
10. Have the client identify and verbalize changes that have occurred during the session. Assess progress toward goals.
11. Assign homework to be done for the next session.

Facilitating the Process of Cognitive Therapy

1. Serve as a guide.
2. Accept the fact that there is no way to predict what will surface, or the meaning that it has to this client.
3. Recognizing that each individual is the best interpreter of his or her own experience, belief, and distortion, assume a nonjudging, reflective listening style.
4. Review the effects of cognitions on health and illness.
5. Review the principles and goals of cognitive therapy.
6. Begin each session with a brief exercise to elicit the relaxation response. Refer to Chapter 23 for information on relaxation.

The Process of Cognitive Therapy

1. In order to facilitate changes, help the client to understand the relationship between thoughts, feelings, behavior, and biology.
2. Monitor the warning signals of stress.
   a. Often, clients have ignored the cues that their body, feelings, thoughts, or behaviors give them.
   b. When asked to monitor their physical/emotional/behavioral/spiritual responses to a particular event, they begin to collect the data that will enable them to be more consciously aware of these cues.
   c. Although it may initially increase a client's perception of physical pain or emotional discomfort, conscious awareness is a necessary first step in recognizing the relationship of thoughts, feelings, behavior, and biology to distorted thinking patterns.
   d. It is important to encourage clients to be aware of stress warning signals as valuable cues that help develop skills to reduce negative mood states, unhealthy behaviors, and physical symptoms and to lead them toward a healthier life.
      1) Have the client identify his or her stress warning signals. Exhibit 17–1 is a sample form for identifying/recording such information.
      2) Have the client identify a stressful experience and his or her physical and emotional reaction to this particular experience. Exhibit 17–2 is an example of a format for recording this information.

Exhibit 17–1 Stress Warning Signals

Physical Symptoms
- ❏ Headaches
- ❏ Indigestion
- ❏ Stomachaches
- ❏ Sweaty palms
- ❏ Sleep difficulties
- ❏ Dizziness
- ❏ Back pain
- ❏ Tight neck, shoulders
- ❏ Racing heart
- ❏ Restlessness
- ❏ Tiredness
- ❏ Ringing in ears

Behavioral Symptoms
- ❏ Excess smoking
- ❏ Bossiness
- ❏ Compulsive gum chewing
- ❏ Attitude critical of others
- ❏ Grinding of teeth at night
- ❏ Overuse of alcohol
- ❏ Compulsive eating
- ❏ Inability to get things done

Emotional Symptoms
- ❏ Crying
- ❏ Nervousness, anxiety
- ❏ Boredom—no meaning to things
- ❏ Edginess—ready to explode
- ❏ Feeling powerless to change things
- ❏ Overwhelming sense of pressure
- ❏ Anger
- ❏ Loneliness
- ❏ Unhappiness for no reason
- ❏ Easily upset

Cognitive Symptoms
- ❏ Trouble thinking clearly
- ❏ Forgetfulness
- ❏ Lack of creativity
- ❏ Memory loss
- ❏ Inability to make decisions
- ❏ Thoughts of running away
- ❏ Constant worry
- ❏ Loss of sense of humor

Do any seem familiar to you?

Check the ones you experience when under stress. These are your stress warning signs.

Are there any additional stress warning signals that you experience that are not listed? If so, add them here.

_____

_____

_____

_____

_____

Source: Reprinted with permission from H. Benson and E.M. Stuart, *The Wellness Book*, p. 182, © 1992, Carol Publishing.

3. Monitor automatic thoughts.
   a. Cognitive therapy encourages clients to see that their stress does not always come from an outside event or situation, but from the way that they interpret these events.
   b. Cognitions, such as the inner dialogue, perceptions, and fantasies that represent the meanings attached to the events, influence moods, feelings, and behaviors in the present.
   c. These thoughts usually occur automatically in response to a situation.
   d. Clients are trained to identify these self-defeating "automatic thoughts."
   e. Negative automatic thoughts have certain characteristics in common:
      1) Reflex or knee-jerk responses to a perceived stressor.
      2) Quick, fleeting, a kind of shorthand.
      3) Usually not in one's conscious awareness.
      4) Frequently unrealistic, illogical, and distorted.
   f. Automatic thoughts are powerful because
      1) The body does not know the difference between things imagined and things actually experienced.
      2) We are always talking to ourselves, and after saying something to ourselves often enough, we begin to believe it.
      3) We rarely stop to question our thoughts or emotions.

4. Identify distortions.
   a. Through years of research and clinical experience, Burns has identified 10 general categories of "cognitive distortions" that lead to negative emotional states:[23]
      1) All-or-nothing thinking: polarized or dichotomous thinking, viewing things in black or white. The person sees himself

Exhibit 17–2 Challenging Stress and Winning—Stop, Take a Breath, Reflect, Choose

Situation	Physical Response	Automatic Thoughts	Moods and Emotions
Briefly describe a situation that caused you stress this week.	Describe how you felt physically in this situation.	Write your automatic thoughts in this situation.	Describe how you felt emotionally in this situation.

Exaggerated Beliefs	Behavior	More Effective Response	Potential Outcome
Write down the exaggerated beliefs behind your automatic thoughts.	Describe how you behaved during or immediately after the situation.	Describe how you might think or act differently that would help you cope more effectively.	Describe how this might make you feel and behave.

Source: Reprinted with permission from H. Benson and E.M. Stuart, *The Wellness Book,* pp. 244–245, © 1992, Carol Publishing.

as a total failure when a performance falls short of perfect. For example, at the end of a performance where the sender got a standing ovation, one person came back stage to congratulate her, and suggest that there was one song he didn't care for. The singer's automatic response was, "I shouldn't have done that song, I can't sing it very well. It ruined the performance."

2) Overgeneralization: viewing a single negative event as a never-ending pattern. For example, "Fixing my car cost twice what they said it would. All mechanics are dishonest and always will be."

3) Mental filter: picking out a negative detail and dwelling on it exclusively, "catastrophizing" or "awfulizing." For example, "I got a lousy grade on that test. I'll probably have to drop out of school. I won't be able to find a decent job and will have to move back in with my parents."

4) Disqualifying the positive. Positive experiences are discounted as if they are not important. The person is unable to accept praise. For example, "You're just saying that because you have to."

5) Jumping to conclusions: reading the minds of others or predicting negative outcomes without sufficient evidence or validation. For example, "He went off to bed without saying anything. He's angry with me for working late again."

6) Magnification: exaggerating the importance of mistakes or inappropriately minimizing the significance of one's assets. For example, "My performance tonight was horrible—I'll never get the lead part."

7) Emotional reasoning: assuming that one's emotions reflect the way things are. For example, "I feel worthless; therefore, I must be worthless."

8) "Should" statements: trying to motivate oneself with shoulds and shouldn'ts. For example, "Good employees should always get to the office early and be willing to stay late."

9) Labeling: name calling; labeling one self "a loser" if a mistake is made; an illogical leap from one characteristic to a category. For example, "She's blond, what do you expect? She's an airhead."

10) Personalization: blaming oneself inappropriately as the cause of a negative event; seeing events only in relation to oneself. For example, "It's my fault that Mary is upset after breaking up with Mike because I introduced them."

b. Helping clients recognize unrealistic, illogical, or distorted negative thoughts is the first step in cognitive therapy. (See Exhibit 17–2.)

5. Recognize silent assumptions and underlying beliefs.

a. Unrealistic, illogical, and distorted automatic thoughts are a result of deeply held silent assumptions and beliefs.

b. A client's vulnerability to a stressor is often dependent upon how absolute these assumptions or beliefs are held.

c. Everyone has a right to beliefs and opinions; problems develop only when these beliefs are held as absolutes and, therefore, provide no room for flexibility in an imperfect world.

d. Because these strongly held assumptions and beliefs are mostly "silent" or out of conscious awareness, it is a challenge to identify them and determine their influence on thoughts, emotions, and behaviors.

e. One technique that is helpful in assisting the discovery of these underlying assumptions and beliefs is the "vertical arrow technique" developed by Burns.[24]

6. Restructure distortions and beliefs.

a. Train the client to recognize personal stress warning signals (thoughts, feelings, or behaviors) and apply a four-step restructuring technique:[25]

1) Stop. The simple act of saying "Stop" can help break a pattern of automatic response before thoughts escalate into the worst possible scenario.

2) Breathe. Physically taking a deep diaphragmatic breath can be important because during times of stress, most people hold their breath. Taking a deep breath can elicit the physiology of the relaxation response, the opposite of the stress response. Be aware of stress warning signs.

3) Reflect. Clients should learn to ask themselves several questions about the automatic thoughts and underlying beliefs: Is this thought true? Is this thought helpful? Apply the vertical arrow technique.

4) Choose. Substituting more realistic, self-enhancing thoughts will reduce the painful feelings. Replace self-defeating "silent assumptions."

b. In addition to the exercise suggested in Exhibit 17–2, journaling can help clients uncover cognitive distortions and irrational beliefs and provide a meaningful way to restructure cognitive distortions and irrational beliefs.

Setting Goals

1. Goals should be specific, concrete, and measurable; in addition, they should be achievable.
2. Outcomes that are mutually agreed upon by both client and provider prior to the initiation of cognitive therapy form the basis for long- and short-term goals. Clients are more likely to accomplish goals if they have had an integral part in establishing those goals.
3. The process of establishing outcomes should take into account the client's
   a. Beliefs about health and illness (i.e., health belief model).
   b. Experience with healthy behaviors (i.e., health behaviors).
   c. Self-awareness, self-monitoring (i.e., self-efficacy theory, self-regulation theory).
   d. Stage of change and readiness to change (i.e., change theory, the transtheoretical model).
   e. Motivation to change (i.e., the dynamics of motivation).
   f. Understanding of the relationship between illness/wellness and behavior (i.e., dynamics of health-wellness-disease-illness).
   g. Preferences (i.e., client rights).
   h. Attitudes, beliefs, and values.
4. Goal setting is a dynamic process that involves both the client and the nurse at each level:
   a. Accumulating a complete bio-psycho-social-spiritual database that is appropriate to the setting and diagnosis.
   b. Using a values clarification exercise (Chapter 7) and picture drawing (Chapter 10) to facilitate a more complete bodymind database.
   c. Reviewing and discussing data from the database and information from the values clarification and picture drawing exercise.
   d. Identifying problems to be addressed in the intervention.
   e. Prioritizing problems.

f. Setting mutually agreed upon long- and short-term goals.

5. To facilitate goal setting, nurses may make a variety of suggestions to clients.
   a. Assess the rewards or secondary gains that you get from illness or ill health. Set goals that allow you to achieve rewards from health rather than from sickness.
   b. Clarify values. Determine what is important, meaningful to you. Begin to focus on those things to sustain meaning and purpose in your life.
   c. Use the 2 × 50 rule of goal setting. State your goal. Then double the amount of time needed to accomplish the goal, or reduce its difficulty by 50 percent. For example, losing 10 pounds in the next month is likely an unrealistic goal; losing 10 pounds in the next 2 months or losing 5 pounds in the next month is probably a more realistic, attainable goal. Smaller, more attainable goals create a sense of achievement, build self-esteem, and foster enthusiasm to set further goals.
   d. Ask yourself the following questions to identify long-term goals:[26]
      1) What would you most like to change about your life right now?
      2) How can you begin the first step in that change?
      3) On what date would you like to achieve that goal?
      4) How can you reward yourself for success?
      5) How will your life be different when you succeed?
6. Rewards can enhance goal attainment.
   a. Clients often find it difficult to identify appropriate rewards. Rewards should be congruent with the difficulty of the goal set. The nurse can help the client keep in mind that rewards need not cost money or even be tangible.
   b. In some circumstances, the nurse may reward a client for successful completion of a goal. Ideally, however, clients learn to self-reward as they gain independence in self-monitoring and self-regulation.
7. Establishing a health contract can increase the quality of communication between the client and nurse and can also help a client become a more willing participant in self-care.[27] Not achieving the goals of the contract opens the

door to a discussion of the reasons and of the best ways to modify behavior(s) to achieve a mutually agreed upon goal.

a. Successful attainment of contract goals is dependent on skills the client learns during the process of developing the contract. This process provides the opportunity to analyze behaviors in relationship to the environment and to choose strategies that facilitate learning, changing, or maintaining a behavior.

b. The contracting process has several steps.[28]

1) Behavioral analysis focuses on events that precede the behavior, small steps that make up the behavior, and consequences that follow the behavior.

2) Self-monitoring is used to collect data for the behavioral analysis. Based on the behavioral analysis, strategies are chosen to support the client's behavioral change. Strategies include rearranging antecedent events, practicing small steps of behavior, and rearranging consequences.

c. Contracts may be verbal, but all parties are more likely to take written contracts seriously. If the contracts are written, both the client and the nurse should sign them.

d. Contracts should always contain these key elements:

1) A concrete, attainable, measurable goal.

2) A time for completion, as well as times to evaluate progress toward goals.

3) The responsibilities of involved parties (e.g., client and nurse, client and spouse).

4) An identified reward for achieving the stated goal.

e. In establishing a contract, the nurse's role is that of facilitator. After introducing the concept of contracting and identifying the reasons that such an approach may be valid in the client's circumstances, the nurse may limit his or her involvement to guidance and support.

Applying the General Principles of Cognitive Therapy[29]

1. Cognitive therapy is useful primarily for individual mood problems, not for relationship or interpersonal conflict.

2. This therapy requires constant shifting between technique and process. It is a combination of resolving problems with cognitive and behavioral techniques while focusing empathically on the client's feelings. The process requires the skills of presence, intention, and communication.

3. Nurses must be imaginative and tenacious. It may take several sessions and several different ways of looking at a situation before a client recognizes the automatic thoughts and underlying beliefs involved.

4. To help change a person's mood, a rational response must be 100 percent valid. Distortions of the truth will not be helpful. The rational response must put the "lie" to the automatic thought.

5. There are two ways of dealing with negative thoughts:

a. Confrontation: proving that the automatic thought or underlying belief is distorted or untrue.

b. Acceptance: finding the truth in the negative thought and accepting it. This is a form of the vertical arrow technique.

6. Cognitive therapy can be used in both the inpatient and outpatient setting, but the goals and process are different and need to be clearly identified.[30]

a. The goal of cognitive therapy in the hospital setting is typically confined to assisting the patient to cope more effectively with the stress of hospitalization and acute illness. Long-standing issues are more appropriately dealt with in follow-up in the outpatient setting.

b. Outpatient cognitive therapy can be provided either individually or in groups.

Evaluation

1. The client outcomes that were established prior to initiating cognitive therapy and the client's subjective experiences can be used to evaluate progress toward long-term *goals*.

2. The client outcomes that were established prior to starting the session and the client's subjective experience can be used to evaluate progress toward short-term goals.

3. It may be necessary to schedule a follow-up session.

REFERENCES

1. A.R. Childress and D.D. Burns, The Basics of Cognitive Therapy, *Psychosomatics* 22, no. 12 (1981): 1017–1027.

2. D. Webster, *Webster's New Encyclopedic Dictionary* (New York: Black Dog and Leventhal Pub., 1994).

3. A.T. Beck, *Cognitive Therapy* (New York: New American Library, 1979).

4. A. Ellis et al., *Handbook of Rational–Emotive Therapy,* Vol. 2 (New York: Springer Publishing Co., 1986).

5. D. Meichenbaum, *Cognitive Behavior Modification: An Integrative Approach* (New York: Plenum Press, 1977).

6. D.D. Burns, *Ten Days to Self-Esteem* (New York: William Morrow, 1993).

7. C. Wells-Federman et al., The Mind/Body Connection: The Psychophysiology of Many Traditional Nursing Interventions, *Clinical Nurse Specialist* 9, no. 1 (1995): 59–65.

8. R.J. Gatchel et al., *Psychophysiological Disorders: Research and Clinical Applications* (Washington, DC: American Psychological Association, 1993).

9. N. Frasure-Smith and R. Prince, The Ischemic Heart Disease Life Stress Monitoring Program: Impact on Mortality, *Psychosomatic Medicine* 47, no. 5 (1985): 431–445.

10. S.C. Kobasa et al., Hardiness and Health: A Prospective Study, *Journal of Personality and Social Psychology* 42, no. 1 (1982): 168–177.

11. R.C. Colligan et al., CAVEing the MMPI for an Optimism–Pessimism Scale: Seligman's Attributional Model and the Assessment of Explanatory Style, *Journal of Clinical Psychology* 50, no. 1 (1994): 71–95.

12. D. Ornish et al., Can Lifestyle Changes Reverse Coronary Heart Disease? The Lifestyle Heart Trial. *Lancet* 336, no. 8708 (1990): 129–133.

13. A.T. Beck, Cognitive Therapy: A 30-year Retrospective, *American Psychologist* (1991): 368–375.

14. P.M. Emmelkamp and P. van Oppen, Cognitive Interventions in Behavioral Medicine [Review], *Psychotherapy and Psychosomatics* 59 (1993): 116–130.

15. G.D. Jacobs et al., Home-Based Central Nervous System Assessment of a Multifactor Behavioral Intervention for Chronic Sleep-Onset Insomnia, *Behavior Therapy* 24 (1993): 159–174.

16. A.D. Domar et al., The Mind/Body Program for Infertility: A New Behavioral Treatment Approach for Women with Infertility, *Fertility and Sterility* 53 (1990): 246–249.

17. A.E. Speckens et al., Cognitive Behavioural Therapy for Medically Unexplained Physical Symptoms: A Randomised Controlled Trial, *British Medical Journal* 311, no. 7016 (1995): 1328–1332.

18. R. Friedman, Behavioral Medicine, Clinical Health Psychology, and Cost Offset [Review], *Health Psychology* 14, no. 6 (1995): 509–518.

19. Burns, *Ten Days to Self-Esteem.*

20. Childress and Burns, Basics of Cognitive Therapy.

21. Ibid.

22. B.M. Dossey et al., *Holistic Nursing: A Handbook for Practice,* 2nd ed. (Gaithersburg, MD: Aspen Publishers, 1995).

23. D.D. Burns, *The Feeling Good Handbook: Using the New Mood Therapy in Everyday Life* (New York: William Morrow, 1989).

24. Ibid.

25. E.M. Stuart et al., Managing Stress, in *The Wellness Book: The Comprehensive Guide to Maintaining Health and Treating Stress-related Illness,* ed. H. Benson and E. Stuart (New York: Fireside, Simon & Schuster, 1993), 177–188.

26. Dossey et al., *Holistic Nursing: A Handbook for Practice.*

27. Ibid.

28. S. Boehm, Patient Contracting, in *Nursing Interventions: Essential Nursing Treatments,* 2nd ed., ed. G.M. Bulechek and J.C. McCloskey (Philadelphia: W.B. Saunders, 1992), 425–433.

29. Burns, *The Feeling Good Handbook.*

30. Stuart et al., Managing Stress.

CHAPTER 18

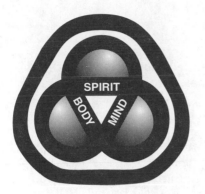

Nutrition

Susan Luck

KNOWLEDGE COMPETENCIES

- Discuss the biochemical effects of nutrition on physiology.
- Describe the effects of dietary fats on health and disease.
- Explore the relationship between nutrient intake and immune function.
- Explore nutrition and the aging process.
- Examine the relationships of nutrition to emotions and mental health.
- Explore nutrition as a key to wellness.
- Describe dietary guidelines for optimal health.
- Explore attitudes, beliefs, and cultural influences on diet and nutrition.
- Explore nutritional interventions for weight management.
- Describe environmental influences that affect nutrition and health.
- Explore self-assessment tools and self-care strategies for enhancing nutrition awareness.
- Explore nutrition as part of the nursing process.

DEFINITIONS

Nutrition: the relationship of foods to the health of the individual.
Nutritional Components: all of the essential nutrients—carbohydrates, fats, proteins, vitamins, minerals, fiber, and water.
Optimal Nutrition: adequate intake of nutrients for health promotion and disease prevention.

 Pause for a moment . . .

❑ *As I study the **AHNA Core Curriculum for Holistic Nursing,** I am better able to promote the education of nurses and the public in the concepts and practice of health of the whole person.*
❑ *I become more aware that holistic nursing embraces all nursing practice that has healing the whole person as its goal.*

THEORIES AND RESEARCH

Physiologic Connections of Nutrition to Health and Illness

1. Good nutrition is essential for normal organ development and functioning; normal reproduction, growth, and maintenance; resistance to infection and disease; ability to repair body damage or injury; and optimal activity and energy levels.
   a. Individuals can be taught how to improve their nutritional intake to produce positive health and enhance the healing process.
   b. Macronutrients are the proteins, carbohydrates, and lipids (fats) that make up the greatest portion of the human diet, providing calories and regulating body heat and energy production.

1) *Carbohydrates* provide the main source of energy for all body functions, aiding in digestion, assimilation, and metabolism of proteins and fats. Carbohydrates are classified as simple and complex.

2) *Proteins* provide the structure for maintaining cellular function and integrity. Complete proteins consist of all of the essential amino acids.

3) *Fats* are concentrated sources of heat and energy. Fats are classified according to their chemical composition: fatty acids, glycosides, phospholipids, glycolipids, sterols, and lipoproteins. The different classifications have different functions, health benefits, and health risk factors.

c. Micronutrients are the vitamins and minerals that are essential for biochemical transformations. Vitamins and minerals in foods are bonded to carbohydrates, proteins, and lipids.

1) Vitamins assist in the regulation of metabolism and in the release of energy from digested foods. They act as catalysts, along with enzymes, and as activators in ongoing chemical reactions. Antioxidant vitamins protect cells from oxidative stress. (See Table 18–1.)

2) Minerals are naturally occurring elements found in earth; they are essential in the formation and integrity of body fluids, blood, bone, and nervous system.

d. Nutritional deficiencies result whenever inadequate amounts of nutrients are provided to cells, tissues, organs, and systems over a prolonged period of time. Metabolic function is dependent on their synergistic effects. (See Table 18–2.)[1]

2. Optimal nutrition is dependent on many different factors, including biochemical individuality, genetic predisposition, enzyme activity, and the body's ability to digest, absorb, and eliminate adequately.

3. Nutritional deficiencies and the disease process are positively correlated.

a. Dietary and nutritional interventions are associated with improved health status in many degenerative disease processes, including heart disease, diabetes, and cancer.[2]

b. New guidelines and research focus on health promotion.

1) New guidelines for nutrition under the food pyramid.[3]

2) Recommended daily allowances (RDAs) and optimal daily allowances (ODAs).[4]

Dietary Fats, Health, and Disease

1. Fats consumed in the diet have a direct effect on maintaining health.[5]

a. Saturated fats, found in animal products, and some plant-derived sources (e.g., coconut) increase the risk of coronary artery disease, diabetes, colon and breast cancer, obesity, and immune dysfunction.

b. Omega 3 and Omega 6 essential fatty acids and immune function.

c. Transfatty acids and the disease process.

d. Elevated cholesterol and high-density lipoprotein levels are risk factors in coronary artery disease.

e. Low-fat/high-fiber diet guidelines are associated with decreased risk of cardiovascular disease.

f. Low fiber intake is associated with increased bile acids in the intestines, constipation, diverticulosis, colon cancer, and other gastrointestinal disorders. Soluble fibers, including guar gum and pectin, have beneficial effects on cholesterol and high-density lipoprotein levels.

g. Reduced consumption of refined and processed sugars and starches decreases the level of tryglycerides.

h. Rancidity in heated fats and oils contributes to oxidative stress and free radical formation.

2. Physiologic changes occur when an individual follows low-fat diet guidelines.

3. Food preparation procedures can lower fat consumption.

4. It is essential to read food labels for fat content and other ingredients.

Nutrition and the Aging Process

1. Nutrient requirements increase with aging.[6]

2. Wellness programs include assessment of nutritional needs for early intervention and prevention.

3. Nutritional status in the elderly is influenced by many factors: economics, behavioral changes, isolation, alterations in taste and appetite, medications, psychologic and physiologic conditions.

4. Antioxidants can protect the body from free radical pathology in the biologic aging process.

Table 18–1 Vitamins

Vitamin	Function	Food Source
Fat Soluble		
Vitamin A (Retinol)	Antioxidant. Maintenance and repair of mucus membranes and epithelial tissue. Growth and development of bones.	All orange and yellow fruits and vegetables; sweet potatoes, squash, yams, carrots, pumpkin, parsley, mango, apricots. Dark leafy greens: kale, spinach, broccoli.
Carotenoids (carotenes)	Antioxidant. Enhances cell communication and immune competence.	Orange, yellow, and dark green fruits and vegetables.
Vitamin D	Transport of calcium. Intestinal and renal absorption of phosphorus. Growth of bones and teeth.	Fish, liver, oils, egg yolk, alfalfa, fatty fish; halibut, salmon, sardines, dairy products.
Vitamin E	Antioxidant. Promotes wound healing. Peroxidation protects cell membranes against lipidpeoxition and destruction. Improves circulation.	Cold pressed vegetable oils, whole grains, dark leafy green vegetables, nuts, seeds, legumes, wheat germ, oatmeal.
Vitamin K	Blood clotting. Maintenance of healthy bones.	Green leafy vegetables. Egg yolks.
Vitamins/Water Soluble		
Vitamin B1 (Thiamin)	Co-enzyme in oxidation of glucose. Assists in production of hydrochloric acid.	Dried beans, brown rice, egg yolks, fish, chicken, peanuts.
Vitamin B2 (Riboflavin)	Red blood cell formation. Aids in metabolism of carbohydrates, fats, and proteins.	Beans, eggs, fish, poultry, meat, spinach, yogurt, asparagus, avocado.
Vitamin B3 (Niacin)	Healthy skin and nervous system. Lowers cholesterol, improves circulation.	Fish, eggs, beef, cheese, potatoes, whole wheat.
Vitamin B5 (Pantothemic Acid)	"Antistress" vitamin. Aids in production of adrenal hormones. Formation of antibodies.	Beans, beef, eggs, mother's milk, fresh vegetables, whole wheat, pork, salt water fish.
Vitamin B6 (Pyridoxine)	Acts as co-enzyme in metabolism of amino acids and essential fatty acids. Production of serotonin and other neurotransmitters. Essential for healthy nervous system. Assists in converting iron to hemoglobin.	Eggs, fish, spinach, peas, meat, nuts, carrots. Poultry, soybeans, bananas, avocado, whole grain cereals, prunes.
Vitamin B12 (cobalamin)	Synthesis of red blood cells. Required for proper digestion and absorption of foods. Prevents nerve damage.	Beef, herring, cheese, sardines, salmon, shellfish, tofu, eggs, dairy products.
Vitamin C (ascorbic acid)	Antioxidant. Collagen formation. Absorption of iron. Interferon production. Capillary integrity. Release of stress hormones.	Citrus fruits, papaya, parsley, watercress, berries, tomatoes, broccoli, brussel sprouts.
Folic Acid	Participates in amino acid conversion. Manufacturing of neurotransmitters.	Dark green vegetables, kidney beans, asparagus, broccoli, whole grain cereals.

5. Digestion, absorption, and elimination are all essential concerns in the evaluation of nutrient intake in the elderly.

Nutrition and Immune Function

1. Diet and nutrition play a key role in the physiology of immune function.[7]
2. Malnutrition and the consequent nutrient deficiencies alter immune function.
3. Immune system integrity is dependent on nutritional factors.
4. HIV infection, AIDS, cancer, and autoimmune diseases require nutritional support.
5. Immune enhancement programs include stress reduction, exercise, and nutrition interventions.

Nutritional Influences on Behavior[8]

1. Nutritional evaluation should include a nursing assessment of emotions and behavior.

Table 18–2 Minerals

Mineral	Function	Food Source
Calcium	Formation of strong bones. Transmission of nerve impulses, muscle growth and movement. Blood clotting. Immune system function.	Dairy products, salmon, sardines, green leafy vegetables, seeds, and nuts, tofu, blackstrap molasses, seaweed.
Chromium (GTF)	Metabolism of glucose. Helps stabilize blood sugar levels. Synthesis of cholesterol, fats, and proteins.	Brewer's yeast, brown rice, cheese, whole grains, beans, mushrooms, potatoes.
Copper	Formation of bone, hemogloblin, red blood cells. Involved in the healing process.	Whole grains, avocado, oyster, lobster, dandelion greens, mushrooms, blackstrap molasses, nuts, seeds, soybeans.
Iodine	Energy production. Body temperature, healthy thyroid gland.	Seaweed, iodized salt, dairy products, salt water fish, garlic, swiss chard, and summer squash.
Iron	Hemoglobin production. Stress and disease resistance. Energy production. Healthy immune system.	Eggs, fish, poultry, dark leafy greens, blackstrap molasses, almond, seaweed.
Magnesium	Formation of bone. Carbohydrate and mineral metabolism. Maintaining proper Ph balance.	Dairy products, fish, seafood, blackstrap molasses, garlic, fish, whole grains, seeds, tofu, green leafy vegetables.
Manganese	Enzyme activation. Sex hormone production, healthy nerves, energy production.	Avocados, nuts, seeds, seaweed, whole grains.
Phosphorus	Bone and teeth formation. Cell growth. Contraction of heart muscle. Kidney function.	Asparagus, brewer's yeast, fish, dried fruits, garlic, legumes, seeds, and nuts.
Potassium	Healthy nervous system. Regulate body fluids with sodium.	Apricots, bananas, potatoes, sunflower seeds, blackstrap molasses, sprouts, broccoli.
Selenium	Antioxidant. Protects immune system.	Brazil nuts, brewer's yeast, brown rice, dairy products, garlic, onions, whole grains.
Sodium	Works with potassium to regulate body fluids, necessary for nerve and muscle function.	Table salt. Seaweed, saltwater fish, miso.
Zinc	Burn and wound healing. Carbohydrate digestion, prostate gland function, reproductive organ growth and development. Healthy immune system.	Fish, legumes, poultry, meat, egg yolks, beans, pumpkin, seeds, sunflower seeds, sardines.

Source: Reprinted from *Holistic Nursing Associates Workbook* by J. Anselmo, S. Luck, B. Schaub, 1996.

---

2. Diet history, food intake, eating patterns, cultural beliefs and attitudes, and lifestyle influences are all part of an evaluation of nutritional status:
   a. Behavioral consequences of prenatal malnutrition and childhood nutrition in early growth and development.
   b. Vitamin deficiencies and excesses and behavioral consequences in adults.[9]
   c. Behavioral disorders triggered by food sensitivities and food allergies.[10]
   d. Nutritional deficiencies associated with drug and alcohol abuse.
   e. Depressive disorders and underlying biochemistry related to nutrient deficiencies.
   f. Eating patterns and disorders: anorexia, bulimia, and obesity.
   g. Environmental factors and effect on emotions and behavior.[11]

Pause for a moment . . .

❑ *As I study the **AHNA Core Curriculum for Holistic Nursing**, I recognize that in holistic nursing there are two views regarding holism:*
   — *Holism involves studying and understanding the interrelationships of the bio-psycho-social-spiritual dimensions of the person, recognizing that the whole is greater than the sum of its parts.*
   — *Holism involves the individual as an integrated whole interacting with and being acted upon by both internal and external environments.*
   — *Holistic nursing accepts both views, believing that the goals of nursing can be achieved within either framework.*

HOLISTIC NURSING PROCESS

Assessment

1. In order to use nutrition interventions, the nurse will assess the following parameters:
   a. The client's relationship to nutrition and diet: biochemical, genetic, cultural, social, emotional, religious, economic, environmental, and physiologic components.
   b. The client's eating habits, food preferences, and nutritional needs.
   c. The client's motivation and ability to make the necessary dietary and lifestyle changes.
   d. It is important for the client to understand that changing foods and eating patterns are part of the wellness process.

Nursing Diagnoses

1. The following nursing diagnoses compatible with nutrition interventions are related to the human response patterns:
   a. Exchanging: Altered nutrition
                    Altered circulation
                    Altered oxygenation
   b. Choosing: Altered coping
   c. Moving: Altered physical mobility
                    Sleep pattern disturbance
                    Altered patterns of daily
                      living
   d. Perceiving: Disturbance in body image
                    Disturbance in self-esteem
                    Potential hopelessness
                    Potential powerlessness
   e. Knowing: Knowledge deficit
   f. Feeling: Pain
                    Anxiety
                    Grieving
                    Depression
                    Fear

Client Outcomes

1. The nurse and the client should establish desired outcomes prior to session.
2. The client will become aware of the impact of nutrition on health and wellness status.
3. The client will be motivated to improve nutrition.
4. The client will demonstrate knowledge of healthful nutrition.

Plan and Interventions

1. Create an environment in which the client feels comfortable discussing physical and nutritional needs.
2. Prepare assessment tools and informational materials.
3. Focus on the client's nutritional, physical, and emotional needs.
4. Use relaxation techniques to assist the client before the nutrition session begins.
5. Have the client document food intake and association between food and feelings: well-being or distress.
6. Assist the client in creating a sample menu.
7. Encourage the client to participate in nutritional goals and action plans.
8. Present specific nutritional guidelines for the client to follow.
9. Direct the client to keep a food journal to present at a follow-up session.

Facilitating the Nutrition Process

1. The nurse serves as guide.
2. Emphasis should be on the connection between nutrition and whole person health.
3. With the nurse's guidance, the client develops strategies for changing nutrition habits, nutrient intake, and eating patterns.
   a. The client should be prepared for issues and problems experienced in changing diet and nutrition.
   b. It is often helpful to explore new ways to prepare foods.
4. The nurse can assist the client in optimizing diet and nutrition by:
   a. Creating an image for food as a healing medicine.
   b. Reframing the nutrition process into a positive action.
   c. Reframing nutrition and food as an empowerment tool.
   d. Illustrating how external nutritional changes promote internal healing responses.
   e. Reinforcing the client's positive changes in nutrition as part of the healing process.
   f. Ending sessions with images of the desired state of well-being.

Ensuring Optimal Nutrition

1. To optimize nutrient intake, the nurse may advise the client to
   a. Adhere to a low-fat/high-fiber diet.

b. Eliminate fried and fast foods.

c. Increase fiber, including fruits, vegetables, whole foods.

d. Increase exercise following evaluation by a trained professional.

e. Practice relaxation techniques.

2. The nurse can share information and research on the health benefits of antioxidants, essential fatty acids, and other nutrients.

3. A daily ideal food plan/menu can be created to fit the client's particular needs:

a. Daily activity status.

b. Current health status.

c. Economic considerations.

d. Emotional state of being.

e. Social and cultural influences.

4. Individual differences include food preferences, religious dietary customs, social situations, and cultural background.

5. The client's physical status (e.g., height, weight), and any physical limitations (e.g., digestive problems, food allergies) must be taken into account.

Helping Clients To Enhance Nutrition

1. To motivate and assist the client, the nurse can

a. Encourage the client to write in a food journal daily.

b. Demonstrate the daily practice of asking the body what it needs to be healthy.

c. Create daily menus using mutually agreed upon healthy choices.

d. Teach the client to self-assess health changes that occur with dietary interventions.

e. Encourage the client, if currently using nutritional supplementation, to organize a routine to optimize compliance and benefits.

2. Open-ended questions, images, journal writing, drawing, and other creative strategies to integrate nutrition into the client's daily life can be used to close the session.

Evaluation

1. It is essential to determine if client outcomes were achieved.

2. The client's subjective experience can be evaluated through open-ended questions about implementing dietary goals.

REFERENCES

1. J. Balch, *Prescription for Nutrition Healing* (New York: Avery Publishing Group, 1990), 5–33.

2. R. Garrison et al., *The Nutrition Desk Reference,* 3rd ed. (New Cannon, CT: Keats Pub., 1995), 287–311.

3. B.M. Dossey et al., *Holistic Nursing: A Handbook for Practice,* 2nd ed. (Gaithersburg, MD: Aspen Publishers, 1995), 257–287.

4. The National Research Council, Recommended Daily Allowances, 10th ed. (Washington, DC: National Academy of Sciences, 1989).

5. U. Erasmus, *Fats and Oils in Health and Nutrition* (Vancouver, Canada: Alive Books, 1986), 34–44.

6. J. Prendergast, *Nutritional Intervention in the Aging Process* (New York: Springer, 1984), 265–280.

7. J. Kaiser, *Immune Power: A Comprehensive Treatment Program for HIV* (New York: St. Martens Press, 1993), 19–30.

8. J. Galler, ed., *Nutrition and Behavior* (New York: Plenum Press, 1984), 207–223.

9. F. Morrow, Assessment of Nutritional Status in the Elderly: Application and Interpretation of Nutritional Biochemistries (Tufts University, Human Nutrition Research Center on Aging, Boston, MA, May 1986, Vol. 5, no. 3, 1986): 112–119.

10. Galler, *Nutrition and Behavior,* 399–400.

11. R. Wurtman et al., Carbohydrates and Depression, *Scientific American* (January 1989), 68–75.

CHAPTER 19

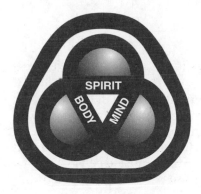

Movement and Exercise

Veda L. Andrus and Jane Yetter Lunt

KNOWLEDGE COMPETENCIES

- Identify movement/exercise as a universal process.
- Discuss the energy principles of movement/exercise.
- Describe the integral energetic effects of movement/exercise.
- Describe the manifestations of body-mind-spirit with movement/exercise.
- Describe the physiologic effects of movement/exercise.
- Identify patterns relevant to choice and commitment to movement/exercise.
- Define motivation to movement/exercise.
- Define commitment to movement/exercise.
- Discuss five different types of movement/exercise.
- Integrate movement/exercise and the nursing process.

DEFINITIONS

Commitment: a conscious, binding decision; a promise to self.
Conscious: aware, cognizant.
Exercise: conscious act of movement.
Frequency: in physics, the number of vibrations or cycles per unit of time.
Gross Energy: energy commonly physically visible.
Holographic Principle: a perspective of energy patterns in which every piece contains information of the whole; the whole is in every part.
Motivation: inner drive based on intention.

Movement: act of passing from one space to another through an energetic flow (subtle/gross, unconscious/conscious).
Pattern: an evolving energetic profile; distinguishing characteristics; a distinct way of being.
Resonance: energy perceived as vibrations or frequency patterns in human/environment.
Subtle Energy: energy not commonly visible as its frequency is faster than light.
Unconscious: not aware or intended.

 Pause for a moment . . .

❏ *The AHNA Core Curriculum for Holistic Nursing serves me as a major reference in my work and life.*
❏ *My studying of the AHNA Core Curriculum has significant value beyond the holistic nursing certification (HNC) examination.*
❏ *Practicing holistic nursing and living a holistic lifestyle bring me joy.*

THEORIES AND RESEARCH

Movement/Exercise As a Universal Process

1. All beings are expressions of the Earth and move in accordance with their own rhythmic patterns.
2. Perception of holographic patterns provides a clear knowledge of the whole.
3. Respecting self-knowledge is vital within this emerging paradigm.

4. The nurse is a resource person who is able to access information to assist client.
5. The caring process is a mutual opportunity for self-reflection/pattern recognition for both the nurse and client.

Energetic Principles Related to Movement/Exercise

1. Energy and matter are the same thing.[1]
2. All matter, physical and subtle, has frequency.[2]
3. The human/Earth community functions as a whole; the movement of one is integral to the other.[3]
4. The human is a pandimensional being within a universe of dynamic energy in many different frequencies and forms.[4]
5. Physical expressions of energy patterns can be viewed as a process of constriction/dilation and building/releasing.[5]
6. Consciousness is a form of energy.[6]
7. Conscious thought participates in formation of reality.[7,8]

Integral Energetic Effects of Movement/Exercise

1. The benefits of movement/exercise for the body-mind-spirit manifest in a variety of ways.[9] Movement/exercise
   a. Reduces depression.
   b. Helps psychologic aspects of disease.
   c. Elevates mood.
   d. Increases energy.
   e. Helps with addictions to cigarettes, alcohol, and caffeine.
   f. Improves self-esteem.
   g. Strengthens immune system.
   h. Improves or increases
      1) Creative energy.
      2) Relaxation.
      3) Awareness of details.
      4) Intimacy with friends and family.
      5) Self-image.
      6) Concentration.
      7) Memory.
   i. Can reduce
      1) Depression.
      2) Addictive behavior.
      3) Emotional fatigue.
      4) Egocentricity.
      5) Boredom.

2. Several physiologic benefits are also possible;[10–12] for example,
   a. Increases the number of small blood vessels to muscles, thereby supplying them with more blood and oxygen.
   b. Increases the number of mitochondria that supply energy inside muscle cells.
   c. Can help decrease percentage of body fat.
   d. Can reduce total body weight.
   e. Can increase bone density.
   f. Can decrease blood clot formation.
   g. Can reduce blood pressure.
   h. Can raise the level of high-density lipoproteins and reduce that of triglycerides.
   i. Increases total blood volume.
   j. Increases lung ventilation and lung diffusion capacity.
   k. Increases ability to metabolize fat for energy.
   l. Increases efficient oxygen extraction from blood at the tissues.
   m. Increases strength in bones, ligaments, and tendons.
   n. Increases insulin sensitivity and glucose tolerance.
   o. Decreases recovery heart rate.
   p. Decreases risk of colon cancer.
   q. Decreases risk of breast and reproductive tract cancer.

Patterns Relevant to Choice and Commitment to Movement/Exercise

1. Conscious participation involves intention, self-awareness (resonance),[13] motivation,[14] and commitment.[15]
2. A variety of vehicles are available for pattern recognition:[16]
   a. Inner advisor.
   b. Presence.
   c. Body scan.
   d. Meditation.
   e. Dreamwork.
   f. Holographic models/profiles
      1) Ayurvedic[17]
         a) Vata
         b) Kapha
         c) Pitta
      2) Rayid[18]
         a) Flower
         b) Jewel
         c) Stream
         d) Shaker

3) Chinese Five-Phase/Element[19]
   a) Earth
   b) Water
   c) Fire
   d) Wood
   e) Metal
g. Body awareness methods
   1) Alexander[20]
   2) Feldenkrais[21]
   3) Trager[22]

Types of Movement/Exercise

1. Universal states of movement for all living beings include breathing,[23] both conscious and unconscious, and moving in stillness.
2. Expressions of gross movement/exercise include the following:
   a. Aerobics.
   b. Tai Chi.
   c. Yoga.
   d. Walking.
   e. Dance.
   f. Sports.
   g. Others (e.g., sex, laughter, singing).
3. Expressions of subtle movement include the following:
   a. Touch (e.g., acupressure, healing touch, reflexology).
   b. Imagery.
   c. Music.
4. In addition to physical challenges,[24] physical diagnoses,[25] and age,[26] there are several other considerations:
   a. Attitudes/values/beliefs.
   b. Transcultural diversity.
   c. Circadian rhythms.
   d. Seasonal changes.
   e. Geographical location.
   f. Environmental sensitivities.

 Pause for a moment . . .

❑ *I am studying the **AHNA Core Curriculum** to be able to better enunciate the knowledge base for holistic nursing.*
❑ *I am studying the **AHNA Core Curriculum** to accomplish my personal goal of successful completion of the HNC examination.*
❑ *I am proud of the goal that I have set for myself.*

HOLISTIC NURSING PROCESS

Assessment

1. Conscious participation in the pre-access phase involves the self, which is centered, present, and respectful; others, who are co-participative; and the environment that they create together as sacred space.
2. Assessment: Pattern Recognition (State of Being): The nine human response patterns can serve as the basis for a holistic assessment and identification of movement and exercise patterns:[27]
   a. Communicating: pattern involving conscious/unconscious interplay of messages and information. The focus is on verbal/nonverbal information that is shared by the person and nurse. A person's self expression is accessed through spoken word, movements, and presence.
   b. Valuing: pattern involving assignment of relative worth; connection. The nurse focuses on connections that exist between a person and what the person values. The actions that the person takes related to values/beliefs are also examined.
   c. Relating: pattern involving the establishment of bonds. The person's role with self/others/universe is accessed; the nurse considers information about relationship patterns, family of origin, connection with other people, the natural world, and the universe.
   d. Perceiving: pattern involving awareness of information. The focus of this pattern is the person's sense of who she or he is and how this translates into a general view of life.
   e. Knowing: pattern involving meaning associated with conscious/unconscious information. The focus here is on body/mind awareness, cognitive functioning, and spiritual remembering. The nurse and person also take into account learning style and willingness/ability to learn.
   f. Feeling: pattern involving awareness of emotional information (state of being: experience, awareness, acceptance, allowance, expression). Questions delve into comfort level and general experience with emotions.
   g. Moving: pattern involving energetic flow/activity. This comprehensive area focuses on patterns of motion and/or current rhythm

in life. The nurse supports the exploration of self-knowledge, self-reverence, and the degree of harmony with one's own energetic profile and environment. Activity is examined in terms of movement/exercise, sleep, and self-care.

h. Exchanging: pattern involving mutual sharing of energy. The perpetual cycles and patterns of sharing intake/output of the living person is accessed.

i. Choosing: pattern involving recognition and selection of options. Addressing the process of choice and change, the nurse serves as a resource person in recognizing, choosing, and encouraging options.

Nursing Diagnoses (Purpose)

1. The nursing diagnoses most compatible and common with movement and exercise and related to the human response patterns of unitary person are as follows: Use unitary person framework as a holographic representation for selection/focus of nursing diagnosis.
2. This is an evolving process of co-participation within an emerging paradigm (Exhibit 19–1).

Client Outcomes

1. The client will participate in identifying movement and exercise outcomes at his or her own pace and desire.

Plan and Intervention (Response/ Influence/Co-Participation)

1. Acknowledge the expanded view of movement/exercise.
2. Act as a guide, facilitator, and resource person, as needed.
3. Refer the client to other professionals, agencies, and resources, when appropriate.
4. Encourage the client/patient to participate in making a personal commitment to a movement/exercise program.
5. Foster relationships with the client/patient, perceived family/community, nurse colleagues, interdisciplinary team members, and the entire Earth community.

Exhibit 19–1 Holistic Movement/Exercise

Old Paradigm	*Emerging Paradigm*
Focus on physical body	Body-mind-spirit integration
Competition with others and self	Self-knowledge and self-reverence
Unaware of environmental rhythms	Conscious co-participation with rhythms of self/Earth (integrality)
Critical and regulated	Expression of spirit
Movement expressed physically	Universal and diverse expression of movement

Evaluation (Reflection)

1. Opportunity for reflection/mirroring
2. Mutual self-acknowledgment
3. Gratitude for shared experience

REFERENCES

1. R. Gerber, *Vibrational Medicine* (Santa Fe, NM: Bear and Company, 1988), 39–69, 119–172.
2. Ibid.
3. B. Swimme and T. Berry, *The Universe Story* (San Francisco: Harper, 1992), 243–245.
4. M. Rogers, Nursing Science Evolves, in *Rogers' Scientific Art of Nursing Practice,* ed. M. Madrid and E.A.M. Barrett (New York: National League for Nursing, 1994), 3–9.
5. D. Johnson, *What the Eye Reveals* (Boulder, CO: Rayid Publications, 1995), 6–54.
6. Gerber, *Vibrational Medicine.*
7. M. Talbot, *The Holographic Universe* (New York: HarperCollins, 1991), 82–118.
8. C. Garfield, *Peak Performance* (Los Angeles: Jeremy P. Tarcher, 1984), 127–153.
9. G. Yanker et al., *Walking Medicine* (New York: McGraw-Hill, 1990), 11, 286–287.
10. D. Ornish, *Program for Reversing Heart Disease* (New York: Ballantine Books, 1990), 330–331.
11. B. Franklin et al., eds., *Exercise in Modern Medicine* (Baltimore: Williams & Wilkins, 1989), 37–38, 44–279.
12. C. Bouchard et al., eds., *Exercise, Fitness, and Health* (Champaign, IL: Human Kinetics Publishers, 1990), 582–583.
13. Swimme and Berry, *The Universe Story.*
14. A. Turock, *Getting Physical* (New York: Doubleday, 1984), 1–22.
15. Ibid.

16. M.A. Newman, *Health as Expanding Consciousness*, 2nd ed. (New York: National League for Nursing, 1994), 73–76, 107–109.

17. D. Chopra, *Perfect Health* (New York: Harmony Books, 1991), 262–267.

18. D. Johnson, *What the Eye Reveals*.

19. H. Beinfield and E. Korngold, *Between Heaven and Earth: A Guide to Chinese Medicine* (New York: Ballantine, 1991), 131–231.

20. J. Leibowitz and B. Connington, *The Alexander Technique* (New York: HarperCollins, 1990).

21. M. Feldenkrais, *Awareness through Movement* (San Francisco: HarperCollins, 1977), 10.

22. M. Trager, *Movement As a Way to Agelessness* (Barrytown, NY: Station Hill Press, 1995), 9.

23. G. Hendricks, *Conscious Breathing* (New York: Bantam Books, 1995), 3–31.

24. K. Lockette and A. Keyes, *Conditioning with Physical Disabilities* (Champaign, IL: Human Kinetics Publishers, 1994), 65–220.

25. Franklin et al., *Exercise in Modern Medicine*.

26. Ibid.

27. P. Wolff and J.Y. Lunt, Nursing in the Nineties: The Holistic Nurse Caring Process, *Journal of Holistic Nursing* 9, no. 2 (1991): 8–16.

CHAPTER 20

Environment

Eleanor A. Schuster

KNOWLEDGE COMPETENCIES

- Discuss the relationship of health to the natural world.
- Name four ways that the natural world is being altered.
- Discuss the concept of infectious disease in relation to the overall sustainability of human activity.
- Name five ways diseases are related to, or caused by, something in the environment.
- Discuss ways in which the by-products and services of health care organizations affect the environment.
- Name four parameters to consider in developing a waste management plan.
- Identify the main intent of the principles developed by the Coalition for Environmentally Responsible Economics (CERES).
- Name 5 of the leading 11 ecologic problems according to the Environmental Protection Agency (EPA).
- Discuss the six key elements of the ecologic paradigm.
- Discuss the concept of the environment as a client.
- Differentiate among the terms *egocentric, homocentric,* and *ecocentric* in relation to world view.
- Identify a major philosophic difficulty with the ecocentric world view.
- Discuss the reasons for conducting an exposure survey.
- Name the main elements of an exposure survey.

DEFINITIONS

Earth Ethics: the development and use of a set of personal and societal principles, and the resulting value systems and behavior patterns, that will sustain a viable life support system on planet Earth.[1]

Ecocentric: having a view of the environment grounded in the cosmos; acknowledging unity and integrality between human and environment.[2] Human beings and their world are not separate.

Ecofeminism: a theory that women and the environment are interconnected, as both share and have been subjected to the same patriarchal domination.[3]

Ecologic Responsibility: the capability to consider and carry out one's actions in light of the needs, feelings, and perceptions of other peoples, other life forms, and of the Earth as a whole.[4]

Ecology: the scientific study of the interrelationships among and between organisms, and between them and all aspects, living and nonliving, of their environment.[5]

Egocentric: having a view of the environment grounded at the personal level; assuming that what is best for the individual is best for society.[6]

Environment: everything that surrounds an individual or group of people: physical, social, psychologic, cultural, or spiritual characteristics; external and internal features; animals and inanimate objects; seen and unseen vibrations and frequencies; climate and not yet understood energy patterns.[7]

Homocentric: having a view of the environment grounded at the social level.[8] Social justice, rather than individual progress, is the key value.

Sustainable Development: the ability to meet the needs of the present without compromising the ability of future generations to meet their own needs.[9]

 Pause for a moment . . .

❑ *I am deepening my understanding that holistic practice draws on nursing knowledge, theories, expertise, and intuition.*

❑ *This understanding guides me in becoming a therapeutic partner with clients in strengthening the clients' response to facilitate the healing process and achieve wholeness.*

THEORIES AND RESEARCH

Health and the Natural World [10]

1. Several factors are profoundly altering the natural world:
   a. Population expansion.
   b. Movement of populations toward cities.
   c. Stressed resilience of land and water systems.
   d. Global shift of climate patterns.
2. Alterations of the natural world make people, along with plants and animals, more vulnerable to infectious diseases.
3. Infectious diseases are a basic barometer of the overall sustainability of human activity.
   a. Key elements of sustainable economic development include the following:
      1) Stabilizing world population.
      2) Reversing the tide of deforestation.
      3) Sustainably managing and cleaning up the world's water supply.
      4) Reducing the 25 billion tons of carbon dioxide added to the atmosphere each year.[11]
   b. Immediate and specific preventive measures available include the following:[12]
      1) Buildup of immunity to stop infection before it starts.

2) Vaccination.
3) Public education.
4) Local stewardship.
5) Attention to simple measures, such as cleansing of drinking water and oral hydration therapy (ORT) to reduce cholera and dysentery deaths by 80 percent.[13]

4. Infectious diseases are still the leading cause of death in the world, killing more persons than cancer and heart disease combined.
   a. Malaria, mumps, diphtheria, and influenza have existed since ancient times.
   b. Since 1973, at least 30 previously unknown diseases (e.g., Lyme disease, Legionnaires' disease, and toxic shock syndrome) have appeared.
5. Both the complexity and diversity of natural ecosystems help to keep infectious organisms and disease vectors in check.
6. Biologic mixing, which is the movement of people, plants, animals, and goods, increases exposure to disease.
7. Many infectious diseases are related to and even caused by something in the environment:
   a. Fire.
   b. Flood.
   c. Deforestation.
   d. Earthquake.
   e. Land use changes: logging, agriculture, migration, and urbanization.
8. All ecologic disruptions tip the balance between people and microbes in favor of microbes.[14]

Health and Chemicals [15]

1. Chemical compounds occur in a vast array of products, including antibiotics, synthetic fibers, dry cleaning solutions, spoil-proof food, pesticides, and contraceptives.
2. Although billions of dollars are spent in product development, marketing, production, and advertising, little is spent on the study of chemical interactions with living things and the environment.
3. There is an indisputable link between exposure to certain industrial substances and serious diseases, particularly cancer (e.g., benzene and leukemia, asbestos and mesothelioma).[16]
4. Many substances cause broad, yet subtle, damage to the nervous system, the reproductive

system, the endocrine system, and the immune system.

5. Federal regulatory agencies have emphasized the prevention of cancer, falsely assuming that protection against cancer is protection against other toxic outcomes.

6. Regulatory agencies must look beyond cancer to assess the effect of chemicals on overall biologic competence.

Economic Impact of Environmental Concerns[17]

1. The relationship between human health and environmental quality indicates that, as environmental quality diminishes, so does human health.

2. Health care institutions generate multiple waste streams: solid, infectious, hazardous, recyclable, and compostable.

3. Health care organizations must ensure that the by-products of their processes and services do not adversely affect environmental quality or integrity.

4. The development and implementation of rigorous pollution control plans can minimize the environmental impacts associated with health care.

5. Whether as citizens, employees, or entrepreneurs, nurses are in positions to influence the systematic management of the waste stream, from manufacture to disposal.
   a. The following questions are important in the evaluation of an item being considered for procurement:
      1) Is is necessary?
      2) What is its life expectancy?
      3) How cost-efficient is it?
      4) What is its environmental impact?
      5) What can be re-used or recycled?
      6) Will the manufacturer assume responsibility for restoration or recycling?
      7) What are the actual or potential health hazards?
   b. There are four parameters to consider in the evaluation of waste management plans:
      1) Cost.
      2) Safety.
      3) Efficiency.
      4) Compliance with regulatory standards.

6. The merging of institutional waste management systems, as health care systems consolidate, reduces operating costs and frees funds to be used elsewhere.

7. Waste management goals include:
   a. Consistent waste management systems.
   b. Pollution prevention plans.
   c. Maximization of cost-effectiveness.
   d. Compliance with regulations.
   e. Safety enhancement and risk reduction.
   f. Consistent sharps management.

8. The CERES principles, formerly the *Valdez* principles in the wake of the Exxon *Valdez* disaster, are a set of guidelines through which corporations and other business entities affirm responsibility for the environment.[18]

9. Voluntary compliance with the CERES principles has several benefits:
   a. Advancement toward a just and sustainable future.
   b. Partnering, rather than exploitation, of business with environment.
   c. Enhanced profits over time.
   d. More credible image as the public and shareholders become more environmentally astute.
   e. Meeting or exceeding of regulatory standards.

10. According to the EPA, the worst world ecologic concerns are (in no particular order)[19]
    a. Global climate change.
    b. Stratospheric ozone depletion.
    c. Habitat alteration.
    d. Species extinction and biodiversity loss.
    e. Particulate air pollutants (e.g., smog).
    f. Toxic air pollutants (e.g., benzene).
    g. Radon gas.
    h. Indoor air pollution.
    i. Drinking water contamination.
    j. Occupational exposure to chemicals.
    k. Application of pesticides.

11. None of the world's environmental problems can be understood in isolation.[20] They are systemic problems, interconnected and interdependent, and need a systemic approach to be understood and solved. *This is a paradigm shift of our perception of world order.*
    a. Shift from objects to relationships. Reality is no longer seen as a collection of separate objects, but as a web of relationships.
    b. Shift from parts to the whole. The nature of any living system, including business organizations, derives from the relationship

among its components, and between the whole system and its environment.

c. Shift from domination to partnership. Cooperative symbiotic relationships are an essential characteristic of the web of life.

d. Shift from structures to processes. The more flexible the system, the greater its stability. Stress is the lack of flexibility.

e. Shift from self-assertion to integration. Effective functioning is derived from a balance between these two essential tendencies.

f. Shift from growth to sustainability. The pursuit of unrestricted growth leads to global environmental destruction. The term *growth* has not only a quantitative meaning, but also a qualitative one: to sustain a web of relationships, defining the system as an integral whole.

The Environment As Client [21]

1. Everything within the planet is living; soils, rocks, atmosphere, space and time, plants, and all creatures make up the living structure of the planet.

2. The environment has many patterns or elements, united into a whole that is greater than its elements.

3. In an interaction, all the elements and patterns existing within the whole are interwoven, interconnected, and interrelated in equilibrium.
   a. Any harm to one pattern affects everything within the whole.
   b. If the balance of the planet is disturbed, illness and disaster result.
   c. The environment has enormous, but finite, recuperative abilities.

4. The perception of a unitary, alive, interacting environment has a personal and professional impact for holistic nurses.
   a. It provides a renewed understanding of the planet and one's place in it.
   b. Any actions taken are globally related and interconnected.

5. Nursing practiced from this ecocentric paradigm makes the community and broader environment a nursing client (e.g., directly addressing the issue of a toxic dump site as well as caring for those affected with leukemia resulting from exposure).

6. The ecocentric approach has some philosophic difficulties. [22]

a. The central problem is finding a philosophically adequate justification for the intrinsic value of nonhuman nature.
b. In mainstream Western thought, only humans have intrinsic worth, while the rest of nature has instrumental value as a resource for humans.

7. A qualitative research study reported that, of 17 nurse scholars interviewed in depth, 15 explicitly reflected the ecocentric paradigm, perceiving the environment to be alive, whole, interconnected, and interacting. [23]

 Pause for a moment . . .

❏ *I am integrating self-care in my own life so that I can practice the best of holistic nursing.*
❏ *My self-responsibility leads me to a greater awareness of the interconnectedness of all individuals and their relationships to the human and global community, and it permits me to use this awareness to facilitate healing.*

HOLISTIC NURSING PROCESS

Assessment

1. Nursing process, with environment as a client, is in the beginning stages of conceptualization and development.

2. It draws from many disciplines and fields of study (e.g., ethics, medicine, law, geography, biology, epidemiology, business, anthropology, education), as well as from nursing.

3. The success of nursing the environment relies on the practitioner's artistry in blending empirical with intuitive data to determine a course of action.

4. Assessment of environmental exposure to hazardous substances is vital for the diagnosis of a variety of diseases. [24]
   a. Many environmental diseases manifest as common health problems or have nonspecific symptoms.
   b. Holistic nurses can play an important role in detecting, treating, and preventing disease due to toxic exposure by taking a thorough exposure history.

1) Exposures
   a) Current and past exposures to metals, dust, fibers, fumes, chemicals, biologic hazards, radiation, noise, vibration, extremes in temperature, light.
   b) Typical work day (e.g., job tasks, locations, materials, equipment, agents used).
   c) Changes in routines or processes.
   d) Affect on other employees or household members.
2) Health and safety practices at worksite.
   a) Ventilation.
   b) Medical industrial hygiene surveillance.
   c) Employment examinations.
   d) Personal protective equipment.
   e) Lockout devices, alarms, training drills.
   f) Personal habits (e.g., smoking in the workplace, eating in work area, washing with solvents).
3) Work history.
   a) Description of all prior jobs, including short-term, seasonal, part-time, and military service.
   b) Description of present job(s).
4) Environmental history.
   a) Present and prior home locations.
   b) Travel, especially abroad.
   c) Jobs of household members.
   d) Home insulating, heating, and cooling systems.
   e) Home cleaning agents.
   f) Pesticide exposure.
   g) Recent renovation/remodeling.
   h) Air pollution, indoor/outdoor.
   i) Hobbies.
   j) Hazardous waste sites exposure.
5. In addition to the exposure survey and environmental history, the nurse assesses exposure to personal stressors (e.g., family, financial, spiritual, social, fears, unfulfilled expectations).

Nursing Diagnoses

1. The most common nursing diagnoses associated with environmental interventions focus on person as client in relation to environment, not environment as client or in relation to person.
2. All nursing diagnoses are potentially congruent with environmental interventions because of the inclusiveness of the environmental perspective.

Client Outcomes

1. The client is aware of being listened to and valued.
2. The client has a sense of personal power to make choices.
3. The client understands self/environment connections and ways that these connections are integral to health.
4. The client knows of appropriate resources for further information or treatment.
5. The client has a sense of addressing his or her particular situation and of formulating with you a specific course of action.

Plan and Interventions

With Person As Client

1. Listen carefully, in a relaxed way, to the client's story.
2. Learn what he or she wants or expects from you.
3. Assure the client that you are interested in and believe what he or she is telling you.
4. Introduce and teach some form of centering and relaxation.
5. Address any immediate presenting problem.
6. Elicit an environmental exposure history, as appropriate.
7. Learn what the client has already done to resolve the problem.
8. Systematically assess what may be addressed within the scope of your practice.
9. Become aware of the various resources for further diagnosis and treatment, as necessary.
10. Refer the client, if he or she needs assistance beyond the scope of your practice.
11. Engage the client as a partner in evolving a plan of action.
12. Offer some form of continued counsel or support, as appropriate.

With Environment As Client

Perspective #1
1. State the problem specifically (e.g., "The well water in the community I visit is being contaminated with fuel").
2. Learn everything possible about the problem (e.g., its level of threat, history, research and popular literature, expert opinions, stories of those affected, what is being done about it, who knows about it).

3. Investigate local, state, and other regulatory guidelines.
4. Find out who has any kind of jurisdiction concerning the problem.
5. Identify the experts in this area of concern.
6. Team up with others whenever possible.
7. Make a commitment regarding your role in addressing the problem.
8. Take necessary immediate steps regarding public safety.
9. The focus is on preventing problems at their inception, not only dealing with their consequences. In 9 of 10 cases of breast cancer, for example, there are no known inherited defects. The disease arises from outside causes, the environment. Research indicates that exposures to hormone-mimicking chemicals explain some increase in breast cancer.[25] These chemicals are found in certain pesticides, drugs, plastics, and fuels.

Perspective #2
1. Acknowledge that you are an integral and wondrous part of the universe, in conscious relationship with all else—present, past, and future.
2. From the center of your being, in silence, listen to what the environment is telling you.
3. Reflect on ways to create your path of simplicity and beauty.
4. Assess what changes, if any, you may want to make in your relationships with the environment.
5. Identify benefits that you have received from the environment, and rejoice.
6. Become aware of ways that the environment needs your partnership, or is threatened, and respond.

Evaluation

1. Explore with the client the following questions:
   a. Are you aware of being listened to and valued?
   b. Do you feel empowered to make choices?
   c. Do you have a sense of self/environment connections and do you believe that these connections are integral to health?
   d. Is there anything else you need to ask about resources for further information or treatment?
   e. Do you have a sense that your particular situation is being addressed?
   f. How do you feel about the specific course of action that you have decided on at this time?
2. Be aware of unspoken clues, such as body language.
3. Listen to your own intuitive sense.

REFERENCES

1. E.A. Schuster, Earth Dwelling, *Holistic Nursing Practice* 6 (1992): 2.
2. D. Kleffel, Environmental Paradigms: Moving toward an Ecocentric Perspective, *Advances in Nursing Science* 18, no. 4 (1996): 4–5.
3. Ibid., 7.
4. Schuster, Earth Dwelling.
5. R. Allaby, *Concise Oxford Dictionary of Ecology* (London, England: Oxford University Press, 1994), 132.
6. Kleffel, Environmental Paradigms, 2.
7. B.M. Dossey et al., *Holistic Nursing: A Handbook for Practice*, 2nd ed. (Gaithersburg MD: Aspen Publishers, 1995), 292.
8. Kleffel, Environmental Paradigms, 3.
9. J. Maughan, Sustainable Communities: An Idea Whose Time Has Come? *Wingspread Journal* 18, no. 2 (1996): 4.
10. A.E. Platt, *Infecting Ourselves: How Environmental and Social Disruptions Trigger Disease*, No. 129 (Washington, DC: The Worldwatch Institute, April 1996), 24–63.
11. Ibid., 60.
12. Ibid.
13. Ibid., 52.
14. Ibid., 31.
15. A. Misch, Assessing Environmental Health Risks, in *State of the World 1994*, ed. L. Brown (New York: W.W. Norton, 1994), 127–136.
16. Ibid., 117.
17. H. Shaner et al., *Managing Wastes in Merger Conditions: Optimizing Systems* (Chicago: American Society for Health and Environmental Services of the American Hospital Association, 1995), 2–48.
18. E. Callenbach et al., *Eco Management: The Elmwood Guide to Ecological Auditing and Sustainable Business* (San Francisco: Berrett-Koehler Publishers, 1993), 161–163.
19. Ibid., 150.
20. Ibid., 70–73.
21. D. Kleffel, Environment As a Domain of Nursing Knowledge, in *Exploring Our Environmental Connections*, eds. E.A. Schuster and C.L. Brown (New York: National League for Nursing, 1994), 1–13.
22. Kleffel, Environmental Paradigms, 5.
23. Ibid., 7.
24. S. Balk, ed., *Taking an Exposure History: Case Studies in Environmental Medicine*, No. 26 (Atlanta, GA: Agency for Toxic Substances and Disease Registry, Department of Health and Human Services, 1992), 1–22.
25. T. Colburn et al. *Our Stolen Future* (New York: Dutton, 1996): 84–86.

CHAPTER 21

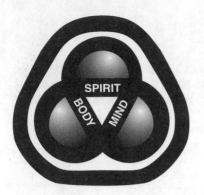

Laughter, Play, and Humor

Patty Wooten

KNOWLEDGE COMPETENCIES

- Explain how humor and laughter affect the body, mind, and spirit.
- Discuss the difference between hoping humor and coping humor.
- Explain three theories about why we laugh.
- Discuss the difference between compassionate humor and caustic humor.
- Discuss ways in which a sense of humor can help in times of stress.
- Discuss the physiologic effects of humor and laughter.
- Describe five steps to finding and creating more humor.
- Explain how to assess someone's sense of humor.
- List eight ways to increase awareness and appreciation of humor.
- Describe and analyze five types of therapeutic humor programs.
- Explain general guidelines for establishing a humor program.
- Discuss guidelines for appropriate use of humor.

DEFINITIONS

Humor: a perceptual and cognitive process involving an ability to recognize and appreciate the absurd and incongruous aspects of a situation.[1,2]

Laughter: a physical and behavioral process that can range from a silent smile to an uproarious guffaw; affects the respiratory, cardiovascular, neurologic, musculoskeletal, and immune system.[3,4]

Mirth: an emotional and spiritual process that stimulates feelings of joy, hope, optimism, and connection with others.

 Pause for a moment . . .

- ❑ *I model wellness in my life.*
- ❑ *I am contributing to the improvement in the quality of health care by promoting education, participation, and self-responsibility for wellness.*

THEORIES AND RESEARCH

Effect of Humor and Laughter [5-7]

1. Illness can damage the body, overwhelm the mind, and break the spirit.
2. Disease causes an imbalance in the energy flowing between the body, mind, and spirit.
3. Humor can stimulate healing in the physical body, bring peace to the emotions, and strengthen the will to live.
4. Daily laughter, especially during difficult or stressful times, can facilitate healing.
5. Laughter strengthens the body; humor engages the mind to perceive new possibilities; mirth lifts the spirit. Individuals begin to feel connected with friends, family, and caregivers.
6. During illness, the body naturally slows down.

a. Sometimes, this inactivity is due to fatigue, sometimes to pain, and sometimes to depression.

b. Immobility punishes the body. Blood no longer moves briskly through the vessels, breathing becomes shallow, and muscles weaken.

7. A vicious cycle begins, spiraling into more serious problems. Illness may require resignation from a job, hospitalization, or cessation of family and leisure activities. These losses may lead to depression, which further weakens the immune system and leaves the person more vulnerable to attack by virus and bacteria.

8. Mirthful laughter stimulates the cardiovascular, respiratory, and musculoskeletal systems. Immune defenses are strengthened. A deep sense of relaxation follows vigorous laughter.

9. Humor and laughter offer a natural catharsis, a kind of "cranial enema," that cleanses the mind of worry and toxic thoughts. It stimulates a person's creative problem-solving ability and initiates new energy and hope.

10. Illness can create feelings of isolation and loneliness.

11. Humor, expressed with compassion and kindness, creates an atmosphere of love and trust, connects people to each other, and strengthens the spirit.

Types of Humor

Hoping Humor and Coping Humor[8]

1. The ability to hope for something better enables human beings to cope with difficult situations.

2. Hoping humor accepts life with all its dichotomies, contradictions, and incongruities. It gives individuals the courage to withstand suffering.

3. Coping humor laughs at hopeless situations. It provides a detachment from the problem and makes it possible to release tension, anxiety, and hostility.

Compassionate Humor and Caustic Humor[9,10]

1. Compassionate humor leaves people feeling relaxed, accepted, and safe. It expresses kindness and connects people in an atmosphere of love and trust.

2. Caustic humor causes feelings of embarrassment, indignation, or threat. It expresses contempt and separates people, creating loneliness and fear.

Specific Theories Related to Laughter, Play, and Humor[11,12]

1. Incongruity theory: Humor involves a sudden and surprising shift in cognitive processing where two concepts normally considered remote from each other are brought together to reveal their similarities (e.g., the surprise ending of a joke).

2. Arousal theory: Laughter occurs when the tension of anxiety or anger needs a release (e.g., nervous laughter or hostile humor).

3. Superiority theory: Laughter comes from the enhanced feelings of self-esteem that occur in response to situations of others more unfortunate (e.g., seeing someone slip on a banana peel).

Usefulness of Humor in Times of Stress[13–15]

1. A sense of humor allows individuals to see new possibilities in difficult situations, feel larger than the problem, and change the perceptions of their circumstances before the circumstances change them.

2. It helps them to cope with the unknown and to communicate more effectively, enhances their ability to recognize the comical aspects of tragic situations, and can be a psychologic strategy that gives them relief from pain, suffering, or tragedy.

3. Gallows humor acknowledges the disgusting or intolerable aspects of a situation and attempts to transform them into something lighthearted and amusing.

a. Caregivers often use gallows humor as a means of maintaining some psychologic distance from the suffering and, thus, protecting themselves from a sympathetic response.

b. Patients or their families may not appreciate gallows humor, so therapeutic for staff.

4. The ability to laugh and find humor in situations helps people adjust better to stress.[16,17]

a. Subjects who value humor most cope better with tension and stress.

b. Those who have the greatest ability to produce humor "on demand" are able to counteract the negative emotional effects of stress.[18]

   c. Subjects with a strong sense of humor have significantly fewer negative mood shifts during stressful life changes than a person with a weak sense of humor.[19]

Physiologic Effects of Humor and Laughter[20]

1. Laughter is a wonderful tonic for the body.
2. The laughter experience has arousal and resolution stages.
   a. Physical activity and physiologic parameters at first increase during the laughter.
   b. After the laughter stops, these physical and psychologic parameter increases subside.
   c. Subjects being monitored while viewing a humorous video had increased heart rate, increased systolic blood pressure, increased respiratory rate and depth, increased minute volume, and decreased residual volume.[21]
   d. Diaphragm, intercostal, abdominal, and facial muscles are activated during laughter.
   e. Peripheral blood vessels dilate, allowing more blood to flow to the extremities.
3. Humor is a cognitive skill that uses both sides of the brain.[22]
   a. The left side of the cerebral cortex is active during the telling of a joke, but as the humor is perceived, the brain wave activity moves toward the right side of the cerebral cortex.
   b. Humor brings together the whole brain, linking the logical left brain with the creative right brain.
4. The experience of mirthful laughter stimulates and strengthens the immune system.[23]
   a. Laughter decreases serum cortisol levels. The cortisol level increase that occurs during the experience of stressful emotions weakens the immune response. Laughter provides an antidote to stress.
   b. Laughter increases the activity of natural killer cells (which release a substance that destroys tumor cells). Among cancer patients, reduced natural killer cell activity is associated with an increase in the spread of tumors.
   c. Laughter increases the number of helper T cells.
   d. Laughter increases the helper to suppresser ratio of T cells.

5. Laughter increased the concentration of salivary immunoglobulin A (IgA) after subjects viewed a humorous video.[24]
   a. Salivary IgA protects against upper respiratory infections such as colds and flu.
   b. Salivary IgA levels have been found to be lower on days when participants were in a negative mood and higher on days when they were in positive moods.
   c. Subjects who had a more developed sense of humor had a larger increase in salivary IgA concentration after seeing a humorous video.

 Pause for a moment . . .

❑ *I am interacting with other health-related organizations to teach about holistic nursing and related healing work.*

❑ *I am encouraging and reporting the research of holistic concepts and practice in nursing.*

HOLISTIC NURSING PROCESS

Assessment

1. Before using laughter, play, and humor interventions, the nurse should assess
   a. The client's attitude toward the ideas of play and laughter.
   b. The client's sense of humor and laughter, as well as their appropriateness.
   c. The client's ability to smile and laugh.
   d. The presence of any physical limitations that would influence the client's ability to engage in play activities.
   e. The frequency with which the client engages in playful activities.
   f. The client's previous experience with play.
   g. The client's ability to enjoy humorous books or videotapes.
2. The client's awareness of the kinds of humor that he or she has enjoyed in the past is also important.

Nursing Diagnoses

1. The following nursing diagnoses compatible with humorous and playful interventions can be related to the human response patterns:[25]

a. Relating: Altered parenting, actual or potential
Social isolation
b. Choosing: Ineffective individual and family coping
c. Moving: Activity intolerance, actual or potential
Deficit in diversional activity
Impaired physical mobility
d. Perceiving: Powerlessness
Disturbance in self-concept
Altered self-esteem, role performance, personal identity
Altered sensory perception: visual, auditory, kinesthetic, gustatory, tactile, olfactory
e. Knowing: Altered thought processes
f. Feeling: Anxiety
Comfort, altered: pain
Fear
Violence, potential for self-directed or directed at others

2. The patient's ability to respond to playful interventions can be categorized in two types:
   a. Expressive—able to create humor
   b. Receptive—able to perceive and understand humorous stimuli

Client Outcomes

1. It is essential to establish client outcomes prior to intervention.
   a. The client will become aware of the health benefits of laughter, play, and humor.
   b. The client will engage in playful activities.
   c. The client will exhibit appropriate spontaneous laughter.
2. The subjective severity of target symptoms will decrease as a result of the play/laughter intervention.

Plan and Intervention [26–29]

1. Guide the client in playful activities; help the client identify amusing puns, jokes, stories, riddles, or other forms of humor.
2. Model appropriate smiling and laughter for the client.
3. Reflect pleasure when the client laughs spontaneously or smiles appropriately when presented with humorous greeting cards, comedy films, audiotapes, jokes, stories, and similar items.

4. Guide the client in grading the severity of a symptom on a 1 to 10 scale before and after the intervention.
5. Use five steps to find and create more humor. [30–32]
   a. Exaggerate and overstate the problem. Making the situation bigger than life restores a humorous perspective. Cartoon caricatures, slapstick comedy, and clowning antics are all based on exaggeration.
   b. Look for the irony—the difference between how things are and how they should be. To spot the little ironies, ask yourself, "Why is it that . . ." or "Have you ever wondered why. . . ."
   c. Recognize the incongruities and the nonsense of a difficult situation.
   d. Learn to play with words. Create puns and spoonerisms.
   e. Learn to appreciate SURPRISE!
6. Assess your own sense of humor, as well as the client's.
   a. What value do you place on your own personal sense of humor?
   b. Do you really believe that humor is helpful?
   c. What makes you laugh?
   d. Do you enjoy cartoons, jokes, toys, stand-up comedy, amusing stories, or the company of funny people?
   e. Has your client given you any indication that he or she is receptive to humor?
   f. Do friends who come to visit or call on the telephone attempt to share humor?
   g. What is your client's ability to perceive and understand humor? Consider any hearing, visual, mental, or reading deficits.
   h. What kind of humor does your client choose to create?
      1) Does it seem to be a natural part of the client's lifestyle?
      2) Is the client physically playful or mentally witty?
      3) Is the client a storyteller?
      4) Is the client's humor sarcastic and cynical, or is it warm and gentle?
      5) Does the client interact with the surroundings in a playful, childlike way?
      6) Are there any humorous topics the client may consider taboo? People are most easily offended by humor centered around religion, sexuality, racism, and politics.

i. Does the client prefer a certain comedy artist?

7. Be careful to choose a style of humor that the person already enjoys. As trust and comfort levels build, introduce other styles of humor.

8. Become aware of the subtle cues a client gives you in response to your initial humorous attempts.
   a. Watch the eyes. Do they become alert and shining? Or does the client furrow the brows and look away?
   b. Listen to the tonal quality of the laugh. Is the laughter sincere or merely a polite response to fill the silence?

9. Avoid laughing at the client or the situation before the client gives you permission to poke fun. This is the aspect of *timing*. Humor about personal or private aspects of a client's life can deeply offend or hurt that client. When you do make a mistake (and we all do, sooner or later), first, forgive yourself for being obtuse or insensitive; then make amends with the patient.

10. Increase your awareness of humor.[33-35]
    a. Create a scrapbook of cartoons.
    b. Develop a file of funny jokes, stories, greeting cards, bumper stickers, poems, and songs.
    c. Collect or borrow funny books, videos, and audiotapes of comedy routines.
    d. Collect toys, interactive games, noise makers, and squirt guns. Keep them available.
    e. Create a humor journal or logbook to record funny encounters or humorous discoveries.
    f. Establish a bulletin board in your facility or on your refrigerator at home to post cartoons, bumper stickers, and funny signs.
    g. Subscribe to a humorous newsletter or journal to collect new ideas and inspiration.
    h. Educate yourself about therapeutic humor. Attend conferences, workshops, and conventions.

11. Become familiar with various types of therapeutic humor programs.
    a. A humor room is a place where patients, their families, and staff can gather to laugh, play, and relax together.
       1) The furniture is arranged in clusters for people to gather.
       2) Book shelves display humorous books, cartoon albums, board games, and stuffed toys.
       3) A volunteer helps patients and families choose a humorous activity.
       4) The humor room setting provides a place for informal patient support, structured group sessions, and even, on occasion, celebrations such as wedding anniversaries, birthdays, and the completion of chemotherapy.
       5) A humor room is ideal for long-term care facilities, rehabilitation programs, psychiatric units, or outpatient clinics.
    b. A mobile unit, a colorful and festive cart, can be wheeled into a patient's room.[36,37]
       1) The comedy cart can contain a wide variety of videos and comedy audiotapes, as well as a portable tape player with headphones; toys; and funny costume items.
       2) Humor volunteers push the cart from room to room, offering a brief but entertaining introduction of the items available. Alternately, there may be a list of the comedy cart items, and patients can make a selection.
    c. Possibly the easiest therapeutic humor program to create, especially with limited time or resources, is a basket of comedy materials to provide a quick access to items with humor potential.[38,39]
    d. Laughter libraries can offer a selection of funny and informative books about humor and health. Audiotapes and videotapes are usually a part of this collection.[40]
    e. Clown visitation programs are attempts to distract patients from their problems to help them forget their pain. Patients are given a chance to watch or participate in some fun and silliness.[41,42]
       1) A clown working in a hospital or nursing home, or on a home visit, is quiet, gentle, and empathetic. These caring clowns are sensitive enough to read nonverbal body language and have good listening skills.
       2) Clowns offer a momentary release from personal burdens, inspire joy, and stimulate the will to live.
       3) All clown visits should be pre-approved by the nursing staff.
       4) Clowns should ask (from the doorway) for each patient's permission before entering the room.
       5) All gifts need to be approved by the nursing staff.
       6) Visits should be limited to 10 minutes per patient, unless the staff permits longer visits.

7) Routines should not depend on the patient's verbal or physical response, but rather, the patient will be allowed to simply observe and be entertained.

12. Adhere to these general guidelines for the use of humor.

a. Establish a "humor advisory" committee, and assign key people to work together in groups to create and implement your program.

1) Assign committee tasks to include writing a mission statement; developing the goals and objectives of the program; formulating and presenting a budget; developing policies and procedures; educating and informing staff about the therapeutic benefits of humor; obtaining supplies; and securing ongoing financial support for the project from community resources.

2) Schedule committee meetings at intervals to update, brainstorm, and gather input from the staff who have seen the results of the program.

3) Have the committee review toys, costumes, videos, and books for their appropriateness, safety, and "funniness factor."

b. Before using humor, establish a relationship with the patient and family that convinces them of your professional competence and sincere caring.

c. Apologize immediately if a patient takes offense to any humor intervention, and indicate the therapeutic intention of your action.

d. Analyze the setting in which the humor intervention is to occur. Assess the degree of "privacy" from other patients or families who may not appreciate the humor.

e. Remember that humor is more likely to be appreciated after the physical and emotional pain has been relieved or after the life-threatening crisis has passed.

Evaluation

1. Evaluate whether the client's outcomes for play, laughter, and humor were achieved.
2. Evaluate the client's subjective experiences with play, laughter, and humor with the client.

REFERENCES

1. P. Wooten, *Compassionate Laughter—Jest for Your Health* (Salt Lake City, UT: Commune-a-key Publishing, 1996).
2. P. McGhee, *How To Develop Your Sense of Humor* (Dubuque, IA: Kendall-Hunt Publishing, 1994).
3. Wooten, *Compassionate Laughter.*
4. McGhee, *How To Develop Your Sense of Humor.*
5. Wooten, *Compassionate Laughter.*
6. L. Nahemow, ed., *Humor and Aging* (New York: Academic Press, 1986).
7. A. Klein, *Healing Power of Humor* (Los Angeles: Tarcher Publishing, 1989).
8. Wooten, *Compassionate Laughter.*
9. P. Wooten, Humor: An Antidote for Stress, *Holistic Nursing Practice* 10(2) (1996): 49–55.
10. Klein, *Healing Power of Humor.*
11. H. Lefcourt and R. Martin, *Humor and Life Stress: Antidote to Adversity* (New York: Springer-Verlag, 1986).
12. McGhee, *How To Develop Your Sense of Humor.*
13. Wooten, *Compassionate Laughter.*
14. K. Buxman and A. LeMoine, eds., *Nursing Perspectives on Humor* (Staten Island, NY: Power Publications, 1995).
15. N. Cousins, *Head First—The Biology of Hope* (New York: Dutton, 1989).
16. McGhee, *How To Develop Your Sense of Humor.*
17. Lefcourt and Martin, *Humor and Life Stress.*
18. Ibid.
19. Ibid.
20. Nahemow, *Humor and Aging.*
21. Ibid.
22. Wooten, *Compassionate Laughter.*
23. L.S. Berk and S.A. Tan, Eustress of Humor Associated Laughter Modulates Specific Immune System Components, *Annals of Behavioral Medicine* 15 (1993): S111.
24. Cousins, *Head First.*
25. B.M. Dossey et al., *Holistic Nursing: A Handbook for Practice,* 2nd ed. (Gaithersburg, MD: Aspen Publishers, 1995).
26. Wooten, *Compassionate Laughter.*
27. McGhee, *How To Develop Your Sense of Humor.*
28. Klein, *Healing Power of Humor.*
29. Dossey, *Holistic Nursing.*
30. Wooten, *Compassionate Laughter.*
31. McGhee, *How To Develop Your Sense of Humor.*
32. Klein, *Healing Power of Humor.*
33. Ibid.
34. Wooten, *Compassionate Laughter.*
35. McGhee, *How To Develop Your Sense of Humor.*
36. Buxman and LeMoine, *Nursing Perspectives.*
37. Wooten, *Compassionate Laughter.*
38. Ibid.
39. F. London, *Whinorrhea and Other Nursing Diagnoses* (Mesa, AZ: JNJ Publishing, 1995).
40. Wooten, *Compassionate Laughter.*
41. Ibid.
42. London, *Whinorrhea and Other Nursing Diagnoses.*

CHAPTER 22

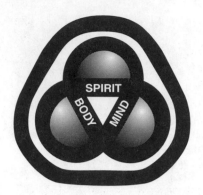

Self-Reflection

Lynn Rew

KNOWLEDGE COMPETENCIES

- Define the concept of self-reflection.
- Discuss theories of self-reflection related to self-identity, intuitive awareness, stress and coping, and health.
- Define intuitive awareness.
- Describe positive outcomes for both clients and nurses associated with self-reflection interventions.
- List five nursing interventions to promote self-reflection.
- Discuss self-reflection as a component of nursing theories.

DEFINITION

Self-Reflection: a way of looking within oneself for solutions to problems; contacting the inner wisdom that can guide the individual (nurse and/or client) toward healing, harmony, and well-being.

 Pause for a moment . . .

❑ *I am empowered when I network with colleagues who are also interested in holistic nursing.*
❑ *I explore, anticipate, and influence new directions and dimensions of health care, especially within the practice of nursing.*

THEORIES AND RESEARCH

Self-Identity and the Crisis of Adolescence

1. In infancy, an individual faces the crisis of trust versus mistrust. Erikson asserted that this crisis must be at least partially resolved before the person can face the crisis of autonomy versus shame and doubt in early childhood.[1]
2. Later in childhood, the individual faces the crises of initiative and industry versus guilt and inferiority.
3. During adolescence, the individual attempts to resolve the crisis of identity versus identity diffusion.
4. The adolescent's identity is formed by resolving previous crises in childhood: trust, autonomy, initiative, and industry. With each stage, the individual becomes a bit more capable of reflecting on the self as separate from others, thus building a self-awareness.
5. How well the adolescent resolves the crisis of identity depends on how well he or she has resolved the previous developmental crises in childhood.
6. The key to resolving these crises is interaction with other human beings and the ability to reflect on how others affect the development of the self.
7. Later in life, the adult faces crises in intimacy, generativity, and integrity, all of which depend on a solid sense of identity, the ability to interact with others, and self-reflection.

8. Crises of earlier stages are faced throughout the life span. Erikson referred to this as developmental residual.[2]
9. Virtues associated with facing the tasks of each stage are hope, willpower, purpose, competence, fidelity, love, care, and wisdom.

Intuitive Awareness and Self-Healing[3]

1. Human beings can learn to expand their awareness beyond ordinary cognition to include higher consciousness experiences.
2. Intuitive awareness is an expansion of knowledge about oneself and one's place in the universe. It is a broader and deeper knowing that goes beyond information available through one's senses.
   a. Intuitive awareness seeks wisdom about wholeness from within. This wisdom or truth is immediately known and is perceived without the usual linear reasoning process associated with cognition.
   b. Developing intuitive awareness requires a willingness to reflect on one's identity and the meaning of one's life.
   c. In the process of self-reflection, the individual learns to recognize and respect an inner voice of wisdom.
   d. Skills in self-reflection and intuitive awareness can be taught and developed through meditation, attention to sensations in the present moment, imagery, creative works of writing and performing, and contemplation of works of art.
   e. Self-reflection skills increase with practice in quieting the chatter in one's mind and listening to the rhythms of nature around and within oneself.
3. Clients/patients and their families, as well as nurses, often experience intuitive awareness as a sense that something is different, wrong, or about to happen but without concrete evidence to support this sense. This "sense" can be brought to conscious awareness through self-reflection.
4. Knowing oneself and what promotes healing are important components of professional health care services.
5. Self-healing includes cognitive awareness of physiologic functioning and intuitive awareness

of what the individual needs to get well and to feel connected with the community at large.
6. Sounds within the environment, including music, verbal suggestions, storytelling, and sounds of nature promote relaxation, self-awareness, and healing.

Stress, Coping, Modeling, and Role Modeling[4]

1. Events (stressors) that are external to the individual are perceived as more or less stressful and, thus, have variable physiologic effects on bodymind functioning.
2. Stressors may also be internal events that have variable effects on physiologic and psychologic functioning.
3. Perception of internal or external events can lead to self-care strategies or to self-destructive strategies.
4. Stressful life events are common to all individuals in diverse cultures. Awareness of one's cultural expectations and place within that culture affect the level of stress experienced.
5. The context of culture influences the meanings assigned to health and illness and affects one's choices and decisions about healthy lifestyle and health care practices.
6. Health, a dynamic state of well-being, is an outcome of continuous adaptation to the stressors of daily living.
7. A person's ability to cope is influenced by the coping resources available to the person and the potential to mobilize these resources.
   a. Learning adaptive coping responses begins with a cognitive awareness of the events that an individual perceives as stressful.
   b. Viewing events as threats or challenges influences the experiences of the individual, even when events are beyond the individual's immediate control.
   c. Becoming aware of choices in perceptions and responses enables the individual to experience and promote self-healing.
   d. Cognitive and emotive coping responses may be positive indicators of self-care, while specific behavioral responses (e.g., excessive drinking and careless driving) are self-destructive.
8. Nurse theorist Helen Erickson asserted that individuals carry with them a personal model of

the world, that is, their view of the world and its unique meaning to them.

9. In the nursing theory known as Modeling and Role Modeling (MRM), Erickson stated that when people are feeling ill or in distress, they know at some level what is out of harmony and what will help them to recover and heal. Self-reflection is one avenue to this self-knowledge (identifying personal strengths).

10. Modeling includes data collection and analysis from which the nurse constructs a model of the client's world. Nursing care is based primarily on the client's view and needs.

11. Role modeling involves the planning and implementation of nursing care based on the client's model.

12. The concept of adaptive potential is central to MRM. It is based on the assumption that individuals have varying abilities to use coping resources based on perceived stressors.

13. The nurse's role is one of nurturer and facilitator. The nurse accepts clients unconditionally and helps them to reach their full potential of optimal health and well-being.

Body-Mind Communication

1. Communication is continuous between the individual's external and internal environments and the unconscious mind.[5]
   a. The unconscious mind hears literally; the conscious mind interprets what is heard within a context of understanding.
   b. Hypnotic suggestion and conversations heard under anesthesia may hinder or promote healing because the unconscious mind does not assign meaning, but rather interprets literally.

2. Dreaming is a source of inner information.
   a. A dream diary may be a powerful documentary of inner wisdom.
   b. Discussing dreams with another person is a self-care strategy that promotes self-understanding and healing.

Health As Expanding Consciousness

1. Margaret Newman's nursing theory explores suffering and illness not as negative entities, but as a process of a dynamic field of energy.[6]

2. This view emphasizes the unity of life and the concept of the pattern of the whole.

3. Nursing interventions are not designed to identify and "fix" what is wrong with a person, but to recognize a person's pattern of information that is related to the whole.

4. Disease is one way for an individual to get in touch with his or her person–environment pattern; disease and disequilibrium may facilitate further growth. Disorder is a necessary predecessor of a new order of consciousness and freedom.

5. Human beings have the capacity for understanding and gaining insight into their person–environment patterns (potential consciousness).

6. As consciousness expands, there are concomitant gains in freedom of action.

7. Action depends on meaning. Nursing requires decisions and action about specific individuals within specific situations.

8. When telling their life stories, persons gain insight into their life patterns. This process of self-reflection leads to heightened self-awareness, integration, and creativity.

9. The nurse and client enter a partnership; they engage in a dialectic conversation that focuses on mutuality. The nurse's intention is to know and to care and to approach the other from a center of truth.

 Pause for a moment . . .

❑ *I operationalize the **AHNA Standards of Holistic Nursing Practice** in my practice and in my life.*
❑ *I understand the standards of care and the standards of practice.*

HOLISTIC NURSING PROCESS

Assessment

1. The nurse–client relationship is one of mutual respect and equality. The approach is subject–subject rather than subject–object.

2. In order to use self-reflection interventions, the nurse will assess the following:
   a. The nurse–client relationship should be purposefully directed toward well-being and more-being (i.e., client's personal motivation to pursue harmony between self and the environment);[7] nursing should be directed toward expanding consciousness.[8]
   b. The client's desire or need for nursing care should be based on self-understanding and

previous experience, awareness of person–environment patterns, and self-care needs.

3. The primary aim of assessment is self-identification of the need and desire to promote well-being and more-being.

4. The client beliefs to be assessed include the client's values, expectations, and self-talk about the meaning of health and the pattern inherent in the health–illness experience.

Nursing Diagnoses

1. The following nursing diagnoses compatible with self-reflection (self-care) are related to the human response patterns:[9]
   a. Exchanging: All diagnoses
   b. Communicating: All diagnoses
   c. Relating: All diagnoses
                       Impaired social
                         interaction
                       Altered role performance
                       Role conflict
                       Altered family processes
   d. Valuing: Disruption of person–
                         environment pattern
                         of the whole
   e. Choosing: All diagnoses
   f. Moving: Activity intolerance:
                         fatigue
                       Sleep pattern disturbance
                       Ineffective breastfeeding
                       Relocation stress
                         syndrome
   g. Perceiving: Body image disturbance
                       Self-esteem disturbance
                       Hopelessness
                       Powerlessness
   h. Knowing: Altered thought processes
   i. Feeling: All diagnoses

Client Outcomes

1. It is essential to establish with the client interventions that focus on encouraging the client's confidence in inner wisdom and ability to be connected to others.

2. The client moves toward the goal of self-understanding at an individual pace.

3. The client develops positive coping and self-protective skills that are congruent with his or her perception of events.

4. The client develops awareness of self as connected to the larger community.

5. The client recognizes freedom to take action and bring order out of chaos through expanded consciousness.

Plan and Interventions

For the Client

1. Plan with the client.

2. Focus on teaching the client to understand what the source of inner wisdom is, how it has helped in the past, what barriers would prevent it from helping in the current situation (e.g., beliefs, fears), and what would facilitate bringing forth inner wisdom.

3. Use relaxation and imagery to elicit the awareness of a deep inner source of knowledge and wisdom.

4. Begin by identifying inner strengths, including past accomplishments and coping resources.

5. Include awareness of fear of competence and self-efficacy.

6. Discuss person–environment patterns of disequilibrium to develop a new consciousness and the freedom to act in new ways.

7. Help the client reconnect with previous experiences and assign meanings to them.[10]
   a. The nurse facilitates self-reflection by encouraging the client to become more aware of self and competence in actions.
   b. Self-awareness in all dimensions of the client's life is not possible at one time; the process is dynamic and may be overwhelming at first.
   c. As the client becomes more familiar with patterns of self-enhancement and self-harm, cognitive awareness may be used to reinforce self-protection. Reinforcement may come from support groups and bibliotherapy.
   d. Guided imagery, meditation, and dream journal keeping can facilitate much of the inner wisdom work.

8. Use specific exercises to facilitate self-awareness and reflection:[11,12]
   a. Those that promote awareness of physical sensations (e.g., listening to sounds of nature, using both hands in new ways, concentrating on a variety of sights and smells).
   b. Those that promote creativity (e.g., drawing with both hands, using metaphors to describe one's life, keeping a scrapbook of things one likes).
   c. Those that promote peace and harmony (e.g., meditation on a mandala or mantra).

d. Those that promote authentic dialogue with others (e.g., writing a personal letter, having a discussion with a nurse).[13]

e. Those that connect the client with past events (e.g., life review or reminiscence therapy used with older adults).

For the Nurse

1. To be effective in helping others with self-healing, be aware of your own inner resources.
2. Give a gift to yourself: self-care and relaxation.[14]
3. Take responsibility for self-care and use power appropriately.[15]
4. As a healer and a helper, be aware of what you can change and what you cannot change.[16,17]
5. Learn to trust your intuition in working with clients.[18,19]
   a. Read about the phenomenon of intuition in nursing.[20]
   b. Discuss intuitive experiences with expert nurses.
6. Adopt for yourself interventions designed for clients for their self-reflection and healing (e.g., journaling, imagery, meditation, bibliotherapy).
7. Extend the transformation in you that comes from working with clients to the clients through energy exchange.[21]

Evaluation

1. The client reports whether aims (desires and needs for nursing) were achieved.
2. The nurse tries to observe objectively the degree of self-awareness reported by the client.
3. The nurse encourages continuous self-reflection to maintain the positive outcomes congruent with the client's view and needs.

REFERENCES

1. E. Erikson, *Identity: Youth and Crisis* (New York: W.W. Norton & Co., 1968).
2. Ibid.
3. L. Rew, *Awareness in Healing* (Albany, NY: Delmar Publishers, 1996).
4. H.C. Erickson et al., *Modeling and Role-Modeling: A Theory and Paradigm for Nursing* (Lexington, SC: Pine Press, 1983).
5. E.L. Rossi and D.B. Cheek, *Mind–Body Therapy: Ideodynamic Healing in Hypnosis* (New York: W.W. Norton & Co., 1988).
6. M.A. Newman, *Health As Expanding Consciousness,* 2nd ed. (New York: National League for Nursing, 1994).
7. J. Paterson and L. Zderad, *Humanistic Nursing* (New York: John Wiley & Sons, 1976).
8. Newman, *Health As Expanding Consciousness.*
9. R.M. Carroll-Johnson and M. Paquette, *Classification of Nursing Diagnoses: Proceedings of the Tenth Conference* (Philadelphia: J.B. Lippincott Co., 1994).
10. L.G. Kolkmeier, Self-Reflection: Consulting the Truth Within, in *Holistic Nursing: A Handbook for Practice,* 2nd ed., in B.M. Dossey et al. (Gaithersburg, MD: Aspen Publishers, 1995), 610–612.
11. Ibid.
12. Rew, *Awareness in Healing.*
13. Rossi and Cheek, *Mind–Body Therapy.*
14. K. Heinrich and M.E. Killeen, The Gentle Art of Nursing Yourself, *American Journal of Nursing* 93, no. 10 (1993): 41–44.
15. L.L. Hay, *The Power Is Within You* (Carson, CA: Hay House, 1991).
16. M.E.P. Seligman, *What You Can Change and What You Can't* (New York: Alfred A. Knopf, 1994).
17. R. Orstein and C. Swencionis, *The Healing Brain: A Scientific Reader* (New York: Guilford Press, 1990).
18. Kolkmeier, Self-Reflection: Consulting the Truth Within.
19. Rew, *Awareness in Healing.*
20. Ibid.
21. Rossi and Cheek, *Mind–Body Therapy.*

Concept IX

Health Promotion

CHAPTER 23

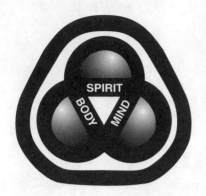

Relaxation

Elizabeth Ann Manhart Barrett and Leslie Gooding Kolkmeier

KNOWLEDGE COMPETENCIES

- Describe five benefits of relaxation training.
- Compare and contrast autogenics and progressive muscle relaxation.
- Compare and contrast hypnosis and self-hypnosis.
- Name ten physiologic responses evoked by the relaxation response.
- Discuss the commonalities of the various types of relaxation interventions.
- Discuss the caveats of the various types of relaxation interventions.
- Discuss key considerations for each phase of the nursing process in relation to the use of relaxation interventions.
- Describe ways for the guide to facilitate the relaxation process.
- Discuss the relationship between the relaxation process and certain types of medication.
- Explain the four stages of hypnosis.
- Discuss the rationale for selecting particular types of relaxation interventions.

DEFINITION

Relaxation: "a psychophysiologic state characterized by parasympathetic dominance involving multiple visceral and somatic systems; the absence of physical, mental, and emotional tension; the opposite of Cannon's fight or flight response."[1]

Pause for a moment . . .

- ❏ *I am increasing my knowledge of the **AHNA Standards of Holistic Nursing Practice** as I study the **AHNA Core Curriculum**.*
- ❏ *I know the two major parts to the **AHNA Standards of Holistic Nursing Practice**.*
  - *— Part I covers the discipline of holistic nursing practice.*
  - *— Part II covers the caring and healing of the client and significant others.*

THEORIES AND RESEARCH

Techniques of Relaxation

1. Relaxation training has a wide variety of benefits:[2,3]
   a. Decreasing anxiety related to painful situations.
   b. Easing muscle tension pain from skeletal muscle contractions.
   c. Reducing fatigue by interrupting the fight or flight response.
   d. Providing a beneficial period of rest.
   e. Assisting the client to fall asleep rapidly.
   f. Increasing the effectiveness of pain medications.
   g. Helping the client to dissociate from pain.

2. The major routes to the meditative state are through the intellect, through the emotions, through the body, and through action.[4]
3. Mantra meditation involves the repetition of specific words or sounds.
4. Progressive muscle relaxation is a technique developed by Jacobson in 1938.[5]
   a. The body responds to stress with increased muscle tension.
   b. Intentional tensing and releasing of successive muscle groups promotes relaxation.
   c. Several studies have shown that progressive muscle relaxation decreases anxiety and increases peak expiratory flow rates in asthmatic clients.[6]
   d. It has also been used successfully with hypertensive patients and those undergoing invasive diagnostic procedures.[7]
   e. It is most effective with moderate to high panic/fear levels.
5. Autogenics is an approach developed by Schultz in 1932.[8]
   a. Brief phrases are used to focus attention on areas of the body for the purpose of inducing change in those areas from within.
   b. Autogenics allows access to homeostatic recuperative mechanisms in the brain.
   c. This approach is effective with disorders involving cognitive functioning.[9]
6. Hypnosis makes it possible to quiet the muscles and direct mental attention to positive statements.
   a. Although hypnosis had been used for centuries, the American Medical Association did not endorse it as part of medical education until the 1950s.
   b. Currently, many medical, dental, psychologic, and holistic nursing practices incorporate hypnosis.
   c. Frequently, the specific purpose of hypnosis is to change behaviors, physiologic functioning, or to ease pain or enhance healing.
   d. Hypnosis and self-hypnosis enhance the client's ability to image through suggestions made when the client is in an altered state of consciousness.
   e. Nurses who personally use self-hypnosis are role models for teaching this modality to clients/patients.

7. Biofeedback is a doorway to sources of feedback that are ordinarily out of awareness (e.g., blood pressure, heart rate, skin temperature).
   a. Learning requires feedback.[10]
   b. Biofeedback enhances the capacity for healing, balancing, and regulating autonomic processes.
      1) Biofeedback research and clinical application have focused on headaches, cardiovascular control, temporomandibular joint disorders and bruxism, motor function disorders, gastrointestinal disorders, Raynaud's syndrome, and chronic pain.[11]
      2) Electroencephalographic biofeedback is being used successfully for addictions and attention deficit–hyperactivity disorder.
      3) Biofeedback can teach relaxation skills to those with type A personalities to modify risks for coronary disease.[12]
8. The open focus technique is an adjunct to biofeedback, especially electroencephalographic biofeedback, that uses phrases to produce alpha waves indicating deep relaxation.[13] It is particularly useful for clients with anxiety, pain, or goal-oriented attitudes.

Relaxation Response

1. The "fight or flight" response that prepares a person to deal with the actual or imagined threat of an emergency is a series of complicated psychophysiologic processes.
2. Benson and colleagues developed a nonreligious type of meditation that requires 20 minutes a day of focused concentration on a word or statement,[14] resulting in changes opposite to those of the "fight or flight" mechanism.
3. This relaxation response brings about changes in the autonomic, immune, endocrine, and neuropeptide systems.
   a. The following increase:
      1) Production of slow alpha waves.
      2) Electrical resistance of the skin.
      3) Peripheral blood flow.
      4) Activity of natural killer cells.
   b. The following decrease:
      1) Oxygen consumption.
      2) Carbon dioxide elimination.
      3) Blood lactose levels.

4) Heart rate.
5) Respiratory rate and volume.
6) Skeletal muscle tension.
7) Gastric acidity and motility.
8) Sweat gland activity.
9) Epinephrine level.
10) Blood pressure, especially in hypertensive persons.[15]

4. Benson's research on the relaxation response has tested a form of meditation similar to transcendental meditation and has been validated in various studies.[16]

Relaxation: Commonalities

1. Success in the use of relaxation interventions requires mindfulness, that is, the ability to focus on one thing only, whatever one is presently doing.
2. Effectiveness requires practice, practice, practice.
3. Clients must be advised of the discipline and self-responsibility required for successful use of relaxation interventions.
4. The sense of timelessness resulting from true relaxation allows for amelioration of anxiety and pain, as well as the regulation of physiologic change.
5. Through timelessness, one goes more deeply into the transpersonal and transcendent levels of creativity, insights, and meditative states.
6. All the interventions share passive attention or passive volition, the opposite state of making a change happen.
   a. Like practitioners of Aikido, clients allow the energy of the image of relaxation to carry them to a calmness state.
   b. Letting go of tension requires the bodymind to step aside and adopt an expectant, but nonstriving attitude.
7. The success of any intervention is enhanced through rapport, openness, and trust between guide and client.
8. Nurses must approach both the client and the teaching of the relaxation skill with a loving, accepting attitude.
9. Relaxation is far from "doing nothing"; it is an active, creative process involving intention and practice and influences other coping skills.

Relaxation: Caveats

1. Some people resist passively "letting go" for fear of losing control of themselves.

   a. These clients need reassurance that they will remain in control throughout the exercise.
   b. Relaxation will allow them to regulate their tension levels more appropriately.
2. Finding time requires creativity in the ways that these skills are incorporated into daily activities.
3. Care must be taken to ensure that relaxation exercises do not become additional stressors for the client.
4. Individualized choices of relaxation interventions require consideration of condition, time available, and personal preferences.
5. Because the need for certain medications may decrease as clients become more adapt at the relaxation process; close monitoring is necessary. If the client discontinues relaxation exercises, it may be necessary to restore the original dosages of medication.

HOLISTIC NURSING PROCESS

Assessment

1. In order to use relaxation interventions, the nurse will assess the following parameters:
   a. The client's perception of tension level and need for relaxation.
   b. The client's readiness and motivation to learn relaxation strategies.
   c. The client's past experience with relaxation, meditation, or hypnosis.
   d. The client's personal definition of what it means to be relaxed.
   e. The client's ability to remain comfortably in one position for 15 to 30 minutes.
   f. The client's hearing acuity.
   g. The client's level of pain, anxiety, fear, or boredom.
2. Because deep relaxation may exacerbate prepsychotic and psychotic symptomatology, it is also important to assess the client's perception of reality and any history of depersonalization states.

 Pause for a moment . . .

❏ *I am increasing my knowledge of the AHNA Standards of Holistic Nursing Practice as I study the AHNA Core Curriculum.*
❏ *I am more aware of the nine conceptual areas of the AHNA Standards of Holistic Nursing Practice:*

— *Holistic philosophy.*
— *Holistic foundation.*
— *Holistic ethics.*
— *Holistic nursing theories.*
— *Holistic nursing and related research.*
— *Holistic nursing practice.*
— *Meaning and wholeness.*
— *Client self-care.*
— *Health promotion.*

Nursing Diagnoses

1. The following nursing diagnoses compatible with and commonly associated with relaxation interventions are related to human response patterns:
   a. Relating: Social isolation
   b. Choosing: Coping, ineffective individual and family
   c. Moving: Activity intolerance: actual or potential diversional activity deficit
   d. Perceiving: Powerlessness
   Self-concept: disturbance in self-esteem, role performance, personal identity
   Altered sensory perception: visual, auditory, kinesthetic, gustatory, tactile, olfactory
   e. Knowing: Altered thought processes
   f. Feeling: Anxiety
   Altered comfort, pain
   Fear
   Violence, potential for: self-directed or directed at others

Client Outcomes

1. It is essential to establish client outcomes prior to the session.
2. The client will participate in relaxation experience at his or her own pace.

Plan and Interventions

1. Focus on baseline feelings/emotions obtained during the assessment.
2. Arrive at mutually agreeable goals for the session.
3. Record baseline vital signs; if using biofeedback equipment, record baseline physiologic parameters.

4. Help the client develop a positive expectation of what is to occur. Imaging a successful outcome facilitates the client's own healing.
5. Modify instructions and strategies to fit the situation; gradually lengthen the exercises.
6. Intersperse instructions with short phrases of encouragement.
7. At the end of the session, initiate a discussion of the experience and engage the client's cooperation in continuing practice until the next session. Review the journal in which the client records symptoms, medications, practice time, and results.

Breath Awareness

1. The nurse guides the client through a basic breathing relaxation exercise as an introduction to deeper relaxation.
2. The client learns to breathe in through the nose and out through the mouth, repeating one of the following breathing exercises slowly for several minutes:
   a. Breathe in blue light and everything needed to nurture oneself; breathe out gray smoke and all the toxins to be removed. Breathe out with long, slow exhalations, longer on the out-breath than the in-breath.[17]
   b. Simply attend to the breath, counting 1 on each exhalation.
   c. Count the breaths sequentially, going up to 4 and starting over.
   d. In the mind's eye, see the breath as a soft relaxing color and breathe that color into all areas of the body.
   e. Imagine the body as hollow, and allow each breath to fill the hollow body slowly with relaxation.
   f. Breathe relaxation up one side of the body and down the other; up the front of the body and down the back; up through the soles of the feet through the inside of the body; down from the top of the head, over the skin, and back into the feet.

Tension Awareness

1. The purpose of the tension awareness exercise is to help the client identify mental tension and anxiety, as well as the accompanying physical tension.
2. If the client becomes aware of internal differences, movement to threshold levels of tension is possible; the client holds just enough

tightness in the muscle group to be aware of beginning tension and then relaxes the group.
3. By moving from strong contractions to very subtle ones, the client can fine-tune the relaxation process.
4. Clients learn to avoid holding their breath as they tighten their muscles.
5. Progressive muscle relaxation is especially effective for clients who feel physically tense, anxious, or agitated; caution should be exercised with clients who have back pain and hypertension.

Body Scanning

1. Body scanning is taking a moment to inventory all parts of the body mentally and identify areas that are full of tension.
2. Clients who have perfected relaxation skills can then allow relaxation to replace tension.
3. Linking a body scan to another frequently performed activity (e.g., entering a patient's room) makes it easier to remember to do a body scan.
4. Doing 20 to 30 body scans a day provides not only insight into tension-triggering events, but also several minutes of relaxation time.
5. By learning to monitor muscle tension levels, one can modify them before they intensify.

Meditation

1. Each of the many different variations of meditation provides a different means to the same end: a relaxed, hypometabolic state, accompanied by a quiet bodymind.
2. Staying with a particular meditation path for 1 month before contemplating a change to another type is usually recommended.
3. Individuals should use the type of meditation that intuitively feels right.

Biofeedback

1. Biofeedback involves the use of instruments that show clients alterations in their physiologic function and allows them to intervene and change their own internal activity.
2. Biofeedback devices do not do anything to the client; they simply record, through skin electrodes, subtle changes in temperature, muscle activity, brain waves, sweat gland activity, cardiac rate and rhythm, along with blood pressure.
3. Feedback of information allows the client to make internal adjustments toward a relaxed state and to receive immediate reward through feedback of changes.

4. The most frequent use of biofeedback is to help clients learn to prevent overactivity of the sympathetic nervous system.

Hypnosis

1. As the bodymind becomes alert, but relaxed, self-talk decreases, and one can communicate with the subconscious.
2. Hypnosis requires motivation, relaxation, and concentration, but it also requires direction by a person trained in hypnosis.
3. The altered state of consciousness achieved through hypnosis is similar to guided imagery.
4. Clients may use the hypnotic trance to rehearse new coping skills, open new possibilities, and gain self-regulation of various aspects of the sympathetic nervous system.
5. There are four stages of hypnosis:
   a. Induction: the beginning stage of the trance, achieved through staring upward, gazing at a point, or fixating on a monotonous action, such as a clock pendulum or waves on a beach.
   b. Deepening: increasing the depth of the trance through spiral images, such as moving down a staircase or elevator.
   c. Plateau: the stage of the trance in which suggestions for positive change are embedded and previously decided goals are reinforced.
   d. Reversing: a return through the process followed in deepening to a state of relaxed alertness.
6. Assurance to clients that they will always remain in control and can enter a hypnotic state only voluntarily will help ease misgivings. Being in a hypnotic state can be compared to being completely engrossed in a book or a movie.

Self-Hypnosis

1. Hypnotic strategies are powerful tools to deal with anxieties, pain, or behavior patterns.
2. Self-hypnosis is safest and most helpful when it is coordinated with other recommendations of health care providers.
3. Clients' willingness to understand the source of their symptoms and to change their mental attitudes, repetitive behaviors, and lifestyles are requirements for letting go of their symptoms.

Evaluation

1. The first priority in evaluation is to determine if client outcomes were achieved.

2. To evaluate the client's subjective experience, the nurse asks open-ended questions about the relaxation experience and the insights gained from relaxation exercises.

REFERENCES

1. B.M. Dossey et al., *Holistic Nursing: A Handbook for Practice,* 2nd ed. (Gaithersburg, MD: Aspen Publishers, 1995), 574.

2. L.G. Kolkmeier, Relaxation: Opening the Door to Change, in *Holistic Nursing: A Handbook for Practice,* 2nd ed., B.M. Dossey et al. (Gaithersburg, MD: Aspen Publishers, 1995), 573–605.

3. M. McCaffery, Relieving Pain with Noninvasive Techniques, *Nursing 80* 10, no. 12 (1980): 57.

4. L. LeShan, *How To Meditate* (New York: Bantam Books, 1975), 32.

5. E. Jacobson, *Progressive Relaxation* (Chicago: University of Chicago Press, 1938).

6. P. Freeberg et al., Effect of Progressive Muscle Relaxation on the Objective Symptoms and Subjective Responses Associated with Asthma, *Heart and Lung* 16, no. 1 (1987): 24–30.

7. N. Pender, Effects of Progressive Muscle Relaxation Training on Anxiety anbd Health Locus of Control among Hypertensive Adults, *Research in Nursing and Health* 8 (1985): 67–72.

8. J. Schultz and W. Luther, *Autogenic Training: A Psychophysiologic Approach in Psychotherapy* (New York: Grune & Stratton, 1959).

9. J. Stoyva and W. Luther, In Memoriam, *Biofeedback and Self-Regulation* 11, no. 2 (1986): 91.

10. E. Green and A. Green, *Beyond Biofeedback* (Ft. Wayne, IN: Knoll Publishing Co., 1977), 24.

11. J. Hatch et al., eds., *Biofeedback: Studies in Clinical Efficacy* (New York: Plenum Press, 1987).

12. C. Moreno, Concepts of Stress Management in Cardiac Rehabilitation, *Focus on Critical Care* 14, no. 5 (1987): 17.

13. L. Fehmi, Paper presented at the Council Grove Conference on Voluntary Control of Internal States, Council Grove, IA, 1975, 2.

14. H. Benson et al., Decreased Premature Ventricular Contraction through the Use of the Relaxation Response in Patients with Stable Ischemic Heart Disease, *Lancet* 2, no. 7931 (1975): 380.

15. H. Benson, *Beyond the Relaxation Response* (New York: Times Books, 1984).

16. H. Benson et al., Decreased Premature Ventricular Contraction.

17. G. Epstein, *Healing Visualizations: Creating Health through Imagery* (New York: Bantam Books, 1989), 16.

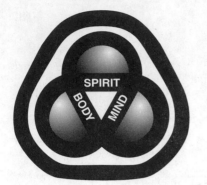

CHAPTER 24

Imagery

Barbara M. Dossey

KNOWLEDGE COMPETENCIES

- Discuss the physiologic effects of imagery.
- Describe the interaction of imagery with state-dependent learning and memory.
- Analyze three major theories on imagery.
- Discuss ten different types of imagery.
- Describe eight different techniques to empower spoken words.
- Explore imagery and the nursing process.
- Describe ways to facilitate and interpret the imagery process.
- Describe guidelines for imagery scripts.
- Analyze concrete objective information and the two components.
- Analyze strategies to empower words and phrases used in guided imagery scripts.
- Discuss how to work with novice and vivid images in the imagery process.
- Discuss ways to enhance the client's imagery skills.
- Explore drawing guidelines and strategies.

DEFINITION

Imagery: internal experiences of memories, dreams, fantasies, and visions; may involve one or more of the senses; serves as a bridge for connecting a person's body-mind-spirit.

 Pause for a moment . . .

❑ *The AHNA Standards of Holistic Nursing Practice provide me with the framework for the AHNA Core Curriculum and the blueprint for the holistic nursing certification (HNC) examination.*
❑ *My study of the AHNA Core Curriculum helps me in articulating and integrating the concepts, knowledge base, and holistic skills in clinical practice and holistic living.*

THEORIES AND RESEARCH

Physiologic Effects of Imagery

1. Images may either precede or follow physiologic changes, indicating that they have both a causative and reactive role.[1]
2. Images can be induced by conscious, deliberate behaviors, as well as by subconscious acts (such as electrical stimulation of the brain, reverie, dreaming, and brainwave biofeedback).
   a. People can be taught how to direct their imagery process to produce positive healing results.
   b. Messages—feelings, attitudes, beliefs, emotions, purpose, and meaning—have to be translated by the right hemisphere into nonverbal terminology before they can be understood by the involuntary or autonomic nervous system.[2]
3. Images can be considered as the hypothetical bridge between conscious processing of information and physiologic change.
   a. Images are preverbal, or without a language base, except through their physiologic connection with the left hemisphere.
   b. If connections between the right and left hemispheres were severed, untranslated im-

ages would continue to affect emotions and alter physiology, but without intellectual interpretation.

4. Images and thoughts are generated in the anterior frontal lobe and are directly connected to the limbic system where emotions are processed.

5. Images and thoughts are transmitted through state-dependent memory learning and emotional areas of the limbic and hypothalamic system by the neurotransmitters that regulate the organ systems of the autonomic nervous system branches.

6. Images can affect the voluntary (peripheral) nervous system, as well as the involuntary (autonomic) nervous system.

7. The neurotransmitters—norepinephrine (sympathetic branch) and acetylcholine (parasympathetic branch)—initiate the information transduction that activates the biochemical changes within the different tissues down to the cellular level.

   a. Neurotransmitters act as messenger molecules.

   b. They cross the nerve cell junction gap and fit into receptor sites found in cell walls, thus changing the receptor molecule structure.

   c. This causes a change in cell wall permeability and a shift of such ions as sodium, potassium, and calcium.

   d. The basic metabolism of each cell is also changed by a series of hundreds of complex activation of cell enzymes that become the second messenger system.

8. With imagery, all sensory modalities may be involved: visual, olfactory, tactile, gustatory, auditory, and kinesthetic. Each individual can learn skills to use his or her dominant sensory modalities with relaxation and imagery exercises.

   a. More than 60 percent of people are visual imagers; these people can see a mental picture of something. Others are predominantly kinesthetic (feeling, sensing) imagers.

   b. Those with highly specialized hearing skills, such as musicians and singers, image primarily with the auditory sense.

   c. With practice, all the senses are used.

9. It is common for affective experiences (e.g., feelings, fears, awe, relief, release) to surface during the imagery process. Sometimes this occurs suddenly or spontaneously and surprises the client. Since the imagery process taps into the subconscious/unconscious mind, emotions are an integral part of the experience. This is why imagery is such a holistic approach to caring and healing. It provides access to the bodymind and connects us to our emotions and spirit/higher self.

State-Dependent Learning and Memory with Imagery [3]

1. What is learned and what is remembered about an experience depend on one's psychologic state at the time of the experience.

2. When a person thinks of a painful memory from childhood (e.g., being reprimanded in front of friends), many different levels of the person's body-mind-spirit remember being severely embarrassed, angry, or shamed (state-bound information) at the time of the experience (state-dependent).

3. Emotions of the body-mind-spirit experience become embedded in memory.

4. Imagery techniques of reframing the experience help to heal the psychospiritual wounds.

5. Dramatic psychophysiologic changes that occur in imagery and hypnosis result from gaining access to state-dependent memory, learning, and behavior systems and creating a condition that makes the encoded information available for problem solving.

6. Every access of information can be seen as an opportunity to gain new meaning, and any nonhelpful behavior or painful state-dependent memory can be reassociated, reorganized, or reframed in a manner that resolves the negative memory and evokes new patterns of wellness and healing.

7. State-dependent learning and memory is the basis for all health education, goal setting, and self-care strategies, such as assessing life stressors, solving problems, and choosing healthy lifestyle behaviors.

Major Theories about Imagery

Eidetic Imagery

1. Ahsen described three unitary, interactive modes of awareness that comprise an eidetic (ISM):[4]

   a. I. The *Image* is the aroused sensation. It is the response to external reality and the objects around a person. Simultaneously, there is an "as if" image that represents an internal reality that is real in its own way.

b. S. Seeing an image produces a *Somatic* response or a neurophysiologic response.

c. M. The *Meaning* is ascribed to the image, and the left hemisphere tries to make verbal sense of a globally perceived experience.

2. Some images create meaning that is superficial, incomplete, or unclear.

3. The behavior in some images may be seen as defensive and self-limiting.

4. A person can have a fixed, frozen image of past events that disrupts thought processes and keeps them from taking on new meaning to evoke more effective behaviors in the present experience.

5. Conversely, a person can have very vivid images that provide profound insight about life processes.

Lexical and Enactive Modes of Imagery

1. According to Horowitz,[5] imagery is encoded, retrieved, and expressed in patterns of thoughts, physical responses, and a person's world view.

2. Images form, express, and evoke emotions that directly affect physiologic response.

3. Information enters the central nervous system, is encoded into images, and is stored in two modes:

   a. The lexical mode is that type of logical and analytic thinking that occurs in the left hemisphere.

   b. The enactive mode of thinking occurs in the right hemisphere, where emotions and kinesthetic experiences evolve.

4. A person has the ability to learn a new solution or develop new sensory-rich imagery patterns to different memories in his or her life.

5. A person can be taught to suspend negative images in a way that allows for a new experience.

6. Using this approach, a client confronts memory images that are having a negative impact on health and well-being in order to associate more healthy, adaptive imagery with new meaning and new somatic responses.

Psychosynthesis

1. In the theory proposed by Assagioli,[6] there are three parts:

   a. The lower unconscious represents the past in the form of forgotten memories and repressed events. It also includes the fight or flight survival mechanism.

   b. The middle unconscious involves the personal self, that is the levels of social awareness such as approval, judging, and so forth. It is the day-to-day processing of logical and intuitive information and daily functioning.

   c. The superconscious (higher unconscious) is the drive and pursuit for meaning and purpose. In this region, individuals touch the higher possibilities for living through inspiration, intuition, philosophy, and contemplation.

2. The greatest challenge for living resides in the superconscious, which is the connection with the higher self and is referred to as the transpersonal self because it transcends the personal self. The higher self is a synthesis of individual and universal connectedness.

3. Transpersonal imagery allows for connections with the transpersonal self.

Types of Imagery [7]

1. Receptive imagery is common when daydreaming, falling asleep (hypnagogic), and immediately upon awakening (hypnopompic). Images seem just to "bubble up" in conscious thought.

2. Active imagery occurs as a person focuses on the conscious formation of an image.

3. Correct biologic imagery implies images of the body as it might appear under a microscope; this type of imagery can help to reverse or stabilize the disease/problem/dysfunction.

4. Symbolic imagery has a quality of "a metamorphosis" in which the individual's unique imagery process creates profound images, often of people, objects, and events; for example, a woman may see her white blood cells as angels carrying bows and arrows around her body to shoot at the cancer cells and then to carry away the fallen cancer cells. This imagery is an unfolding process that cannot be forced.

5. Process imagery is a step-by-step rehearsal of any procedures, treatment, surgery, or other events related to health problems or life's challenges prior to the event. It may also be referred to as imagery rehearsal.

6. End-state imagery is the rehearsal of being in a final, healed state.

7. General healing imagery includes events rather than a process. It may involve colors or sounds; an inner guide, a wise person, animal, or object; a felt sense of unity, universal power, spirit, or God.

8. Packaged imagery is the use of tapes, such as self-hypnosis, relaxation, and imagery scripts,

sold commercially or prepared by the health care practitioner.

9. Customized imagery arises from an individual's unique imagery process after listening to packaged imagery tapes.

10. Interactive guided imagery goes to an even deeper level by eliciting and using a person's own images, both positive and negative.[8]

   a. A practitioner facilitates this process by guiding a person to bring to mind an image of something and then directly interacting with this image, often in dialogue. For instance, talking with the image of something that is healing may uncover what is needed to heal.

   b. This technique is often the most meaningful and self-empowering way to use imagery, because it taps into the individual's inner resources.

Pause for a moment . . .

❑ *The IPAKAHN Survey (Inventory of Professional Activities and Knowledge of a Holistic Nurse, see Appendix B) helped me to define and validate the professional activities statements and knowledge statements requisite for competent holistic nursing practice in various practice environments.*

❑ *I am excited about my goal of certification in holistic nursing.*

HOLISTIC NURSING PROCESS

Assessment

1. In order to establish rapport and mutual understanding about what will be done during the imagery session, the nurse assesses the client's

   a. History for organic brain syndrome, psychosis, or prepsychotic disease. If present, general relaxation techniques should be used instead of imagery techniques.

   b. Anxiety/tension levels.

   c. Experience to be gained from the session, why help has been sought, and what he or she wishes to change.

   d. Wants, needs, desires, or recurrent/dominant life themes.

2. When preparing to use the imagery interventions themselves, the nurse assesses the client's

   a. Primary sensory modalities.

   b. Experience with the imagery process.

   c. Ability to work with the eyes closed. If the client's eyes are to remain open, the client should gaze at a fixed point about 1 or 2 feet in front of him or her to help work with the imagery process.

   d. Knowledge and presence of relaxation skills.

   e. Uses of any daily medications (nitroglycerin, bronchial inhaler), as these medications can trigger some physiologic responses.

Nursing Diagnoses

1. The following nursing diagnoses compatible with imagery interventions are related to the human response patterns:

   a. Exchanging: All diagnoses

   b. Relating: Social isolation
   Altered role performance

   c. Valuing: Spiritual distress

   d. Choosing: Altered effective coping

   e. Moving: Sleep pattern disturbance

   f. Perceiving: Altered self-concept
   Disturbance in body image
   Disturbance in self-image
   Potential hopelessness
   Potential powerlessness

   g. Feeling: Pain
   Anxiety
   Fear
   Post-trauma response

Client Outcomes

1. It is essential to establish the client's desired outcomes prior to the session.

2. The client will participate in imagery experience at his or her own pace.

Plan and Interventions

1. Focus on the baseline feelings/emotions of the client obtained during the assessment.

2. Review with the client the basic structure of an imagery session.

3. Help the client develop a positive expectation of what is to occur. Positive imagery that is directed toward a successful outcome helps to focus and organize the client's own efforts to facilitate healing.

4. Be aware of individual differences with the imagery process.

a. Differences include images, colors, symbols, and meanings in relationship to the cultural diversity of individuals.

b. The use of each person's individual characteristics assists in the discovery of unique inner healing capacity of personal imagery patterns.

c. This awareness helps the nurse to recognize when the patient is ready for the more in-depth imagery and to avoid flooding the patient with too many imagery suggestions.

5. Use a relaxation exercise to assist the client in deep relaxation prior to an imagery session. A basic exercise is to have the client go to a special, safe place in his or her mind, using as many sensory experiences as possible.

6. Determine the length of the session based on the individual's needs, body responses, and session outcomes. The sessions can last from 10 to 15 minutes to an hour or longer.

7. Use the imagery assessment tool (Exhibit 24–1) to enhance the effectiveness of the client's imagery process after the session.

8. If it is an interactive imagery session, ask questions in a manner to keep the client in the imagery experience.

a. The unique power of the interactive process lies in the dialogue and interaction between the client and the images that arise.

b. Having the client describe what he or she is experiencing seems to deepen the process and engage the right and left hemispheres of the brain at the same time.

c. Interactive imagery cannot be scripted, because it depends on what is happening moment by moment in the process.[9,10]

Facilitating and Interpreting the Imagery Process[11]

1. Explain to the client that there is absolutely no way to predict what will surface in the client's imagination, for every experience is different.

2. Guide the client through the imagery process with the following steps:

a. Identify the problem or disease or goal of imagery. Have a basic understanding of the physiology involved in the normal healing process.

b. Begin with 5 to 10 minutes of relaxation or breathing exercises.

c. Encourage the client to explore the following images:[12]

1) The problem/disease.
2) Inner healing resources (strengths, faith, belief systems, and coping strategies).
3) External healing resources (treatments, medication, tests, and surgery).

d. End with images of the desired state of well-being.

3. Choose words/phrases to empower guided imagery.[13]

a. Metaphors: implied comparisons (e.g., relaxation as a "warm waterfall").

b. Truisms: statements that the intellectual mind accepts as accurate or as true (e.g., "As you take in the next breath, oxygen is flowing into your lungs and into every cell in your body").

c. Embedded commands: short phrases that stand out in a sentence because of changes in quality of voice, pitch, and tone (e.g., "You can . . . relax more deeply . . . if you want to").

d. Linkage: diversion of intellectual thoughts by connecting certain statements, behaviors, and actions with thoughts (e.g., "Once more . . . relax more deeply . . . and really sink into the surface of the chair . . . feeling yourself being supported by this surface").

e. Therapeutic double-bind: relaxation of the body-mind-spirit through involvement in the intellectual process of making different choices (e.g., "As you are stretched out in the chair . . . you might be able to relax more deeply by changing the position of your arms . . . or your head . . . or your feet. . . .").

f. Synesthesia: cross-sensing, combination of several senses simultaneously (e.g., "Can you *hear* the *color* of the wind?" or "Can you *see* the *sounds* your shoulders are making?").

g. Reframing: ability to contact the part of a behavior/s that may be preventing or prohibiting healthier behaviors or thoughts (e.g., "I dread the pain" to "I am opening and softening around the discomfort and it is floating away").

h. Mirroring: repetition of the client's words or descriptions rather than using your own.

4. Encourage client to discuss the meaning of his or her symbols and images. Often more insights will come.

a. Symbolic information that surfaces in the imagination is rich with personal meaning and is the most powerful type of imagery.

b. It is always best for the client to determine the meaning and interpretation of his or her

Exhibit 24–1 Imagery Assessment Tool

Clarity of imagery: How vivid, cohesive, and complete is the imagery overall? Does the story make sense to you?

0	1	2	3	4
not clear at all		moderately clear		extremely clear

Clarity Score _____

Imagery of disease/problem: How serious and curable is the disease or problem? Or is it incurable, vulnerable, and weak?

0	1	2	3	4
very serious, incurable		moderate severity		curable, no problem

Imagery of Disease Score _____

Imagery of inner healing forces: How powerful, righteous, pure, directed, and intense are the internal healing forces? How active and controllable are they?

0	1	2	3	4
none		moderately strong		extremely powerful

Imagery of Healing Forces Score _____

Imagery of external healing forces: How effective, comprehensive, curable, positive, and helpful is your treatment? Do the images depict a powerful therapy or one that is destructive? If several types of external healing forces are used, evaluate them separately.

0	1	2	3	4
harmful		helpful		curative

Imagery of Treatment Score _____

Symbolism of imagery: How symbolic is the imagery? Is it more factual or concrete? High amounts of symbolism are usually associated with a personal or mythic story.

0	1	2	3	4
no symbols		mixed or some		highly symbolic

Imagery Symbolism Score _____

How To Use Your Scores
- Evaluate each score independently. Do not add them up.
- Identify areas where you had the highest scores. These are your strengths.
- Identify what could be strengthened or clarified—the areas where you had low scores.
- Think about your emotional response to each component.
- Modify your imagery, if you wish. Take the IAT again after you've experienced your new imagery for about a week.
- If any of the IAT areas are unclear to you, you might benefit by gaining more information about the actual nature of the component—such as details about how your external healing forces are supposed to work.

Source: From *Rituals of Healing: Using Imagery for Health and Wellness,* by Jeanne Achterberg, B. Dossey, and L. Kolkmeier. Copyright © 1994 by Jeanne Achterberg, Barbara Dossey, and Leslie Kolkmeier. Used by permission of Bantam Books, a division of Bantam Doubleday Dell Publishing Group, Inc.

images. The guide should not interpret for the client.

5. Recommend that clients use imagery skills 20 minutes twice a day as well as incorporate "mini-practice" sessions on their own to enhance their skills.

Using Imagery Scripts

1. Guide the client in flowing with the flow of images and feelings from the imagery realm. It is not necessary for the guide to know the images during the session.
2. If the client has a question, answer briefly to avoid disrupting the free flow of images.
3. Insert the client's name at the beginning of each script and occasionally during the script.
4. To lengthen the scripts, pick up cues from the client's behavior and insert key words, such as "good . . ." and "relax even more."
5. Repeat key words that increase the client's relaxation response.
6. Speak slowly and pace the script as you watch the client's breathing patterns and other body responses. This increases the guide–client rapport and, thus, the effectiveness in the guiding process.
7. Use metaphors and phrases to enhance the imagery process.

8. Provide continuous encouragement for novices and less vivid imagers. A person with less vivid imagery may need more guidance as well as time to find the image. Positive statements can guide the client in positive self-talk following the session.

9. Do not distract vivid imagers with unnecessary encouragement. Suggest that the extremely vivid imager keep the eyes partially open to avoid feeling overwhelmed.

10. Close an imagery session with a brief general relaxation script. Have client connect from the inner world of personal images to the outer world of everyday life. (Example: "As you prepare to bring your attention to this room, remaining relaxed and calm, become aware of the chair, etc. . . .).

Providing Concrete Objective Information [14]

1. Include both subjective and objective experiences of events such as treatments, procedures, or recovery.
   a. For example, information about a surgical patient's subjective experience may include what is felt, heard, seen, heard, or tasted before, during, or after a procedure; the sensory experiences of a postsurgical healing incision (e.g., pressure, smarting, tingling); sensations over time (e.g., those that travel from the incisional area, fleeting sharp sensations when turning in bed or when coughing).
   b. Information on the surgical patient's objective experiences may focus on those that can be observed and verified by someone other than the person going through the procedure; information about the visits, the timing of events, and the environment of the procedure; when and where the surgeon, anesthesiologist, and presurgical nurse will visit; what information will be discussed in the visit; how and when the preoperative skin preparation is done; the procedure of being placed on the stretcher to go to surgery; awakening in the recovery room or critical care unit; what to expect about any tubes, sensations, and so forth.

2. Identify the sensory features of the procedure to be used.

3. Determine the individual's perception of the procedure/treatment/test to be experienced.

4. Choose words that have meaning for the client.

5. Use synonyms that have less emotional impact, such as "discomfort" instead of "pain."

6. Select specific experiences when giving examples rather than abstract experiences.

7. Help individuals reframe negative imagery if elicited in the previous steps.

Intervening through Drawing [15,16]

1. Use drawing to help clients externalize internal mental images and emotions and to ground their experience.
   a. The clients need not know how to draw.
   b. Most people are inhibited about drawing stick figures or just using colors, but stick figures and colors can reveal significant information to them about their rich imagery patterns.
   c. Using the nondominant hand helps clients get past the "I can't draw"; it is fascinating how the images come forward and are meaningful when done in this manner.
   d. Drawing is helpful with all clients who are not verbally sophisticated.

2. When working with a client's specific disease/symptoms, encourage the client to draw the disease/symptoms in the way that has self-meaning. [17]
   a. Two examples are as follows:
      1) Draw a picture of yourself, the disease, the treatment. [These drawings can be separate or interactive. The client's interpretation of the drawings often provides new insight.]
      2) Draw a picture of symptom/pain at its worst, at its best (usually tolerable), and gone. Then imagine the process in imagery.
   b. Drawing the imagery process often reveals how a client is sabotaging recovery. When an individual has a constricted view of healing possibilities or has a misunderstanding of the disease/symptoms, recovery is impaired.

3. Explain how drawing may help the client learn how to join the disease process, to let go of the inner struggle, and overcome resistance in order to achieve desired outcomes.

Evaluation [18]

1. The nurse and client should refer to Exhibit 24–1 to clarify the following areas:[19]
   a. Disease or disability: the vividness of the client's views of the disease, illness, or disability; if the disease or disability process is chronic, the client's strength or ability to overcome the barriers and create conditions to lessen the struggle.
   b. Internal healing resources: the vividness of the client's perception of the healing ability and effectiveness of this ability/action to combat the disease.
   c. External healing resources: the vividness of the treatment description and the effectiveness of some positive mechanism of action.
2. The nurse should explore with the client the following questions:
   a. Was this a new kind of imagery experience for you? Can you describe it?
   b. Did you have a visual experience? Of people, places, or objects? Can you describe them?
   c. Did you see colors while being guided? Did you see colors change as the guided imagery continued?
   d. Were you aware of your surroundings? Were you able to let the imagery flow?
   e. Did you like the imagery? Can you describe it? What is your dominant sensory mode/s?
   f. Did the imagery produce any feelings or emotions? Can you describe them?
   g. Did you notice any textures, smells, movements, or taste while experiencing the imagery?
   h. What is your next step (or your plan) to integrate imagery into your life?

REFERENCES

1. B.M. Dossey, Imagery: Awakening the Inner Healer, in *Holistic Nursing: A Handbook for Practice,* 2nd ed., by B.M. Dossey et al. (Gaithersburg, MD: Aspen Publishers, 1995), 606–667.
2. E. Rossi, *The Psychobiology of Mind–Body Healing: New Concepts of Therapeutic Hypnosis,* rev. ed. (New York: W.W. Norton & Co., 1993), 47–68.
3. Ibid., 51–54.
4. A. Ahsen, Imagery, Dreams, and Transformation, *Journal of Mental Imagery* 8 (1984): 53–78.
5. M. Horowitz, *Image Formation and Cognition* (New York: Meredith Corp., 1970), 73–79.
6. R. Assagiolo, *Psychosynthesis: A Manual of Principles and Techniques* (New York: Hobbs, Doorman and Co., 1965), 17–18.
7. J. Achterberg et al., *Rituals of Healing: Using Imagery for Health and Wellness* (New York: Bantam Books, 1994), 38–48.
8. S. Ezra and T. Miller, *Nurse Certificate Program in Interactive Imagery Workbook* (Mill Valley, CA: Nurse Certificate Program in Interactive Imagery, 1996).
9. K.H. Shames, *Creative Imagery in Nursing* (Albany, NY: Delmar Publishers, 1996).
10. Ezra and Miller, *Nurse Certificate Program in Interactive Imagery Workbook.*
11. B.M. Dossey et al., *The Art of Caring: Holistic Healing Using Relaxation, Imagery, Music, and Touch* (Boulder, CO: Sounds True Audio, 1995).
12. Achterberg et al., *Rituals of Healing,* 77–83.
13. Dossey et al., Imagery: Awakening the Inner Healer, 619–622.
14. N. Christman et al., Concrete Objective Information, in *Nursing Interventions,* 2nd ed., ed. G. Bulechek and J. McCloskey (Philadelphia: W.B. Saunders, 1992), 140–149.
15. Dossey et al., Imagery: Awakening the Inner Healer, 650–658.
16. H. Wadeson et al., *Advances in Art Therapy* (New York: John Wiley & Sons, 1989).
17. Achterberg et al., *Rituals of Healing,* 71–83.
18. Dossey et al., Imagery: Awakening the Inner Healer, 663.
19. Ibid., 651–652.

CHAPTER 25

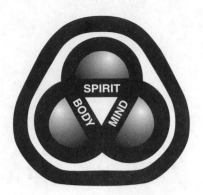

Music Therapy

Cathie E. Guzzetta

KNOWLEDGE COMPETENCIES

- Discuss the principles of sound.
- Analyze the psychophysiologic theories that explain why music therapy works as a bodymind modality.
- List the factors involved in choosing music selections that are relaxing for clients.
- Outline the recommendations for assisting clients to select appropriate music to achieve the desired therapeutic response.
- Discuss the development of a music library for use with clients.
- Examine the variables that a nurse would assess before guiding a client in a music therapy session.
- Compare and contrast the types of patients who may benefit from music therapy sessions.
- Outline the role of the guide in a music therapy session.
- Compare and contrast the uses for various music therapy scripts.
- Explore the ways in which the nurse and the client may evaluate the subjective and objective outcomes of a music therapy session.

DEFINITION

Music Therapy: behavioral science concerned with the systematic application of music to produce relaxation and desired changes in emotions, behavior, and physiology.[1]

Pause for a moment . . .

- ❑ *My successful completion of the holistic nursing certification (HNC) examination offered by the AHNA is both a personal and a professional mark of achievement.*
- ❑ *I will pass the HNC examination and will have the honor of writing the prized HNC after my name.*

THEORIES AND RESEARCH

Origin of Sound

1. Sounds result from the vibration of some object in a random or periodic repeated motion.
2. The human ear hears sound when it vibrates between 16 and 25,000 cycles per second.
   a. Within this vibratory range, 1,378 different tones are heard.[2]
   b. Sound is also perceived through skin and bone conduction, as well as through sight, smell, and touch.
3. The interrelationship between wave forms and matter is understood by rendering vibrations into physical forms.
   a. When scattered liquids or powders are placed on a metal disk with a vibrating crystal, repeatable patterns form on the disk.
   b. As the pitch changes, the harmonic pattern formed on the disk also changes. Thus, mat-

ter assumes certain shapes or patterns based on the vibrations or frequency of the sound to which it is exposed.

   c. The study of patterns of shapes evoked by sound is called cymatics.[3]

4. Waves are a series of advancing impulses set up by a vibration or impulse.
   a. In the heart, for example, the pressure produced by aortic distension after the ejection of blood from the left ventricle causes a pressure wave to travel down the aorta to the arterial branches.
   b. The pressure wave travels faster than the flow of blood and creates a palpable pulse called the pressure pulse wave.
   c. The pressure pulse wave is composed of a series of waves that have differing frequencies (i.e., number of vibrations per unit of time) and amplitude.
   d. In the arterial branches, there is one fundamental frequency and a number of harmonics that usually have a smaller amplitude than the fundamental frequency.
   e. Because the arterial vessels resonate at certain frequencies (fundamental frequency), some waves intensify while other waves disappear.
   f. This phenomenon is called resonance.

5. The human body vibrates, from the aorta and arterial system, down to its atoms.
   a. Atoms, molecules, cells, glands, and organs have a characteristic vibrational frequency that absorb and emit sound.
   b. Thus, the human body is a vibratory transformer that gives off and takes in sound.

6. Sympathetic vibration or sympathetic resonance is the reinforced vibration of an object exposed to the vibration at about the same frequency as another object.[4]
   a. For example, if two tuning forks are designed to vibrate at approximately the same pitch, striking one of the tuning forks produces a sound that spontaneously causes the second tuning fork to vibrate and produce the same sound as if the second fork was physically struck.
   b. The sound wave from the first fork physically strikes the second fork, causing the second to resonate responsively to the tune of the first.
   c. This sympathetic resonance occurs because the two forks contain similar vibratory characteristics that allow an energy transfer from one to the other.

7. When two objects have similar vibratory characteristics that allow them to resonate at the same frequency, they form a resonant system.

8. The atomic structure of the body's molecular system is also a resonant system.
   a. As long as the atom, cell, or organ contains an appropriate vibrational pattern, it can be "played" by outside stimuli in harmony with its vibrational make-up.[5]
   b. Environmental sounds may be capable of stimulating or producing sympathetic vibrations in the molecules and cells of the body.
      1) Some sounds assault the body because they are not in harmony with its fundamental vibratory pattern.
      2) Others are in tune with the body's fundamental vibratory pattern and may have a profound healing effect on emotions and organs, enzymes, hormones, cells, and atoms.

Therapeutic Use of Music

1. Musical vibrations can help restore regulatory function to a body out of tune (e.g., during times of stress) and help maintain and enhance regulatory function to a body in tune.
2. The therapeutic appeal of music may lie in its vibrational language and its ability to align the body-mind-spirit with its own fundamental frequency.
3. Music therapy complements traditional therapy, providing clients with integrated body-mind experiences and encouraging them to become active participants in their health care and recovery.
   a. Music can be helpful in reducing psychophysiologic stress, pain, anxiety, and isolation. It also is used to help clients develop self-awareness and creativity, improve learning, clarify personal values, and cope with a variety of psychophysiologic dysfunctions as well as cope with dying.[6,7]
   b. Appropriate music serves as a vehicle in achieving the relaxation response by remov-

ing one's inner restlessness and quieting ceaseless thinking.[8]

    1) It can be used to stop the mind from running away to achieve inner quietness.

    2) The healing capabilities of music are intimately bound to the personal experience of inner relaxation.

4. Music elicits a variety of different imagery experiences.

    a. Clients may visualize settings, peaceful scenes, images, or may experience various sensations or moods.

    b. Music passages can evoke scenes from fantasy to real life.

    c. Melodic patterns can evoke love, joy, and deep peace.

    d. During music therapy and relaxation, individuals can experience synesthesia or a mingling of the senses. Musical tones can evoke color and movement, or tastes can evoke shapes.

Shifting States of Consciousness

1. Music can be a vehicle for reaching nonordinary levels of human consciousness.

2. With music therapy, individuals are able to perceive two types of time:[9]

    a. Virtual time is perceived in a left brain mode and is characterized by hours, minutes, and seconds.

    b. Experiential time is perceived through the memory because of a state of tension and resolution.

3. Tensions and resolutions are perceived by the memory in a linear sequence that is called an event.

    a. An emotion or a sound, for example, is an event that can produce tension (producing psychophysiologic effects), which is followed by a return to equilibrium or resolution.

    b. The rate of these linear sequences or events influences the perception of time. For example, slow-moving music lengthens the perception of time because the memory has more time to experience the events (tensions and resolutions) and the spaces between the events. Thus, clock time becomes distorted, and clients can lose track of time for extended periods, allowing them to better cope with stress, anxiety, and pain.

Psychophysiologic Responses

1. Music alters a client's psychophysiologic status. The goal of music therapy and the type of music played (i.e., soothing or stimulating) determine the direction of the psychophysiologic changes.

2. Soothing music can produce a hypometabolic response that is characteristic of relaxation and alters autonomic (i.e., lowers heart rate, blood pressure, and respiratory rate, and increases peripheral temperatures), immune, endocrine, and neuropeptide systems. Likewise, music therapy produces desired psychologic responses such as reductions in anxiety and fear.

3. Some of these responses have been linked to the effects of music on the hemispheric functioning of the brain.

    a. Left brain functioning involves the rational, analytic, and logical way of processing information.

    b. Right brain functioning, in contrast, is concerned with the intuitive, melodic, creative, and imaging way of processing information.

    c. Music may activate the flow of stored memory material across the corpus callosum and provide a means of communication between the right and left brain.[10]

    d. Because music is nonverbal in nature, it appeals to the right hemisphere.

    e. In a relaxed state, individuals can let go of preconceived ideas about listening to music and its patterns, instruments, and rhythm and shift their thinking to the right side of the brain to alter their states of consciousness.

4. Some psychophysiologic responses result from music therapy's influence on the limbic system.

    a. Musical pitch and rhythm influence the limbic system, affecting emotions and feelings.

    b. The quieting and calming effect of music can produce other desirable autonomic, immunologic, endocrine, and neuropeptide changes.

5. The immediate influence of music therapy is on the mind state, which in turn influences the body state, producing a psychophysiologic response and a balance of body-mind-spirit.

Selection of Appropriate Music

1. Musical selections can influence the outcomes of music therapy.[11] Thus, it is important to choose the appropriate music for the desired response.

2. No one musical selection or any one type of music works best for all people in all situations. Musical selections that are relaxing and meditative to one client can be disruptive and annoying to another.

3. A variety of selections at least 20 minutes in length (e.g., nontraditional, classical, popular, country, operatic, folk, jazz, chorals, hymns) should be available because it is difficult to predict a client's music preference and response to any particular selection.

4. Musical selections without words are recommended. When the music has words, clients may concentrate on the words, their messages, and their meaning rather than allowing themselves to concentrate and flow with the music.

5. The iso-principle matches the individual's mood to the appropriate music so that the mind and feelings, which are vibrating at a certain frequency, are in resonance with the frequency of the music.

6. The nurse may guide clients to create their own tapes to match their moods and their musical preference.
   a. If the mood is tense or angry and a quiet outcome is desired, it is wise to start out with a short selection (3 minutes or less) of music that resonates with the mood.
   b. Then musical selections that increasingly move the individual to a more relaxed state can be added.
   c. Clients may enjoy spending some time experimenting with music and evaluating what happens to their body and mind when they listen to specific selections.
   d. Based on the response, they may create their own relaxation music tape 20 to 30 minutes in length.
   e. The more regularly they use the tape, the more effective they will become in achieving the desired outcomes.

7. Music has its greatest effect when the listener is appropriately prepared to experience the sounds.
   a. The four elements of relaxation should be applied to music therapy sessions:
      1) Find a quiet environment.
      2) Find a comfortable position.
      3) Maintain a passive attitude (i.e., neither force nor resist the experience).
      4) Focus all concentration on the music.
   b. Some form of relaxation exercise is recommended before the music experience.
   c. With a relaxed and receptive bodymind, music has the potential to enter the body and play through it rather than around it.
   d. The therapeutic effect of music decreases when individuals are angry, distracted, critical, analytic, or resistant.

Development of an Audio Cassette Library

1. An audio cassette library for use in inpatient or outpatient settings should include tapes on relaxation, imagery, and music therapy.
2. The suggestions in Exhibit 25–1 can facilitate the establishment of a successful tape library.

 Pause for a moment . . .

❑ *When I receive the HNC, I will be recognized as having the distinction of excellence in the area of holistic nursing.*
❑ *I will attain my HNC goal as an achievement of proficiency defined by the AHNA Certification Board.*

HOLISTIC NURSING PROCESS

Assessment

1. Before using music therapy interventions, the nurse will assess the following parameters:
   a. The client's music history and the types of music that the client prefers (e.g., classical, popular, country, folk, hymns, jazz, rock, blues, other).
   b. The types of music that the client identifies as making him or her happy, excited, sad, or relaxed.
   c. The types of music that the client identifies as being distasteful and making him or her tense.
   d. The importance of music in the client's life. Is music played at home? In the car? At work? For relaxation? For enjoyment? During times of stress? As a means of coping with stress?
   e. The frequency (per day or per week) with which the client listens to music.
   f. The client's past participation in relaxation/imagery techniques combined with music. How long? How regularly?

Exhibit 25–1 Establishing an Audio Cassette Library

Tapes and Recorders
- Have several tape recorders with comfortable headsets per unit.
- Place all equipment in a safe and convenient location.
- Have a variety of music tapes available. Commercial tapes are relatively inexpensive and readily available. A complete tape library will include music, relaxation, imagery, stress management tapes, and specific tapes for smoking cessation, pre- and postsurgery, weight reduction, pain management, insomnia, self-esteem, subliminal learning, etc. Consider different types of music such as easy listening, light and heavy classical, popular, jazz, operatic, folk, country, hymns, choral, and nontraditional selections.
- Ask staff members to donate one favorite relaxation tape to the library.
- Write the different tape companies . . . and request a catalog of their tape selections and descriptions. (See Resources at the end of this chapter.)
- Encourage nurses to develop tapes for specific client/patient problems that can help with procedures, tests, and treatments. The tapes may or may not have soothing background music.
- Have brochures and catalogues of recording companies available upon request from the patient.
- Encourage use of different tapes for further relaxation, imagery, and stress management training.

Tape, Recorder, Headset Check-Out Procedure
- If tapes are checked out on an outpatient basis, have the client make a deposit for the tape. It is suggested that the deposit cover the cost of the tape in case it is not returned.
- Establish who will have authority to check out the tapes and recorder. If in the hospital, a volunteer could assist in checking out the equipment for the patient after the nurse has assessed the patient's needs and selected the appropriate tape.
- Prepare a sign-out log that records the patient's name, room, date, and check-out time.
- Instruct the patient in the use of the recorder and specific tapes, if required.
- Allow 20 to 30 minutes of listening without interruption twice a day. Place a sign on the patient's door stating, "Relaxation Session in Progress—Please Do Not Disturb."
- Following the listening session, evaluate the patient's response to the tape and answer any questions.
- Chart the patient's specific response to the therapy. For example, were the desired outcomes achieved (e.g., lowered respiratory rate, decreased heart rate and blood pressure, decreased muscle tension and anxiety)? Identify the client's subjective evaluation of the experience (e.g., found the experience relaxing, helped with sleep, assisted in coping with pain, assisted with painful procedure).
- Return the tape/recorder/headset to the library and record the check-in information in the log.

Source: C.E. Guzzetta, "Music Therapy: Hearing the Melody of the Soul," in *Holistic Nursing: A Handbook for Practice,* B.M. Dossey, L. Keegan, C.E. Guzzetta, L. Kolkmeier (Gaithersburg, MD: Aspen Publishers, 1995), 686–687.

g. The client's use of some type of music for relaxation purposes.

h. The bodymind responses evoked by music.

i. The client's insight into the use of music to produce psychophysiologic alterations.

2. The client's mood (iso-principle) determines the appropriate type of music and the goals of each session.

Nursing Diagnoses

1. The following nursing diagnoses compatible with music therapy interventions are related to the human response patterns:[12,13]
   a. Exchanging: All diagnoses
   b. Relating: Social isolation
   c. Valuing: Spiritual distress
   d. Choosing: Ineffective individual coping
                   Noncompliance

   e. Moving: Sleep pattern disturbance
   f. Perceiving: Alterations in self-concept
                   Disturbance in body image
                   Disturbance in self-esteem
                   Hopelessness
                   Powerlessness
   g. Feeling: Alterations in comfort: pain
                   Anxiety
                   Fear

2. Based on the identified nursing diagnoses, outcomes and interventions are planned.

Client Outcomes

1. It is essential to establish the desired psychophysiologic outcomes with the client prior to the session.

2. The client will participate in music therapy at his or her own pace.

3. The client or family will select music of their choice.

Plan and Interventions

1. Explain that the purpose of music therapy is to facilitate relaxation and self-healing.
2. Discuss the length of the session, which is usually 20 to 30 minutes, generally two times a day (e.g., morning and afternoon).
3. Ask the client to remove eyeglasses or contact lenses. Dim the lights, and close the drapes.
4. Ask the client to sit or lie in a comfortable position. It is sometimes helpful to place a small pillow under the knees to relieve lower back strain. Have a light blanket available for warmth, if needed.
5. Suggest closing the eyes, if the client wishes, and finding a comfortable position with the hands at the side of the chest or on the body—whichever is most comfortable. Explain that they may change positions, scratch, or swallow. There may be noises around, but these will not be important if the client concentrates on your voice.
6. Spend a few moments centering yourself to be fully present with the client.
7. First guide the client in a few exercises to relax. Use breathing exercises and a head-to-toe relaxation script. (Refer to Chapters 23 and 24.)
8. Then, prior to turning on the music, guide the client in how to listen to the music (of their choice).
   a. Instruct the client to listen to the music and to let the music take him or her wherever the music wants to go.
   b. Advise the client to follow the music and let the music suggest what to think and what to feel.
   c. Ask the client not to analyze the music or the melody. Suggest that if distracting thoughts occur, the client should simply let go of the thought and come back to concentrating on the music.
9. Encourage the client to allow the music to relax him or her even more.
10. Inform the client that the music will play for 20 minutes, that you will be leaving the room, and that you will quietly come back into the room before the music is over.
11. In closing the session, guide the client back into the room by counting from 5 to 1. Suggest that the client will come back into the

room easily and quietly, feeling relaxed, calm, and peaceful.

12. While the client is in a self-reflective state, lead him or her in further guided imagery exercises, or journal entries, if desired.
13. If a client does not perceive any beneficial effects of the therapy after the first or second sessions, allow him or her to express that feeling.
    a. Explain that there is no right way to experience a music therapy session.
    b. Encourage the client to continue to practice the technique a few more times.
    c. Explain that relaxation is an acquired skill and the effectiveness of such therapy is usually a function of practice.
    d. Have two, three, or more sessions with the client to ensure that he or she acquires the skills to practice the technique at home.
       1) Some clients may wish to make an audio cassette tape of the guide's voice during the session or record a personal script.
       2) The audio cassettes then serve as the guide.

Music Bath Script

1. Explain that the purpose of the session is to prepare for a balanced day, prevent stress, and reduce stress.
2. Conduct a general relaxation session with the client before proceeding with this script.
3. Turn on the music and begin the following Music Bath script slowly, pacing the words with the client's increased relaxation:
   a. *As the music begins, you will begin a music bath. Allow the sound to wash over you, letting the music touch every surface of your body. Permit the sound to rinse off any tension, unpleasant emotions, and any sound pollution to prepare for the day. . . .*
   b. *Allow yourself to be immersed in the musical sounds as if you were in a warm, relaxing tub of water or standing under the warm water in a shower. Imagine the water filled with soothing, relaxing sounds. The sounds are cleansing your body and calming your emotions. . . .*
   c. *As you allow your entire body to become immersed in the sounds, notice how the music resonates in different parts of your body. As you become more relaxed, notice how much more you are enjoying the music* (pause).
   d. *As the music rinses away your tension, permit yourself to feel refreshed. The music bath has*

reached every part of your body. You have renewed and refreshed energy (pause).

e. *Allow any remaining tension to be washed away, permitting you to feel balanced, calm, and refreshed.*

f. *Continue listening to the music now for 20 minutes. As the music ends, gradually come back into a wakeful, relaxed, and refreshed state.*

Expanding the Senses Script

1. Explain that the purpose of the session is to expand awareness, open up the senses, and participate in a mingling of the senses.

2. Conduct a general relaxation session with the client before proceeding with this script.

3. Turn on the music and begin the following Expanding the Senses script slowly, pacing the words with the client's increased relaxation:

a. *Let the music take you to a soothing, peaceful place that is filled with various textures, sights, colors, and sounds. . . . Take a moment to find this place (pause). You feel comfortable and relaxed in this peaceful place. Slowly begin to explore the surface and texture of your surroundings. Permit the music to help you experience softness, smoothness, and gentleness (pause).*

b. *As you continue to explore, discover the colors associated with the shape, texture, and feelings of things. Let the music suggest the sound of the colors and textures.*

c. *Touch the things in your environment. Let your fingers, tongue, and cheeks experience the textures. Take time to enjoy each feeling. Do not feel rushed as you explore (pause).*

d. *As you touch each thing in your surroundings, take time to investigate its source. Where did it come from? Why does it feel as it does? And why is it here?*

e. *With each surface, explore its color, its sound. The deeper you travel into the essence of your surroundings, the richer the experience will be. . . .*

f. *Continue this experience for another 10 to 20 minutes. Gradually come back into the room awake, alert, and ready to continue the day.*

Merging the Bodymind with Music Script

1. Explain that the purpose of the session is to have a quiet listening experience, mingle the senses, and induce relaxation.

2. Conduct a general relaxation session with the client before proceeding with this script.

3. Turn on the music and begin the following Merging the Bodymind with Music script slowly, pacing the words with the client's increased relaxation:

a. *Image your ears. Explore your ears. Feel your ears expanding and becoming larger. Permit your ears to become channels in the sides of your head that open and lengthen throughout your body and into your feet. Allow these channels to hear all parts of your body.*

b. *Think of the sounds you are hearing as something more than a pleasant hearing sensation. The sounds are nourishment and energy for your body, your mind, your spirit. . . . Let the sound of the music move in you, around you, above you, below you. The sound is everywhere and you can hear it throughout your body. . . .*

c. *See the sound, taste it, feel it, smell it, hear it. Turn the sound into light and color and see it. Concentrate your attention on the sounds and the silences between them (pause).*

d. *Open your ears. You have beautiful, big ears—channels throughout your body. Let the sounds pass through these channels to totally experience the event. Merge with the music. There will no longer be music and a listener, rather a state of total experiencing of the sound. Total concentration of the sound—moment by moment and on the silences between (pause). You can go beyond. . . . You will experience the soundless sound, the state where sound becomes silence, silence becomes sound, and they merge together.*

e. *Continue the experience for another 10 to 20 minutes. Gradually come back into the room awake, alert, and ready to continue the day.*

Toning and Groaning Script

1. Explain that the purpose of the session is to release intense emotions, prepare for meditation, or induce an altered state of consciousness for music listening.

2. Instruct the client to lie comfortably on the back.

3. Use the following Toning and Groaning script, pacing the session based on the client's needs:

a. *Lie comfortably on your back. Begin with an audible groan such as "Ohhh" or "Ahhh." Let the groan be as deep as possible without forcing* it. *Let it give you a feeling of release, of emptying out any tension. Feel your skin and bones vibrate with the sound.*

b. *Many people spontaneously groan when they have taken off a tight belt or tight shoes. Your groaning should be a comparable release of and freedom from constraint. Let it be loud and natural without forcing the sound (pause). You might even feel a bit silly about groaning. You might giggle or laugh. That's OK. Just let it out. . . .*

c. *Stretch your arms and legs now. Then let your body relax and groan again. Notice the sound becoming effortless, relaxing, and deeper. . . . Be sure to let the groan come from deep down in your feet. Notice the vibrations starting up your body. As you continue to groan, feel a weight being lifted from you. Heaviness is being lifted while a sense of lightness sets in (pause). Groaning is a healing process. Allow it to happen. Enjoy the feeling of release. . . .*

d. *You will notice a tendency for your voice to rise as your tensions are allowed to leave. Let your voice do what it wants as you continue to groan. It will find its natural place. When your body reaches its tune, it will be satisfied, and you will sigh a deep satisfying sigh.*

e. *At this point, you are toning. You have found your tone. You are sounding your tone. You are resonating with your body. This is your own music.*

4. End session or prepare for imagery scripts, meditation, or music listening.

Training for Skillful Listening Script

1. Explain that the purpose of the session is to improve the art of listening and train oneself to hear sounds clearly and consciously.
2. Instruct the client to lie or sit comfortably.
3. Use the following Training for Skillful Listening script, pacing the session based on the client's needs:
   a. *Concentrate on the sounds around you. Let your ears hear every possible sound. Explore the subtle sounds, breathing, distant cars, wind blowing, hum of the lights. . . .*
   b. *Limit your sensations. Keep your eyes closed. Avoid touching. Heighten and isolate your perception of sound. Listen to the parts of sound. Listen to a sound. Imagine the sound makes a*

line. *Bend the line that the sound makes. Does it go up? Does it go down? Does it curve or have humps? The word* bend *itself has a bend. Notice the height of the bend. Image the top and bottom of the bend. . . . Image the grain of the sound. Is it rough or smooth? Rough like sandpaper or smooth like silk or something in between? What is the volume? High or low? What is the intensity? Loud or soft? What color do you associate with the sound? What emotions do you notice as you listen to this sound?*

c. *Now use your voice to imitate sound. Imitate the sound of a jet flying high through the air. . . . Now imitate the sound of a helicopter flying through the air. . . . Imitate the sound of a soft wind. . . . Imitate the sound of an autumn leaf falling. The point of this exercise is not to become an expert jet imitator, but to realize there is more to the art of listening and hearing than we think. When you practice focused and conscious hearing, you will recognize subtle differences in sound. You will expand your skills in the art of listening.*

Evaluation

1. To evaluate the client's subjective responses to specific types of music, the nurse asks the following questions:
   a. Was this a new kind of music listening experience for you? Can you describe it?
   b. Did you have any visual experiences? Of people, places, or objects? Can you describe them?
   c. Did you see any colors while listening? Did the colors change as the music changed?
   d. Did you notice any textures, smells, movements, or taste while experiencing the music?
   e. Were you less aware of your surroundings? Were you able to flow with the music?
   f. Did you like the music?
   g. Did the music produce any feelings or emotions?
   h. Was the experience pleasant?
   i. Did you feel relaxed and refreshed after the experience?
   j. Would you like to try this again?
   k. What would be helpful to make this a better experience for you?[14]

2. Sharing helps evaluate the experience and clarify any misconceptions.
   a. Clients may worry if they cannot image, see colors, or feel relaxed.
   b. They need reassurance that there is no right response and that all people do not experience the same type of sensations, feelings, sights, or sounds in the same way.
3. Some people may share that their experience was totally different from anything else they had ever experienced.

REFERENC ES

1. C. Schulbert, *The Music Therapy Sourcebook* (New York: Human Sciences Press, 1981), 13.

2. R. Leviton, Healing Vibrations, *Yoga Journal*, January–February (1994): 59–60.

3. H. Jenny, *The Structure and Dynamics of Waves and Vibrations* (Basel, Switzerland: Basilius Press, 1967).

4. S. Halpern and L. Savary, *Sound Health: Music and Sounds That Make Us Whole* (New York: Harper & Row, 1985), 33.

5. Ibid., 37.

6. P.M. Hamel, *Through Music to the Self* (Boulder, CO: Shambhala Press, 1979), 166.

7. H. Bonney and L. Savary, *Music and Your Mind* (New York: Harper & Row, 1973), 15.

8. C.E. Guzzetta, Music Therapy: Hearing the Melody of the Soul, in *Holistic Nursing: A Handbook for Practice*, by B.M. Dossey et al. (Gaithersburg, MD: Aspen Publishers, 1995), 669–698.

9. R. McClellan, Music and Altered States of Consciousness, *Dromenon* 2 (1979): 3–5.

10. D.G. Campbell, *Introduction to the Musical Brain* (St. Louis: MMB Music, 1984), 14–65.

11. G.C. Mornhinweg, Effects of Music Preference and Selection on Stress Reduction, *Journal of Holistic Nursing* 10, no. 2 (1992): 101–109.

12. B.J. Crowe, Music—The Ultimate Physician, in *Music: Physician for Times to Come*, ed. D. Campbell (Wheaton, IL: Quest Books, 1991), 111.

13. D. Aldridge, The Music of the Body: Music Therapy in Medical Settings, *Advances* 9, no. 1 (1993): 17–35.

14. Guzzetta, Music Therapy: Hearing the Melody of the Soul, 693.

RESOURCES

Relaxation, Music and Imagery Tapes

Awakening Productions
4132 Tuller Avenue
Culver, CA 90230

Bodymind Systems
910 Dakota Drive
Temple, TX 76504
(817) 773-2337

Catalog Services
P.O. Box 1244
Boulder, CO 80306
(303) 443-8484

Conscious Living Foundation
P.O. Box 9
Drain, OR 97435
(1-800) 752-CALM

Steve Halpern Sound Rx
P.O. Box 1439
San Rafael, CA 94915
(415) 491-1930

Institute for Music, Health, and Education
Don G. Campbell, Director
P.O. Box 1244
Boulder, CO 80306
(303) 443-8484

Magna Music
10370 Page Industrial Blvd.
St. Louis, MO 63132
(800) 543-3771

Mind/Body Health Sciences
393 Dixon Road, Goldhill
Salina Star Route
Boulder, CO 80302
(303) 440-8460

Music Design
4650 N. Port Washington Road
Milwaukee, WI 53212
1-800-862-7232

New Era Media
425 Alabama Street
San Francisco, CA 94110
(415) 863-3555

Sources Cassette
Dept. 99, P.O. Box W
Stanford, CA 94305
(415) 328-7171

Windham Hill Records
P.O. Box 9388
Stanford, CA 94305

Music Therapy Tapes Designed for Hospital Use

Music RX
P.O. Box 173
Port Townsend, WA 98368
(206) 385-6160

Steven Halpern (Hospital Suite)
P.O. Box 1439
San Rafael, CA 94915
(415) 491-1930

Additional Resources

American Association of Music Therapy
P.O. Box 80012
Valley Forge, PA 19484
(215) 265-4006

Institute for Consciousness and Music
7027 Bellona Ave.
Baltimore, MD 21212

International Society for Music in Medicine
Dr. Ralph Springe, Executive Director
Sportkrankenhaus Hellersen
Paulmannshoher, Strasse 17
D-5880 Ludenscheid, Germany

Mid-Atlantic Institute for Guided Imagery and Music
Sara Jane Stokes, Director
Box 4655
Virginia Beach, VA 23454

National Association of Music Therapy
8455 Colesville Road, Suite 930
Silver Spring, MD 20910
(301) 589-3300

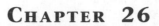
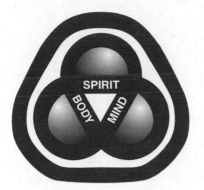

Touch

Karilee Halo Shames

KNOWLEDGE COMPETENCIES

- Discuss the physiologic effects of touch.
- Compare and contrast various types of touch therapies.
- Describe subjective and objective changes in a client after a touch therapy session.
- List uses for touch therapies by nurses in clinical settings.
- Identify ways to prepare for a touch therapy session.
- List two important nursing actions immediately after the session.

DEFINITIONS

Acupressure: the application of finger and/or thumb pressure to specific sites along the meridians of the body to relieve tension and enhance flow of energy along meridian lines.

Centering: a process of entering a state of balance where one can feel unified, integrated, and focused.

Energy Meridian: according to Eastern theories, an energy circuit or lines of flow vertically through the body, with culminating points in hands, feet, ears.

Foot Reflexology: a system of applying pressure with the hands or a blunt instrument to points on the feet that correspond to various organs and areas of the body.

Intention: motivation for touching as established by the healer when working with the client.

Shiatsu: a healing system that was developed in ancient Japanese culture and is widely used today. It involves the use of the thumb and/or heel of hand (occasionally, the feet) for deep pressure work along energy meridian lines.

Therapeutic Massage: the use of the hands to apply pressure and motion on the skin and underlying muscle of the recipient for purposes of physical and psychologic relaxation, improvement of circulation, relief of sore muscles, and other therapeutic effects.

Therapeutic Touch: a specific technique of centering intention used while the practitioner moves the hands through the recipient's energy field to assess and treat imbalance.

Touch Therapy: a broad range of hand techniques that a practitioner can use on or near the body to support the client's movement toward balance, wholeness, and optimal function.

 Pause for a moment . . .

- ❑ *It is exciting to be part of a historic time in the history of the AHNA and holistic nursing.*
- ❑ *I will emerge on the doorstep of the twenty-first century with my holistic nursing certification (HNC).*
- ❑ *I am empowered to join with other nurse healers as we reclaim what has always been at the core of nursing and healing.*
- ❑ *My healing journey is rich with life experiences.*
- ❑ *I am achieving my goal of certification in holistic nursing.*

THEORIES AND RESEARCH

History of Touch Therapies

1. Rubbing, pressing, massaging, and holding are natural manifestations of the desire to heal and care.
2. The oldest written documentation of the use of touch therapies is from the Orient; it was written 5,000 years ago.
3. Egyptians used poultices, touch, and manipulation.
4. Ancient Indian Vedas, Polynesian Lomi, and native American Indians all described healing massage.
5. There have been cultural prohibitions around touch.
   a. The rise of the Puritan culture during the 1600s correlated with a decline in use of touch therapies.
   b. Scientific medicine associated early touch therapies with superstition and primitive healing.
   c. Touch as a therapeutic intervention in U.S. health care remained undeveloped until research into its benefits began in 1950s.
6. All cultures, both ancient and modern, have developed some form of touch therapies, but specific attitudes about touch vary from culture to culture.
   a. Nurses must be aware of personal and cultural views of touch.
   b. The Oriental world view is founded on energy.
      1) Qi, chi energy, or vital force is the center of body function.
      2) A meridian is an energy circuit or line of force that runs vertically through the body.
      3) Magnetic or bioelectrical patterns flow through our bodies as magnetic patterns flow through the earth.
      4) Pressure placed on points along those lines influences meridian lines and zones; hence, acupuncture or Shiatsu direct healing energy via a flow through the body and out through the hands.
   c. The Western world view is based on reductionism of matter.
      1) The physical effect of cellular changes influences healing.
      2) Massage stimulates cells to aid in waste discharge, promotes dilation of vascular system, and encourages lymphatic drainage.

Modern Concepts of Touch

1. Current research is documenting what healers have known intuitively.
2. In the 1950s, Harlow's studies with monkeys and surrogate mothers demonstrated the significance of touch in normal growth and development.[1]
3. Studies of human development have likewise demonstrated the importance of touch to healthy maturation.
   a. In a study of abandoned infants and infants whose mothers were imprisoned, babies held by nurses thrived; those who were left alone became ill and died.[2]
   b. Other studies have shown that touch has a positive effect on the immune system.[3]
4. As these early studies awakened scientific interest in the uses of touch for healing, Grad investigated the laying on of the hands through a series of double-blind experiments with renowned healer Oskar Estebany.[4]
   a. Studies on wounded mice and damaged barley seeds in control and experimental groups demonstrated a significantly accelerated healing rate in those touched intentionally by Estebany.
   b. In another study, an enzymologist worked with Grad in using the enzyme trypsin in double-blind studies; the activity of the enzyme was significantly increased after exposure to Estebany's treatments.[5]

Nursing Studies

1. In the area of critical care, studies have shown that the use of touch enhances verbal interaction between nurses and patients.[6]
2. Touch slows heart rate, decreases diastolic blood pressure, and reduces anxiety.[7]
3. Despite growing evidence that touch is beneficial, Schoenhofer found that touch was seldom used as a nursing comfort measure in 30 nurse–patient dyads in hospital critical care units.[8]
4. Poverty of touch is acute among the elderly.[9]
   a. Older patients are likely to receive the least amount of touch.[10]
   b. Less mobile elderly patients respond more positively to touch than do mobile patients.[11]

5. Therapeutic touch has been shown to reduce time needed to calm children after stressful experiences.[12]
6. In obstetrical nursing care, touch helps women cope with labor.
7. The process of touch involves more than skin contact. It involves many aspects of connecting with others, including nonverbal interaction and response.

Touch Techniques

1. Most general touch therapies have basic, intermediate, and advanced levels. The complexity used can depend on the amount of time that the practitioner has spent studying the multiple variations of the therapy and whether it is being used in conjunction with other therapies.
2. The various techniques of therapeutic massage are similar, involving the use of effleurage, petrosauge, and tapotement.
   a. All are classic nursing back rub strokes designed to enhance circulation of blood and lymph.
   b. Therapeutic massage increases the dispersion of nutrients, promotes the removal of metabolic wastes, and increases lymphatic and blood flow.
3. In continuing education seminars on therapeutic touch, experienced practitioners from beginning to advanced levels teach
   a. Assessment.
   b. Hand scan.
   c. Intuition.
   d. Energy field reading and mapping.
      1) Recording.
      2) Pattern comparison.
      3) Verbal information.
      4) Stress levels.
      5) Relaxation levels.
      6) Meditation.
   e. Synergistic therapies.
      1) In a therapeutic touch session, the practitioner may ask the client to visualize clearly the part of the body that is to be influenced.
      2) Practitioners must develop an awareness of events that normally occur below the level of consciousness to come in contact with these subtle energies. The imagery and visualization process is one way to contact subtle energies.
      3) It is time to stop the therapeutic touch process when there are no longer notable differences in body symmetry relative to density or temperature variation.
      4) Common responses to therapeutic touch are flushed skin, deep sighs, physical relaxation, and verbalized relaxation.
      5) It is advisable to limit the amount of time or energy sent to the very young, very old, and the infirm. When the client's field is full, the nurse can feel pushed away.
4. Transformational Healing is a process of using one's personal journey as a healer for purposes of growth, education, health promotion, and environmental enhancement.
   a. It provides the nurse with an opportunity to explore the personal meaning of his or her personal healing process and to use a variety of healing approaches, including energy interventions, to maximize wellness.
   b. This deepened understanding can then be applied to support the empowerment and transformation of clients.
5. Healing touch is a collection of noninvasive, energy-based techniques intended to make energy available to the client. It involves working from a centered state, applying localized and systemic techniques to enhance relaxation and balance energy.
6. Acupressure and Shiatsu treatments range from basic to advanced, working with points and energy flow.
7. Reflexology is a system of pressing points on the hands or (more commonly) feet to evoke bodymind relaxation. Some practitioners believe that specific areas represent nerve or meridian endings for specific vital body parts.
8. There are numerous other systems and therapies involving touch and energy field maneuvers:
   a. Somatic/therapeutic/musculoskeletal therapies.
      1) Swedish massage.
      2) Esalen massage.
      3) Neuromuscular therapy.
      4) Myofascial release.
      5) Lymphatic massage/drainage therapies.
      6) Aston patterning.
   b. Oriental/Meridian-based/point therapies.
      1) Acupressure.
      2) Amma therapy.

3) Jin Shin Jyutsu.
4) Shiatsu.
5) Myotherapy.
6) Reflexology.
7) Touch for health.
c. Energy-based therapies.
1) Therapeutic touch.
2) Reiki.
3) Polarity.
4) Barbara Brennan chelation.
5) Leonard Laskow HoloEnergetics.
6) SHEN therapy.
d. Emotional bodywork.
1) Lomi.
2) Network chiropractic.
3) Reichian.
4) Hellerwork.
5) Rolfing.
6) Structural integration.
e. Manipulative therapies.
1) Chiropractic.
2) Osteopathic.
3) Physical therapy.
f. Other holistic touch-related therapies.
1) Trager.
2) Craniosacral therapy.
3) Feldenkrais.
9. Related Programs, Therapies, and Organizations
a. Programs (some of which lead to specialization and certification)
1) Alexander Technique—using gentle hands-on guidance and verbal instruction, teaching simple ways of moving to improve balance, posture, and coordination.
2) Amma Therapy®—techniques working with physical body, bio-energy, and emotions working with "qi" (energy) to restore to optimal balance.
3) Barbara Brennan School of Healing Science—multidimensional healing program based on teachings of Barbara Brennan; chelation work through the layers of the human energy field.
4) Chiropractic—alternative form of medical care with extensive training program; manipulations create spinal alignment.
5) The Crucible Program—multidimensional healing program based on teachings of Reverend Rosalyn Bruyere.
6) Feldenkrais—gentle manipulations to heighten awareness of body.

7) Healing Touch—multilevel energy healing program combining techniques from a variety of sources.
8) Jin Shin Jyutsu—"art of compassionate spirit"; gentle acupressure-type self-healing approach.
9) Lomi—aids learning of postural alignment to enhance flow of energies; directs attention to muscle tension.
10) Leonard Laskow's Healing with Love Foundation—uses HoloEnergetics®.
11) National Association of Nurse Massage Therapists—for nurses specifically trained in massage therapy.
12) Nirvana School of Enlightenment—advanced healing program in energy mastery.
13) Osteopathic—alternative form of medical care working with soft tissue, skeletal manipulations, and pulses.
14) Reiki—"universal life energy"; techniques to direct healing to specific sites.
15) Robert Jaffe Advanced Energy Healing—"heart-centered awareness," clairvoyant perception, and various techniques to transform energy patterns thought to cause disease.
16) Rolfing—helps client establish structural relationships deep within; manipulation of muscles for balance and symmetry.
17) Touch for Health—uses kinesiology (muscle-testing) and points to strengthen.
18) Trager—rhythmic rocking to aid relaxation and optimal flow.
19) Transformational Pathways—comprehensive energy-based healing program with focus on development of healership; includes nursing theory, communication skills, and exposure to the transpersonal perspective.

Pause for a moment . . .

❑ I have the capacity to be exceptional in holistic nursing and holistic living.
❑ I am future oriented.
❑ My personal goals for studying for the HNC examination are _____.

HOLISTIC NURSING PROCESS

Assessment

1. In order to use touch therapy interventions, the nurse will assess the following parameters:
   a. The client's perception of his or her body-mind challenges and needs.
   b. The client's potential pathophysiologic problems that may require referral to a physician for evaluation.
   c. The client's history of psychiatric disorders. The nurse must modify the approach when clients exhibit present or previous psychiatric disturbance. Touch itself may present a problem, as the deeply relaxed state that feels enjoyable to a healthy balanced person may frighten an imbalanced client.
   d. The client's cultural beliefs and values about touch.
   e. The client's past experience with body therapies. The approach must be modified according to previous experiences.

Nursing Diagnoses

1. The following nursing diagnoses compatible with touch interventions are related to the human response patterns:
   a. Exchanging: Altered circulation
   Impairment in skin integrity
   b. Relating: Social isolation
   c. Valuing: Altered spiritual state
   d. Moving: Physical mobility impaired
   e. Perceiving: Altered meaningfulness
   f. Feeling: Altered comfort
   Anxiety
   Grieving
   Fear

Client Outcomes

1. The client is relaxed following touch therapy session.
2. The client has improved circulation.
3. The client receives touch therapy to maintain/enhance health.

Plan and Interventions

1. Prepare the hospital bed, therapy table, or other working surface.
2. Control the room environment so that it is warm, dimly lit, and quiet. If using a hospital room, draw the curtains, and turn off televisions, radios, and noisy equipment when possible. Soft music may be used to enhance and soothe.
3. Use relaxation and breathing techniques, imagery, or music to elicit the relaxation response.
4. After talking with the client, take time to center yourself, focus on your healing intention, and begin.
   a. Explain the steps in the touch process to the client. The first session requires more time for explanations and adjustment. The length of the remaining sessions may be 15 to 60 minutes.
   b. If working on the client's entire physical body, have the client disrobe completely and cover up with a towel from chest to thighs. The client lies on a padded surface (therapy table or bed) that is covered with cotton blanket and sheet. Sides of the sheet can be wrapped over the client so that he or she feels protected and warm (not always necessary, though with energy therapies clients can easily become cool).
   c. Unwrap only the body area that is being massaged as therapy proceeds. Cover the client appropriately for maximum comfort.
   d. In most situations, begin with the client lying on the back. When therapy on medial aspect and limbs of the body is complete, lift wraps and reapply after the client turns over.
   e. Encourage the client to take slow, deep, releasing breaths. When he or she lets go of tension through breath, affirm in a soft tone, "Ah, feel how relaxed you are becoming."
   f. When turning the client, slide the towel around the client's body, ensuring that the client will not be exposed. As the client lies prone, continue therapy on the dorsal aspect of the body.
5. Be aware of the client's responses to treatment. This awareness will build trust and help the client achieve optimal relaxation.
6. In the initial sessions, continue to explain to the client what can be expected to increase comfort with the continued direction of the touch sessions. After trust has been established and the relaxation response learned, the client will relax more quickly and move to deeper levels in subsequent sessions.
7. In subsequent sessions, proceed the same as in the initial sessions, perhaps with shorter explanations, if any at all.

8. When you have completed the session, verbally let the client know that it is time to return gradually to an awareness of the present; encourage the client to move around slowly and fully reawaken.

   a. Anticipate that the client will require a few minutes to become oriented again to time and place after deep states of relaxation.

   b. Allow silence for the client to experience the wisdom of the relaxed bodymind.

   c. Stay in the room while the client rouses and sits up. Give the assistance necessary to ensure a safe transfer to an ambulatory position.

   d. Allow time to receive the client's verbal feedback about the value of the session, if this need arises. Sometimes, it is beneficial to elicit feedback if it is not offered. The insight gained provides guidelines for further sessions or ideas for the client to consider in daily living.

   e. When touch therapy is used for relaxation or sleep induction for hospitalized patients, close the session by softly pulling bed covers up over the patient and quietly turning off the light as the patient moves into sleep.

9. Schedule a follow-up session.

Evaluation

1. The client outcomes established before the session and the client's subjective experience can be used to evaluate the session.

2. The client willingly accepted touch therapy.

3. The client

   a. exhibited decreased fear and anxiety.

   b. demonstrated a decrease in pulse and respiration rate.

   c. reported muscle relaxation.

   d. exhibited satisfaction through facial expression and expressed inner calmness.

   e. reported greater satisfaction in individual coping patterns.

4. Clients with white skin have reddened color in area where nurse had used massage strokes. Skin in massaged area is warmer than before therapy.

5. The client asked for touch therapy.

REFERENCES

1. H. Harlow, Love in Infant Monkeys, *Scientific American* 200 (1958): 68–74.

2. R. Spitz, *The First Year of Life* (New York: International Universities Press, 1965).

3. L.L. Roth and J.S. Rosenblatt, Mammary Glands of Pregnant Rats: Development Stimulated by Tickling, *Science* 151 (1965): 1403–1404.

4. B. Grad, Some Biological Effects of the Laying on of Hands: A Review of Experiments with Animals and Plants, *Journal of the American Society for Psychical Research* 59 (1965): 95–127.

5. M.J. Smith, Enzymes Are Activated by the Laying on of Hands, *Human Dimensions* (February 1973): 46–48.

6. D.C. Aguilera, Relationship between Physical Contact and Verbal Interaction between Nurses and Patients, *Journal of Psychiatric Nursing* 5, no. 1 (1967): 5–21.

7. S.J. Weiss, Effects of Differential Touch on Nervous System Arousal of Patients Recovering from Cardiac Disease, *Heart and Lung* 19, no. 5 (1990): 474–480.

8. S. Schoenhofer, Affectional Touch in Critical Care Nursing: A Descriptive Study, *Heart and Lung* 18, no. 2 (1989): 146–154.

9. H. Rozema, Touch Needs of the Elderly, *Nursing Homes* (September/October 1986): 42–43.

10. K. Barnett, A Survey of the Current Utilization of Touch by Health Team Personnel with Hospitalized Patients, *International Journal of Nursing* (1973): 2060–2066.

11. E. Duffy, An Exploratory Study: The Effects of Touch on the Elderly in a Nursing Home (Master's thesis, Rutgers State University, 1982).

12. N. Kramer, Comparison of Therapeutic Touch and Casual Touch in Stress Reduction of Hospitalized Children, *Pediatric Nursing* 16, no. 5 (1990): 483–485.

CHAPTER 27

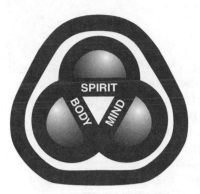

Weight Management

Sue Popkess-Vawter

KNOWLEDGE COMPETENCIES

- Discuss biologic, behavioral, psychologic, and cognitive theories of weight control.
- Describe four basic tenets of reversal theory, and list the four pairs of metamotivational states.
- Contrast unidimensional and multidimensional treatments for permanent weight control.
- Discuss the basic principles of the holistic self-care model for permanent weight control, and describe the three holistic components.
- Name the five assessment parameters and two nursing diagnoses and related outcomes for clients desiring weight control prescriptions.
- Discuss four of the seven baseline knowledges for the holistic self-care model for permanent weight control.
- Discuss ways to accommodate eating within the food pyramid and the American Diabetic Association diet using the four steps to stop overeating.
- Describe two types of aerobic exercise and strength training and sample prescriptions for both types.
- Describe the four steps for dealing directly with unpleasant feelings, instead of eating to cope.
- List the four steps of Fighting Fair.
- List one positive self-talk statement for each of the eight metamotivational states.
- Name the purpose of the personal daily calendar and describe its use to examine patterns of exercise avoidance and overeating.

DEFINITIONS

Obesity: body weight greater than 20 percent above ideal or body mass index ranging from 30 to 38.

Overeating: eating when not hungry.

Overfat: percentage of body fat greater than recommended for client's gender and age; 28 percent for women and 20 percent for men.

Overweight: body weight 10 to 20 percent above ideal or body mass index ranging from 25 to 29.

Weight Cycling/Yo–Yo Dieting: repeated weight loss greater than 10 pounds followed by weight gain, repeated three or more times over the past 2 years.

 Pause for a moment . . .

❑ *I am a critical thinker.*
❑ *I am caring.*
❑ *I manage my time and resources wisely.*

THEORIES AND RESEARCH

Types of Theories

1. Biologic theories are usually aimed at reducing the number of available calories to prevent the deposit of excessive fat and to encourage the use of fat stores.
   a. According to the chronic positive energy balance theory, excessive calories beyond metabolic expenditure result in excessive body weight.
   b. Genetic factors theory suggests that people have a genetic predisposition to the excessive accumulation of fat (genetic predisposition).

c. The adipocyte tissue cell size and number theory is based on the idea that the number of fat cells at birth determines lifetime adiposity.

d. Set point theory suggests that the body attempts to keep weight constant so that despite dieting, body weight goes back to a set point at the original weight.

2. Behavioral theories are based on the notion that behaviors such as overeating are learned responses.

a. They suggest that individuals who wish to lose weight must alter their behaviors and eating patterns.

b. Clients monitor themselves by keeping records for understanding situations surrounding eating.

c. Stimulus control strategies (such as distraction) for new eating behaviors replace old habits that perpetuate excess body weight.

d. Behavioral therapy seems effective on a short-term basis and is most appropriate for mild to moderate overweight conditions.

3. Psychologic theories generally focus on decreasing stress-induced eating and finding ways to control eating in the presence of stressful situations.

4. Cognitive theories address the need to recognize and change negative thoughts and self-statements concerning the roles that food plays in individuals' lives.

a. Negative and faulty self-evaluations rather than feelings of hunger are thought to be the stimulus for eating and overeating.

b. Emphasis is placed on teaching individuals to think about themselves more realistically and optimistically as a means of gaining the self-control necessary to stop overeating.

c. Coping skills models suggest that, although situational antecedents may trigger relapse crises, relapse resulted from ineffectual coping with these situations.

d. The combination of cognitive and behavioral coping is most strongly associated with survival of relapse crises.

e. The cognitive–behavioral approach teaches changing negative self-views and self-monitoring of new eating habits.

5. Apter's theory of psychologic reversals, commonly referred to as reversal theory, provides a framework to explain factors related to weight cycling.[1]

a. An individual's motivation to stay on a diet or abstain from eating varies according to the individual's metamotivational states and amount of tension stress experienced.

b. Reversal theory is a phenomenologic theory of arousal, motivation, and action.

c. Personality is inherently inconsistent, and individuals reverse between opposing states called metamotivational states.

d. States are called metamotivational because they are not, in themselves, concerned with motivation but with the way in which motivation is experienced. A new diet, for example, may be perceived as necessary restrictions for weight loss or as dreaded deprivation.

e. Four pairs of opposing states have been identified (Exhibit 27–1).

1) Telic and paratelic. In the telic state, individuals are serious-minded and goal-oriented; in the paratelic state, they are playful and spontaneous.

2) Conformist and negativistic. In the conformist state, people prefer to go along with rules and regulations; in the negativistic state, they want to be rebellious or noncompliant and to break rules.

3) Mastery and sympathy. In the mastery state, individuals feel that being tough and being in control are important; in the sympathy state, they feel that being tender and not competing are important.

4) Alloic and autic. In the alloic state, people think of others first and put themselves last; in the autic state, they think of themselves first and put others after themselves.

f. Healthy individuals reverse between states easily and often throughout the day.

g. At a given point in time, individuals are in combinations of the different states, consisting of one state of each of the four pairs, but never in both states of a pair at the same time.

h. Dominance, defined as spending relatively more time in one of the pairs of metamotivational states than the other, is a kind of personality characteristic.

i. Each metamotivational state has pleasant and unpleasant feelings and self-described responses associated with it, as Exhibit 27–1 indicates.

j. Tension stress, according to reversal theory, is the uncomfortable experience of a discrepancy between the preferred and actual level of some variable.

Exhibit 27–1 Apter's Reversal Theory Metamotivational State Characteristics

TELIC
Serious-minded
Goal-oriented
Plan ahead
Try to accomplish something
Future-oriented
*anxiety **calmness

CONFORMIST
Don't make waves or disagree with others
Follow the rules
Feel embarrassed/guilty if I break a rule
Compliant
Agreeable
Stay in line
Do what others do
Worry about what others think
*unprotected **protected

MASTERY
Do your best
Give it your all
Be strong & don't show feelings of weakness
Be tough, stay strong
Compete
Be in control
*soft **hardy

ALLOIC
Think of others first
Put self last
Others are most important
*shame **modesty
*guilt **virtue

PARATELIC
Playful
Spontaneous
Emphasize good feelings
Have fun for fun's sake
Present-oriented
*boredom **excitement

NEGATIVISTIC
Stick up for what I think when I disagree with others
Bend/break the rules
Feel angry
Stubborn
Rebellious/defiant
Want to be difficult
*trapped **free

SYMPATHY
Let my feelings tell me what to do
Deserve a break
OK to show & tell feelings of weakness
Be tender, OK to not be strong
Don't compete
Be nurturing
*insensitive **sensitive

AUTIC
Think of self first
Put others after self
I am most important
*humiliation **pride
*resentment **gratitude

Note: *unpleasant feelings/responses (tension stress) associated with specific metamotivational states
  **pleasant feelings/responses associated with specific metamotivational states
Source: Used with permission from Sue Popkess-Vawter, "Apter's Reversal Theory Metamotivational State Characteristics," © 1996.

1) Tension stress is a feeling of unease or discomfort, an impression that things are not as they should be and that something needs to be done.
2) The level of tension stress can be reduced by taking actions within the same metamotivational state or spontaneously reversing to the opposing state within the metamotivational pair.

Types of Treatments

Unidimensional Treatments

1. Two major reasons for the failure of weight reduction programs is the lack of multifaceted programming and the lack of sensitivity to the complicated forces influencing behaviors.
2. Examples of unidimensional treatments include the following:
   a. Fasts and/or calorie restrictions.
   b. Specific food supplements.
   c. Regular exercise to reduce calorie intake or metabolize stored fat.
   d. Behavior modification and psychotherapy.
3. Medical treatments to reduce amounts of ingested foods include the following:
   a. Surgical reduction of the gastrointestinal tract.
   b. Placement of stomach expansion devices to simulate feeling full.

c. Administration of drugs to suppress the appetite.

Multidimensional Treatments

1. Overweight is a multifaceted condition that involves biologic, psychologic, and social factors.
2. Comprehensive approaches that address all these factors hold greater promise for long-term weight loss than the singular approaches.
3. The most successful, long-term physical treatment is a program that combines controlled amounts of healthy food intake and aerobic exercise.
4. Psychologic treatments must accompany comprehensive physical treatments concurrently for permanent life changes to occur.

Holistic Self-Care Model for Permanent Weight Control[2]

1. The basic principles on which the holistic self-care model for permanent weight control is based include the following:
   a. There are continual feedback lines among the three dimensions of eating, physical exercise, and self-talk, as there are integrations among mind, body, and spirit.
   b. Both counselors and weight cyclers must give equal consideration to the mind, body, and spirit trinity as the weight cycler develops permanent life changes.
   c. Clients are in charge of redesigning lifestyle patterns in these three areas, consistent with self-care tenets.
   d. Making permanent life changes takes a very long time. Small steady efforts to modify old habits can be more successful than drastic changes that lead to feelings of deprivation, burnout, relapse, and eventual failure.
2. Dieting only causes feelings of deprivation that set dieters up for failure and can reduce metabolic rate.
3. A four-step strategy to stop overeating replaces dieting.[3]
   a. Eat only when you are hungry after rating your hunger on a scale from 1 to 10:
      1) Ravenously starved = 1.
      2) Uncomfortably stuffed = 10.
      3) Feeling nothing = 5.
      4) Eating to satisfy hunger = between 4 and 6.
   b. Eat exactly what your body wants.
      1) Your body has the natural ability to know what it wants and needs.
      2) When you crave "unhealthy, junk, and forbidden" foods, ask yourself if it is truly a craving; if so and you are hungry, go ahead and eat it.
      3) If the food does not taste good, do not eat it.
   c. Eat slowly, enjoying every bite.
      1) Eating slowly helps you fully experience the pleasure of eating the food.
      2) Eating slowly allows time for your brain to get the messages of your satisfaction and feeling nothing (usually about 20 minutes).
      3) Conscious eating satisfies cravings so that they will not come again for a while.
   d. Stop eating when your hunger is gone and you feel nothing.
      1) Eating to a 5 is like drinking water until your thirst is gone.
      2) If hunger is still present, take three more bites slowly and then stop.
4. When people do not overeat, although not a diet, a caloric deficit results over time to reduce overall intake and, thereby, promote weight loss.
5. Regular, challenging exercise is an important part of the holistic self-care model.
   a. Aerobic exercise provides the cardiorespiratory fitness necessary for general good health and eventual reduction of the percentage of body fat.
   b. Resistance exercise/strength training/weight lifting enhances muscle building, which demands greater energy and over time can increase metabolic rate so that the percentage of body fat declines.
   c. The American College of Sports Medicine recommends 2 days of resistance exercise and 3 days of aerobic exercise per week.[4]
6. Positive self-talk
   a. Parents and other authority figures often emphasize and place great value on the telic, conformist, mastery, and alloic states.
   b. Less emphasis and value are placed on the paratelic, negativistic, sympathetic, and autic states; consequently, these ways of being are not as comfortable, and people have fewer skills in being these ways.
   c. When people naturally reverse to the lesser valued ways of being or experience the unpleasant emotions associated with each metamotivational state, they may develop tension stress.

d. People have learned to deal with their tension stress by eating; thus, when uncomfortable and unpleasant feelings arise, overeating often occurs.

e. Their beliefs and values dictate the way people behave. Behaviors and their underlying meanings can be tapped through self-talk, or the words that automatically come to mind prior to, during, and after life situations.
   1) Self-talk often is learned from parents and other authority figures.
   2) People often do not question whether their automatic thoughts are truly what they believe in as part of their personal belief system; thus, their self-talk and consequential behaviors may have been programmed by their past modeling rather than their own operating systems.

f. Re-programming, or cognitive restructuring, is the technique used first to examine negative self-talk and then to replace unrealistic and implausible beliefs with realistic, new beliefs that will drive new behaviors intended to deal directly with emotional discomfort and thereby eliminate eating to cope.

 Pause for a moment . . .

❑ *I place my hands comfortably in my lap.*
❑ *I allow myself to focus on my relaxed breathing.*
❑ *I breathe in and out, slow, easy, and relaxed.*
❑ *I repeat this relaxed breathing 10 times.*
❑ *I then proceed with my important studying.*

HOLISTIC NURSING PROCESS

Assessment

1. In order to use weight management interventions, the nurse will assess the following parameters:
   a. The client's body composition.
      1) Body mass index.
      2) Percentage of body fat.
   b. The client's resting heart rate and blood pressure.
   c. The client's blood profile.
      1) Cholesterol.
      2) High- and low-density lipoproteins.
      3) Sugar.
   d. The client's physical fitness.
      1) Exercise testing by means of submaximal bicycle ergometer or maximal treadmill.
      2) Strength testing by means of repetition maximum.
   e. The client's psychologic profile.
      1) Biographical inventory and dieting history.
      2) Bulit scale to screen for bulimia.[5]
      3) Body image.[6]

2. It is helpful in assessment to ask the client to keep a personal daily calendar—a daily report of physical exercise, one episode of overeating or not overeating, and reversal theory metamotivational state, associated feelings, and tension stress (Exhibit 27–2).

Nursing Diagnoses

1. The following nursing diagnoses compatible with weight management interventions are related to the human response patterns:
   a. Exchanging: Altered nutrition (more than body requirements)
   b. Valuing: Spiritual distress
   c. Choosing: Ineffective individual coping
   d. Moving: Decreased physical mobility
   e. Perceiving: Disturbance in body image
      Disturbance in self-esteem
      Hopelessness
   f. Knowing: Knowledge deficit
   g. Feeling: Anxiety

2. Specific nursing diagnoses related to the holistic self-care model and reversal theory include
   a. Overeating related to tension stress.
   b. Decreased aerobic/resistance exercise related to poor self-worth and no time for self.
   c. Infrequent episodes of play related to earlier modeling that work is more valuable.
   d. Lack of skills expressing anger/disagreement related to belief that it is unacceptable behavior.
   e. Lack of skills expressing feelings related to earlier self-protective mechanisms.
   f. Inability to put self first related to earlier teaching that others have higher value.

Client Outcomes

1. The client will report fewer overeating episodes.
2. The client will report less tension stress during daily eating.

Exhibit 27-2 Personal Daily Calendar

DATE _____ DAY _____ # _____

Special Thoughts & Comments About Today

Did I exercise today?

____ **Yes Congratulations!**

Check below what exercises you did:

EXERCISE OR ACTIVITY	MINUTES PLANNED	MINUTES ACTUALLY DID

____ **No**   Circle why: Free day   No time

Other (explain) _____

Did I overeat today?

____ **No   Congratulations!**

Think about one time today when I ate & circle only 1 box below that best represents me then; in that box circle only 1 feeling word for each of the 4 word pairs that best matches how I was feeling at the time.

____ **Yes   How many times?** _____

Think about the time I overate *the most* & circle only 1 box below that best represents me then; in that box circle only 1 feeling word of each of the 4 word pairs that best matches how I was feeling at the time.

WORK/GOALS		PLAY/FUN	
unsettled	— settled	bored	— excited
uneasy	— at ease	unstimulated	— stimulated
anxious	— calm	uninterested	— interested
nervous	— composed	indifferent	— enthusiastic

FOLLOW RULES/AGREEABLE		BREAK RULES/ANGRY	
embarrassed	—not embarrassed	trapped	— free
foolish	— sensible	held back	— released
isolated	— belonging	caught	— liberated
uncomfortable	— comfortable	restricted	— unrestricted

TOUGH WITH SELF		TENDER WITH SELF	
out of control	— in control	resentful	— appreciated
humiliated	— proud	deprived	— cared for
wimpy	— sturdy	offended	— grateful
disrespected	— respected	hurt	— pleased

PUTTING OTHER FIRST		PUTTING SELF FIRST	
ashamed	— satisfied	guilty	— virtuous
dishonorable	— honorable	bad about self	— good about self
burdensome	— useful	heavy conscience	—clear conscience
disloyal	— loyal	blameworthy	— praiseworthy

Referring to the time above:

1. **Circle** the number that best describes **MY HUNGER** when I **STARTED** to eat & put an "**X**" on the number that describes **MY HUNGER** when I **FINISHED**.

   starving 1...2...3...4...[feel nothing 5]...6...7...8...9...10   stuffed

2. **Circle** the number that best describes my **TENSION STRESS.**

   least   0...1...2...3...4...5...6...7...8...9...10   most

Source: Used with permission from Sue Popkess-Vawter, "Personal Daily Calendar," © 1996.

3. The client will report exercising more frequently.
4. The client will have a lower percentage of body fat and more pounds lost.
5. The client will have lower resting heart rate and blood pressure.
6. The client will have lower levels of total cholesterol and low-density lipoproteins, and a higher level of high-density lipoproteins.
7. The client will have blood sugar levels within normal limits.
8. The client will have greater maximum oxygen consumption and muscle strength.

Plan and Interventions

1. Have the client stop dieting, stop counting calories, stop weighing daily/weekly; explain that the percentage of body fat is a more accurate way to determine if a person weighs too much, because weight can be normal when the percentage of body fat is high and vice versa.
2. Provide baseline knowledge for holistic self-care for permanent weight control. Explain that the model combines stopping overeating, getting challenging exercise four to six times every week, and re-programming negative, self-destructive self-talk to realistic and personally valued self-talk.
3. Address the physical and psychologic reasons that clients are not losing excess pounds so that they can learn to control their weight for the rest of their lives.
   a. Most people with weight problems have lost weight successfully, are very knowledgeable about food and exercise, and are somewhat in touch with the psychologic reasons that they "go off" of their weight reduction programs.
   b. Active lifestyles keep many people from having an overweight problem until they reach their adult years when greater responsibilities, increasing stressors, short-term bouts of weight gain (e.g., because of pregnancy, loss of a job), and a sedentary lifestyle put extra pounds on their bodies.
4. Disconnect eating from the emotions felt, and re-connect it with hunger.

Stopping Overeating

1. Discuss the food pyramid and healthy eating.
   a. The food guide pyramid daily food choices include the following:
      1) Bread, cereal, rice, and pasta group, 6 to 11 servings.
      2) Fruit group, 2 to 4 servings; vegetable group, 3 to 5 servings.
      3) Meat, poultry, fish, dry beans, eggs, and nuts group, 2 to 3 servings; milk, yogurt, and cheese group, 2 to 3 servings.
      4) Fats, oils, and sweets, sparing use.
   b. Minimum daily requirements may be met over 2 or 3 days rather than every day. When clients take in all of their calories to meet minimum daily requirements from foods that they "should" eat, the extra calories eaten to satisfy natural cravings will be beyond their needs and result in stored fat.
2. For the client with diabetes, consider recommending the American Diabetic Association Diabetic Diet, which consists of taking in six small feedings at regular intervals throughout waking hours.
   a. The purpose is to keep blood sugar at a relatively stable level, preventing dramatic peaks and valleys.
   b. The pattern simulates eating between a 4 and 6 on the hunger scale, so there are no dramatic swings in hunger and fullness.
3. Find out if the client has old eating habits that may need to be broken, as represented by the following statements:
   a. I always eat a "good breakfast"—even when I'm not hungry.
   b. I had better eat now since I may not have time later.
   c. I always finish my meals with a little something sweet.
   d. I always clean my plate (for the starving children).
   e. I cannot stand to throw away perfectly good food.
   f. I eat it whether it tastes good or not.
   g. I can't eat the foods I want until I eat the healthy foods I should eat first.

Getting Regular, Challenging Exercise[7]

1. Explain the differences between aerobic and anaerobic exercise to the patient.
   a. Aerobic exercises (e.g., walking, slow jogging, swimming, biking) use more oxygen, large muscle groups, and are at lower intensities and of longer duration.
   b. Anaerobic exercises (e.g., running, swimming, stair climbing, biking, and weight lifting at a very fast/vigorous pace) use more glucose stores, usually use isolated muscle

groups, and are at higher intensities and of shorter duration.

2. Help the client get ready to exercise.
   a. The client's physical health should be good, and physician approval should be sought.
   b. The client should wear loose-fitting, environmentally proper clothes, and supportive shoes.
   c. The client should be knowledgeable about and plan for physical and environmental safety.
3. Make an exercise schedule with the client.
   a. Frequency.
      1) Aerobic exercises: 3 or 4 times per week.
      2) Strength training/weight lifting exercises: 2 or 3 times per week.
   b. Duration.
      1) Aerobic: 20 to 60 minutes.
      2) Strength: 30 to 60 minutes.
   c. Intensity.
      1) Aerobic: 70 to 80 percent of the maximum heart rate.
         (a) A quick method to calculate working heart range (the range within which rate should be kept to gain aerobic benefit) is 220 – your age × 70% (lower end) and × 80% (upper end).
         (b) Example: $220 - 40 = 180 \times 70\% = 126$; $180 \times 80\% = 144$; working heart range = 126–144.
      2) Strength: 1 to 2 sets of 12 to 15 repetitions.
      3) Sample workout plans may be prescribed in four levels:
         (a) Level 1: Exercise 3 days, 1 strength day and 2 aerobic days.
         (b) Level 2: Exercise 4 days, 2 strength days and 2 aerobic days.
         (c) Level 3: Exercise 5 days, 2 strength days and 3 aerobic days.
         (d) Level 4: Exercise 6 days, 3 strength days and 3 aerobic days.
4. Establish an exercise workout routine with the clients.
   a. Stretch arms and legs in a static stretch without bouncing.
   b. Warm up 3 to 5 minutes, slowly increasing heart rate.
   c. Follow a varied, interesting, and increasingly challenging weekly workout plan, alternating aerobic and strength exercises and including 1 to 2 days off for muscle repair and rest.

d. Cool down by continuing slow-paced aerobic exercise.
   e. Stretch arms and legs in a static stretch without bouncing.
5. Explain the processes of burning fat and building muscle
   a. A slight soreness 12 to 24 hours after exercise indicates an energy-expending repair to build muscle and an increased excess post-exercise oxygen consumption (EPOC).[8]
   b. Often called "after-burn," EPOC helps clients lose excess fat even at rest, particularly with resistance exercise.
   c. For maximum benefit, it is necessary to challenge the body; repeating the same workout does not challenge the body, because the body adapts.
6. Teach the client to schedule exercise ahead of time.
   a. Scheduling weekly exercise ahead develops a new habit.
   b. Committing workout days and time in the personal calendar also helps build new habits.
   c. Arranging variability in workouts from day to day prevents boredom and maximizes use of different muscles.
   d. Working out with friends and family adds interest and challenge.

Changing Negative Self-Talk Triggers

1. Explain that feeling bored, nervous/stressed/anxious, lonely, tired, angry, and overwhelmed frequently triggers overeating.[9]
2. Describe the steps for dealing directly with the feelings without eating/overeating to cope:
   a. Feel the feelings self-talk.
      1) It is OK to let go and feel this way without being ashamed or afraid.
      2) My feelings are a part of me, and I choose to feel them.
   b. Accept the feelings self-talk.
      1) I am entitled to feel this way.
      2) I am a worthy human being who has natural feelings like these.
   c. Understand the feelings self-talk.
      1) Are these feelings ones that I received strong messages about in earlier years?
      2) What is the voice inside my head saying to me?
   d. Deal with the feelings self-talk.
      1) Am I feeling worthless, unloved, ugly, unacceptable? Why? Is this real or something that seemed real in past years?

2) What do I personally believe about the reasons I'm feeling this way?

Evaluation

1. Use the client outcomes that were established prior to initiating weight management strategies.
2. Use the client outcomes and the client's subjective experience to evaluate progress toward short- and long-term goals.
3. With client, review the client's personal daily calendar and listen to the meaning inherent in the story being told (see Exhibit 27–2).
   a. Examine the client's exercising over the last months of daily sheets by asking the following questions:
      1) What is the total number of days that the client reported?
      2) What is the average number of exercise days per week?
      3) What is the client's major trigger for not exercising?
   b. Examine the client's overeating over the last months of daily sheets by asking the following questions:
      1) What is the client's average number of overeating days per week?
      2) What is the client's major trigger for overeating?
      3) On the days the client overate, did he or she exercise or not?

4) On the days the client exercised, did he or she overeat or not?
5) On the days the client did not exercise and overate, what was the reversal theory state and how high was the tension stress?
6) What way of being human does the client need to work on?

REFERENCES

1. M. Apter, *Reversal Theory: Motivation, Emotion, and Personality* (London: Routledge, 1989), 18–32.
2. S. Popkess-Vawter, Holistic Self-Care Model for Permanent Weight Control, *Journal of Holistic Nursing* 2, no. 4 (1993): 341–355.
3. B. Schwartz, *Diets Still Don't Work* (Houston, TX.: Breakthru Publishing, 1990), 58–62.
4. American College of Sports Medicine, *ACSM Position Stand: The Recommended Quantity and Quality of Exercise for Developing and Maintaining Cardiorespiratory and Muscle Fitness in Healthy Adults* (1990), 265–274.
5. M. Smith and M. Thelen, Development and Validation of a Test for Bulimia, *Journal of Counseling and Clinical Psychology* 52 (1984): 863–872.
6. S. Popkess-Vawter and N. Banks, Body Image Measurement in Overweight/Obese Females, *Clinical Nursing Research* 1, no. 4 (1992): 402–417.
7. C. Bailey and L. Bishop, *Fit or Fat Woman: Solutions for Women's Unique Concerns* (Boston: Houghton Mifflin Co., 1989), 25–31.
8. American College of Sports Medicine, *ACSM Position Stand.*
9. S. Popkess-Vawter et al., Reversal Theory and Overeating: A New Paradigm To Study Weight Control (Unpublished manuscript, 1996), 8.

CHAPTER 28

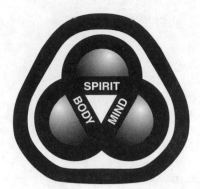

Smoking Cessation

Christine A. Wynd

KNOWLEDGE COMPETENCIES

- Discuss the physiologic effects of smoking.
- Discuss the physiologic effects of smoking cessation.
- Explore the rationale behind an individual's smoking habit (nicotine addiction/dependence, psychosocial aspects, and habitual cues).
- List at least ten symptoms of nicotine withdrawal.
- List five common psychosocial reasons for smoking.
- Cite two examples of habitual smoking cues.
- Explore smoking cessation and the nursing process.
- List the mechanisms available for assessing nicotine dependence, psychosocial and habitual cues.
- Describe six nursing interventions for assisting clients/patients with smoking cessation.
- Cite three factors influencing relapse prevention.

DEFINITIONS

Smoking: inhalation of tobacco burned in cigarettes, cigars, and pipes resulting in nicotine absorption through the lungs.

Smoking Cessation: discontinuation of the use of cigarettes, cigars, and pipes.

 Pause for a moment . . .

❑ *I watch my rhythmic breathing.*
❑ *I allow myself to go inside the breath.*
❑ *I flow into the edges of the moment.*
❑ *I am with this process for ten complete breaths.*
❑ *I then proceed with my studying.*

THEORIES AND RESEARCH

Physiologic Effects of Smoking

1. Tobacco use contributes to more than 400,000 deaths in the United States each year.[1]
2. Smoking is a factor in three of the five leading causes of death in the United States:
   a. Heart disease.
   b. Cancer.
   c. Chronic obstructive pulmonary disease.
3. It is estimated that 25 percent of people in the United States smoke.
4. More than 3,000 children and adolescents become addicted to smoking each day.
5. Nicotine is the addicting drug used in tobacco. Smoking and tobacco use can be as addicting as heroin and cocaine.[2]
6. Nicotine increases the heart rate 15 to 25 beats per minute and increases blood pressure by 10 to 20 points.
   a. Nicotine causes a repetitive release of epinephrine and norepinephrine, simulating an adrenergic state that increases heart rate, cardiac contractility, and myocardial oxygen demand.
   b. Vascular constriction follows the use of nicotine, and platelet aggregation increases the risk of thromboembolic problems.
7. Nicotine triggers hypercholesterolemia by increasing the number of plasma-free fatty acids,

resulting in an increase in low-density lipoproteins and decreased high-density lipoproteins. The end result is high cholesterol levels.[3]

8. Carbon monoxide from cigarette smoke decreases oxygen transport and, thus, the oxygen available for the body's use, by binding hemoglobin and other hemoproteins.

9. Smoking irritates the large pulmonary airways and causes greater production of mucous secretions with accompanying cough. In the smaller airways, smoking causes inflammation, ulceration, fibrosis, and loss of ciliary function.

Physiologic Effects of Smoking Cessation

1. Nonsmokers have a 1.0 mortality ratio for coronary artery disease, and smokers (smoking less than one-half pack per day) have a 1.24 mortality ratio. Smokers who quit reduce their mortality ratio to 1.02 after 10 years of remaining smoke-free.[4]

2. Smoking cessation reduces the risk for lung cancer. After 10 years of remaining tobacco-free, the lung cancer risk for former smokers was the same as the risk for nonsmokers.[5]

Rationale behind the Smoking Habit

1. The 1988 report of the Surgeon General describes the terms *addiction* and *dependence* as scientifically synonymous in reference to the repetitive and purposive use of a mood-altering substance. In the case of smoking, this substance is nicotine.[6]

2. A physical addiction occurs when an individual requires incrementally higher doses of the drug to produce the same effects and when stopping intake of the drug causes a withdrawal period. Nicotine produces a physical addiction through its effects on the central nervous system.

3. Treatment of nicotine addiction must address the drug and its influence on the physical health of individuals.
   a. Nicotine withdrawal symptoms (e.g., insomnia, fatigue, irritability, headaches, coughing, tension, hunger, dry mouth, constipation, confusion, impaired concentration) must be addressed during any attempts at therapeutic intervention.
   b. Most withdrawal symptoms subside within 2 to 3 weeks; however, an intense craving for a cigarette and the urge to smoke may last for months.

c. The severity of withdrawal symptoms is often related to the extent of the nicotine addiction.

4. Common psychosocial reasons for smoking include relaxation, enhancement of pleasure and enjoyment, stress reduction, socialization, a reward system.

5. Habitual cues, habits and behaviors strongly linked to cigarette use, reinforce nicotine dependence.
   a. These links are difficult to break because it is difficult for the smoker to separate the cue from smoking.
   b. Some smokers automatically light a cigarette when dialing a number on the telephone, for example.

Pause for a moment . . .

❑ *I focus on being relaxed.*
❑ *When I am relaxed, I feel _____ .*
❑ *I can increase my relaxation skills by _____ .*
❑ *I use relaxed breathing and imagery to be more in the moment.*

HOLISTIC NURSING PROCESS

Assessment

1. Smoking status should be considered "the new vital sign"[7] and should be assessed for every client/patient with the four traditional vital signs—blood pressure, pulse, respiratory rate, and body temperature.

2. This assessment not only helps nurses and other health care professionals recognize smoking as a chronic disease requiring long-term, intensive attention and follow-up, but also establishes a basis for interventions.[8]

3. Every client's status as a current, former, or never smoker should be documented in the chart.

4. A smoker's motivation and readiness to change smoking behavior falls into one of five stages of smoking cessation (behavioral change):[9]
   a. Precontemplation. The smoker is not considering quitting and will not be interested in advice about cessation.
   b. Contemplation. The smoker is considering quitting and has had thoughts about quit-

ting within the last 6 months; this client is receptive to advice about cessation.

c. Preparation. The smoker intends to stop smoking within the next 30 days; this client is ready and open to interventions for smoking cessation.

d. Action. The smoker actively endeavors to promote cessation and abstinence for 6 months.

e. Maintenance. This client has abstained from smoking 6 months to 3 years or longer. Smokers frequently move through the earlier stages three or four times before entering the maintenance stage and becoming successfully abstinent.

5. The nurse should help the smoker do a self-assessment of reasons and benefits for quitting smoking. Interventions for smoking cessation that are tailored to the individual smoker's needs and desires will result in better outcomes.

a. The smoker should list five personal benefits.

b. Many smokers find a smoking (cigarette) diary useful in self-assessment. The smoker records each cigarette smoked during a 24-hour (or longer) period along with the date, time, activity, and the perception of urgency related to the desire for the cigarette (i.e., 1= highly urgent, 2 = not as urgent, 3 = smoked automatically, like a reflex). The diary helps smokers become aware of patterns for smoking.

6. The Fagerstrom Nicotine Tolerance Test relates the frequency of smoking as a factor in nicotine dependence (e.g., cigarettes smoked upon waking in morning, difficulty refraining from smoking in places where it is forbidden).[10]

Nursing Diagnoses

1. The following nursing diagnoses compatible with the interventions for smoking cessation relate to the human response patterns:[11]

a. Exchanging: Altered circulation
              Altered oxygenation
b. Valuing: Spiritual distress
              Spiritual well-being
c. Choosing: Ineffective individual coping
              Effective individual coping
d. Moving: Self-care deficit
e. Perceiving: Disturbance in body image
              Disturbance in self-esteem

            Hopelessness
            Powerlessness
f. Knowing: Knowledge deficit
g. Feeling: Anxiety
            Fear

Client Outcomes[12]

1. The client will keep a smoking diary to examine patterns of cigarette usage.

2. The client will make a list of five reasons for quitting smoking and five benefits.

3. The client will establish a quit date for "cold turkey" cessation of smoking through use of a contract.

4. The client will adhere to the contract and will become a "former" smoker; that is, the client will achieve and maintain a zero smoking rate.

Plan and Interventions

1. Carry out interventions with smokers during other routine health care tasks, such as taking traditional vital signs, providing routine treatments, and collecting specimens.

a. Smokers are likely to visit health care settings frequently throughout the course of a year.

b. Nurses should incorporate counseling into the care plan, especially when a smoker is hospitalized for a smoking-related illness. Such an illness may motivate the patient to receive smoking cessation advice.

2. Following a thorough clinical assessment and smoker self-assessment, target interventions to the individual smoker's unique situation. Interventions can be geared toward problems of actual nicotine addiction/dependence, psychosocial needs for change, the need to break long-established habits, or a combination of any of these factors.

3. Ensure that all interventions should follow the "4 Rs."[13]

a. Relevance. Consider the intervention's relevance to the smoker's illness or health status, family situation, age, gender, etc.

b. Risks. Review potential risks related to smoking cigarettes, especially risks directly related to the individual's conditions and characteristics.

c. Rewards. Review the potential benefits already assessed by the smoker (e.g., improves health, sharpens senses, saves money, builds self-control and self-esteem).

d. Repetition. Continuously repeat helpful interventions and motivational factors as needed.

4. Encourage the individual client/patient/smoker to designate a "quit date." The smoker needs to understand that, although the nurse can suggest and guide smoking cessation interventions, the smoker must commit to the "hard" work and intense follow-through required for success. The most successful cessation strategy is to set a "Quit Date," make a self-contract to respect that date, and complete the contract by quitting "Cold Turkey" on the "Quit Date," that is, stopping all cigarettes and/or smoking, forever, on that date.

5. Explain to the smoker that the greater the intervention intensity (e.g., the number of weeks the intervention is used plus the length and number of treatment sessions), the greater the success rate for smoking cessation. Recommended guidelines are
   a. Length of intervention in weeks—at least 2 weeks.
   b. Session length—at least 20 to 30 minutes in length.
   c. Number of sessions—at least 4 to 7 sessions.[14]

6. Assist the client/patient with preparation for quitting cigarettes/smoking. Advise client/patient to
   a. Inform family, friends, and co-workers of the effort to quit and ask for their support.
   b. Remove cigarettes, ashtrays, and other smoking paraphernalia from home, car, and workplace.
   c. Purchase no-calorie substitutes for cigarettes (oral stimulation), such as sugarless gum, lollipops, candies, swizzle sticks, paper clips and safety pins for making chains, lip gloss, and toothpicks.
   d. Do not think in terms of never smoking again—just think in terms of 1 day at a time.
   e. Get in the habit of drinking lots of water (eight 8-oz glasses per day).

1) Nicotine policrilex/gum is available in 2- and 4-mg doses; the 4-mg dose is intended for those smokers who are highly dependent on nicotine (smoke more than 25 cigarettes per day, or score 6 or higher on the Fagerstrom Tolerance Test).
2) One piece of gum per hour is advised for maintaining appropriate blood levels. The nicotine must be absorbed through the buccal mucosa; therefore, the gum should be chewed periodically, but, for most of the time, "parked" along the buccal mucosa.
3) The gum needs an alkaline environment for successful absorption; thus, acidic beverages (e.g., coffee, cola, juices) should be avoided.
4) The client should not drink or eat immediately before or during the use of the gum, and should delay using gum at least 15 minutes after ingesting food or fluids.[15]
5) Clients chewing nicotine gum must not smoke cigarettes, or the dosage of nicotine can have deleterious effects, especially to the cardiac system.

b. Nicotine transdermal patches provide a 24-hour delivery of nicotine to maintain constant blood levels and, thus, avoid fluctuations of nicotine levels in plasma levels.
1) The patches are used to reduce nicotine withdrawal symptoms.
2) The client applies a clean patch to a dry, nonhairy area of the outer arm or upper torso for the prescribed time period (16 to 24 hours).
3) The patches should be reapplied at the same time during each period of wear.
4) Like those who chew gum, clients who wear patches must not smoke.

2. Because this therapy is time-limited and temporary, teach the client/patient lifestyle, behavioral changes for long-term smoking cessation and abstinence.

Interventions for Nicotine Addiction/Dependence

1. If the assessment reveals an actual nicotine addiction/dependence, suggest nicotine replacement therapy.
   a. Nicotine replacement therapy includes the use of nicotine gum (policrilex).

Interventions for Psychosocial Aspects of Smoking

1. Suggest substitutes for smoking/use of cigarettes as a form of relaxation and/or stress reduction.
   a. Relaxation and imagery (see Relaxation, Chapter 23, and Imagery, Chapter 24). The client may find it helpful to purchase relax-

ation and imagery tapes or to create an audiotape that focuses on the physiologic and psychologic images of being smoke-free.[16] The imagery should be designed specifically to assist the client in breaking the cigarette and nicotine habit, or reducing stress related to situations in which cigarettes used to suffice.

   b. Deep breathing. The client should close the eyes and gently relax the shoulders. The nurse should instruct the client to

     1) Breathe in slowly and deeply through the nose.

     2) Expand the abdomen and lower the diaphragm.

     3) Hold the breath for a few seconds, and feel it cleanse the lungs.

     4) Exhale slowly through the open mouth.

     5) Empty the lungs, raising the diaphragm.

     6) Repeat five times.

2. Suggest substitutes for cigarettes and smoking as confidence boosters.

   a. Affirming self-talk (positive self-talk). The client must become aware of the little voice inside the head that sabotages or facilitates the adoption of new and healthier behaviors. Negative talk must be immediately replaced with positive affirmations.

   b. Tips for building self-confidence include the following:

     1) Avoid negative people, especially those who are irritating and overly competitive.

     2) Concentrate on one task at a time.

     3) Do something positive and self-nurturing at least once per day.

     4) Plan for time to relax each day.

     5) Exercise each day (e.g., take a walk).

     6) Express emotional feelings directly and verbally, and/or in writing through letters and journals.

     7) Chew sugarless gum.

     8) Have a "safe" place for retreat.

     9) Find a support person.

    10) Recognize accomplishments and provide self-rewards.

    11) Listen to music.

    12) Stretch arms and legs.

    13) Laugh.

    14) Get a therapeutic massage, facial, manicure, pedicure.

Interventions for Habitual Cues of Smoking

Habitual Links to Smoking	Substitute Activities
1. Morning wake-up routines.	Stretch. Exercise. Drink a big glass of ice water or juice. Take a cool or cold shower.
2. Mealtime	Get up from the table immediately. Brush teeth. Get involved in another activity. Go for a walk.
3. Coffee	Drink an alternative hot beverage: tea, hot chocolate, hot apple cider.
4. Social situations	Drink something nonalcoholic or limit self to one drink. Say affirmations; use relaxation and imagery to build self-confidence. Ask friends for support.
5. In the car	Listen to motivational or informational audiotapes. Take several long, deep breaths. Change the route taken to work; view new scenery.
6. Anger	Roll up windows in car and give a long, loud yell. Take a walk. Pound a pillow; stomp feet. Take deep breaths. Write an angry letter (but do not send it). Write in journal.

Evaluation

1. Follow-up contacts (person-to-person or by telephone) are essential to assist smokers with long-term maintenance.

a. First follow-up: within 2 weeks of quit date, preferably during the first week.
b. Second follow-up: within the first month.
c. Further follow-up contacts as needed.
2. Activities during follow-up should include
a. Congratulations on success.
b. Active discussion of personal benefits from being smoke-free to encourage continued cessation.
c. Relapse prevention.
1) If lapse has occurred, the nurse should ask for recommitment to total abstinence.
2) Lapse is only a temporary distraction from goal.
3) Circumstances contributing to the lapse can be reviewed and used as a learning experience.
d. Weight gain prevention.
1) Some weight gain is common (5 to 10 lbs) and is a minor risk compared to the dangers of continued smoking.
2) The nurse can make recommendations for dietary, exercise, and lifestyle changes.
3) The client/patient can participate in a program that focuses on these issues.
4) The client can deal with the weight gain after smoking cessation maintenance is established.

REFERENCES

1. M.C. Fiore et al., *Smoking Cessation: Information for Specialists.* Clinical Practice Guideline. Quick Reference Guide for Smoking Cessation Specialists, No. 18. (Rockville, MD: U.S. Department of Health and Human Services, Public Health Service, Agency for Health Care Policy and Research and Centers for Disease Control and Prevention, AHCPR Pub. No. 96-0694, 1996), 1–3.

2. S.A. Brunton and J.E. Henningfield, *Nicotine Addiction and Smoking Cessation* (New York: Medical Information Services, 1991), 3–4.

3. M.H. Criqui et al., Frequency and Clustering of Nonlipid Coronary Risk Factors in Dyslipoproteinemia: The Lipid Research Clinics Program Prevalence Study, *Circulation* 73 (1986): I-40–I-50.

4. E. Rogot and J.L. Murray, Smoking and Causes of Death among Veterans: 16 Years of Observation, *Public Health Reports* 95 (1980): 213–222.

5. J.H. Lubin et al., Modifying Risk of Developing Lung Cancer by Changing Habits of Cigarette Smoking, *British Medical Journal* 288 (1984): 1953–1956.

6. U.S. Department of Health and Human Services, *The Health Consequences of Smoking: Nicotine Addiction. A Report of the Surgeon General* (Rockville, MD: U.S. Department of Health and Human Services, Public Health Service. Office on Smoking and Health, 1988).

7. M.W. Edmunds et al., *Smoking Status: The New Vital Sign* (Baltimore: The University of Maryland School of Nursing, Office of Professional Development and Services, Division of Business and Industry, 1993).

8. M.C. Fiore, The New Vital Sign: Assessing and Documenting Smoking Status, *JAMA* 266 (1991): 3183–3184.

9. J.O. Prochaska and C.C. DiClemente, Stages of Change in the Modification of Problem Behaviors, *Progress in Behavior Modification* 28 (1992): 183–218.

10. K.O. Fagerstrom et al., Nicotine Addiction and Its Assessment, *Ear, Nose, and Throat Journal* 69 (1991): 763–765.

11. B.M. Dossey, Smoking Cessation: Breathing Free, in *Holistic Nursing: A Handbook for Practice*, 2nd ed., eds. B.M. Dossey et al. (Gaithersburg, MD: Aspen Publishers, 1995), 483–510.

12. Ibid.

13. Fiore et al., *Smoking Cessation: Information for Specialists.*

14. Ibid.

15. Brunton and Henningfield, *Nicotine Addiction.*

16. Dossey, Smoking Cessation: Breathing Free.

CHAPTER 29

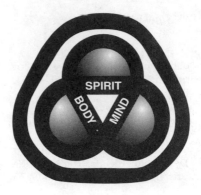

Overcoming Addictions

Lynette W. Jack

KNOWLEDGE COMPETENCIES

- Examine current research and theories related to the etiology of addiction.
- Apply the bio-psycho-social model to the development of addictive behavior.
- List factors that increase the risk for addiction.
- Describe protective factors that contribute to resiliency.
- Identify strategies for reducing risks and increasing resiliency in order to help clients avoid addictions.
- Describe the process of screening all clients for actual or potential problems related to addictive substances and/or behaviors.
- Explain key components of a nursing assessment with a client experiencing problems related to addictive substances/behaviors.
- List nursing diagnoses that are useful in directing interventions for the client with addiction problems.
- Identify nursing interventions helpful in assisting clients and families to overcome addictions.
- Conduct a personal lifestyle inventory related to use of addictive substances/behaviors and make changes as needed to achieve wellness.
- Provide support and appropriate referral for treatment to colleagues who may be experiencing problems related to addiction.

DEFINITIONS

Addiction: an illness characterized by compulsion, loss of control, and continued patterns of abuse despite perceived negative consequences; obsession with a dysfunctional habit. Dysfunctional patterns of behavior are associated with alcoholism, drug abuse, cigarette smoking, eating disorders, excessive gambling or spending, and compulsive sexual disorders.[1]

Codependence: unhealthy patterns of relating to others, accompanied by low self-esteem, an excessive need to be needed, a strong urge to change and control others, and a willingness to suffer as a result of being closely involved with someone who has an addiction.

Dependence: condition that may be physical or psychologic, or both. Physical dependence is a state of physiologic adaptation to the presence of a psychoactive substance, indicated by the presence of tolerance and the occurrence of withdrawal symptoms after the cessation of consumption of that substance. Psychologic dependence is a subjective feeling of need for the substance in order to avoid unpleasant feelings or to create positive feelings.

Enabling Behavior: any actions, either knowingly or unknowingly, that make it possible for the person's addiction to continue.

Misuse: the inappropriate use of drugs that were meant to be used therapeutically.

Problematic Use: the use of alcohol and/or drugs that has resulted in one or more problems, but does not meet the criteria for diagnosis as dependence or abuse. Examples may be drunk driving, early medical consequences, family problems, or other behavioral consequences.

Recovery: restoration of health; return to a normal state in which the individual no longer engages in problematic behavior, can feel good about himself or herself, and is able to accomplish goals.

Relapse: recurrence of use of addictive substance or behavior in an individual who had previously achieved some degree of sobriety or wellness.

Spirituality: the motivating force in the self that gives a sense of meaning and purpose to life.

Substance Abuse: the harmful use of a psychoactive substance.

Treatment: intervention with planned strategies to assist the person to change maladaptive or injurious behaviors in order to restore health and effective functioning.

 Pause for a moment . . .

❏ *I become aware of my breathing.*
❏ *My inbreath and my outbreath are balanced.*
❏ *As I stay with my breathing, I find a deeper place of inner peace.*

THEORIES AND RESEARCH

Theoretical Models Used To Explain the Development of Addiction [2,3]

1. Neurobiologic theory describes an underlying predisposition to develop the addictive disease, resulting from the interaction of many factors. Genetic deficiencies and imbalances in neurotransmitters, neuropeptides, and receptors, and the chemical changes that result, lead to cravings for mood-altering substances and compulsive behaviors.

2. Intrapersonal theory describes addiction as a result of personality traits and developmental failures. Current research has limited the usefulness of this theory, although many people in the general public still view addiction as a personality flaw.

3. Behavioral theory addresses the antecedents of addictive behavior, expectations regarding the effects of the substances or behaviors, prior experiences, and reinforcement provided by the addictive behaviors or substances themselves.

4. Learning theory suggests that people who are dependent on addictive substances or behaviors have learned to use them as maladaptive coping strategies, because they have not yet learned healthy coping strategies.

5. Sociocultural theory relates the development of addiction to prevailing cultural values and social norms within the person's experience, such as family or cultural rituals, racism, loss of ethnic heritage, lack of education and job skills, poverty, and spiritual crisis.

6. Those who study the ultradian stress syndrome suggest that binge behavior of any kind becomes an addiction when it interferes with an individual's normal ultradian and circadian rhythms.

Consequences of Addiction

1. Approximately 67 percent of the population in the United States consumes alcohol.
   a. Of that group, approximately 10 percent can be classified as dependent on alcohol, and a substantially larger group have occasional problems resulting from their consumption of alcohol.
   b. Total social cost of alcohol-related problems is estimated to be $98.6 billion.[4]

2. Approximately 29 percent of the population smokes nicotine-containing cigarettes. In 1993, the medical costs associated with treatment for smoking-related illnesses were estimated to be $50 billion.[5]

3. Problems with gambling may affect 1.5 to 4 percent of the population, at a cost to society of $80 billion.[6]

4. Estimates of the number of people experiencing a drug-related disorder range from 1 to 9 percent of the population, depending on which type of substance is being considered.

5. For the individual, the results of addiction can be many and varied:
   a. Addiction may lead to decreased coping skills repertoire; physical health problems, such as cancer, heart disease, pulmonary disease, hypertension, liver disease, increased risk of infections (including infection with the human immune deficiency virus [HIV]), increased exposure to trauma and accidents; irreversible brain damage; fetal alcohol syndrome; psychiatric syndromes, such as paranoia, depression, and anxiety.
   b. Legal problems may develop following criminal activity or excessive drinking and driving or fights.
   c. Work performance may be altered, leading to job loss.

6. For the family, chaos develops, with inconsistency of rules, lack of routines and rituals, lack of nurturing, increased levels of conflict, enabling behavior, and isolation.

a. The spouse is at higher risk for physical and emotional problems.

b. Children also display physical and emotional problems, as well as school performance difficulties.

c. Financial difficulties mount because of missed time at work, money spent on addictive substances, and job loss.

7. For society, addictions bring increased accidents and injury, increased crime, higher rates of violence, child abuse, increased rates of suicide (particularly in children and adolescents), prostitution, risky sexual behavior, increased rates of HIV infection, excessive health care costs, decreased work productivity, and community deterioration.

Application of the Bio-psycho-social Model to the Etiology of Addictions

1. Research has shown that some risk factors put people at higher risk for developing alcohol and other addiction problems, while other factors protect people.

2. Predictable stages of use by the predisposed individual include contact, experimental use, excessive use, addiction, and recovery.

3. The enabling system is the group of persons around the user whose actions encourage the addiction to progress. They may encourage use through overt modeling and approval of addictive behavior, denial that addiction is occurring, or removal of consequences that may deter use.

Risk Factors That Contribute to Addiction[7]

1. Personal risk factors for addiction are inherent to an individual, such as a genetic predisposition to alcoholism, relationship with family members, school, and peers.

   a. Alienation, withdrawal from conventional groups and activities, excessive rebelliousness, strong influence by peer group rather than parents (particularly if those peers are using alcohol, tobacco, and other drugs), and first use of any substance during the early teen years increase the risk.

   b. The children of substance abusers; victims of physical, sexual, or psychologic abuse; school dropouts; adolescents who have become pregnant; those who are economically disadvantaged; perpetrators of a violent or delinquent act; those who have a mental health problem; those who have attempted suicide; those who have experienced long-term physical pain due to injury; and gay and lesbian youth with poor support systems are all at particularly high risk.

2. Family-based risk factors include the following:

   a. Unclear expectations for behavior.
   b. Lack of monitoring and supervision.
   c. Inconsistent or harsh discipline.
   d. Lack of bonding and caring.
   e. Conflict with parents/caregivers.
   f. Parent's use/abuse of alcohol or drugs.
   g. Low expectations of children's success.
   h. Family history of alcoholism.
   i. Parental involvement of children in parents' use or misuse.

3. School-based risk factors include the following:

   a. Negative school climate.
   b. Expectations of schoolteachers and others that child will not succeed.
   c. Inconsistent policies.
   d. Transitions between schools, such as the transition from elementary to junior high.
   e. Consistent school failure.
   f. Lack of student involvement in curricular and extracurricular activities.
   g. Truancy and suspension.

4. Community-based risk factors include the following:

   a. Extreme economic and social deprivation, which includes poverty, lack of adequate housing, poor health care, and a sense of no future or quality of life.
   b. Extreme wealth.
   c. Low neighborhood attachment and community disorganization.
   d. No involvement with others in geographic region.
   e. Little or no community leadership.
   f. Lack of employment opportunities.
   g. Lack of opportunities for youth to become involved in the community.
   h. Easy availability of alcohol, tobacco, and other drugs.
   i. Attitudes, practices, policies, or laws that are favorable toward use and misuse.

Protective Factors That Increase Resiliency

1. Individual-based factors that provide some protection against addiction include:

   a. Involvement in healthy drug and alcohol-free activities.
   b. Respect for authority.
   c. Bonding to conventional groups, such as church.

d. Appreciation of the unique talents of each person.
2. Family-based protective factors include the following:
   a. Prenatal care.
   b. Strong parent bonding with children.
   c. Education valued and encouraged.
   d. Good stress management.
   e. Quality time spent together.
   f. High degree of warmth and low degree of criticism within family, rather than overly authoritarian or overly permissive style.
   g. Nurturing family that is able to provide safety.
   h. Clear expectations for behavior.
   i. Supportive relationships with caring adults beyond the immediate family, such as minister or teacher.
   j. Shared responsibility for family tasks according to age and developmental abilities.
3. School-based protective factors include the following:
   a. High expectations and encouragement of goal setting.
   b. Encouragement of achievement of goals.
   c. Nurturing school staff.
   d. Encouragement of a sense of doing good for others and a sense of cooperation.
   e. Leadership and decision-making opportunities.
   f. Encouragement of active involvement by students.
   g. Training of teachers in social development and techniques for encouraging learning.
   h. Involvement of parents in a meaningful way.
   i. Provision of alcohol and drug-free activities.
   j. Encouragement of student participation and autonomy.
4. Community-based protective factors include the following:
   a. Shared responsibility for prevention.
   b. Access to resources such as housing, health care, child care, job training, employment, and recreation facilities.
   c. Social networks readily available.
   d. Involvement of youth in community service.

Efforts To Prevent Addiction

1. Prevention activities are aimed at reducing known risk factors and providing or enhancing protective factors.
2. Effective prevention planning addresses risk factors at the appropriate developmental stage and intervenes early, before the individual has any contact with substances or problematic behavior becomes established.
3. Prevention strategies should be gender-specific and culture-sensitive, and they should address multiple risks throughout the life span.
4. Prevention programs should provide individuals with opportunities to make healthy choices, should assist in the development of skills needed to make these choices, and should provide positive recognition.
5. Caregivers have a variety of prevention strategies available to them. For example, they can
   a. Offer parenting skills classes.
   b. Disseminate information about healthy lifestyle.
   c. Strengthen family interactions.
   d. Provide information about prevention services and availability.
   e. Develop coping skills such as decision making, refusal skills, critical analysis, problem-solving abilities, goal setting, and stress management techniques.
   f. Strengthen connections to and expressions of spirituality.
   g. Increase sense of empowerment and self-responsibility.
   h. Increase self-esteem through success experiences.
   i. Provide and strengthen relationships with healthy adult role models/mentors.
   j. Participate in community partnerships to decrease risk factors within the community.
   k. Provide anticipatory guidance when clients are facing transitions and other known stressful periods of life.
   l. Create recreational programs/facilities and ensure access for all members of the community.
   m. Convey and reinforce consistent norms of nonsmoking, nondrinking, non–drug use. Convey zero tolerance for intoxication or hazardous behavior while under the influence.
   n. Provide outlets and activities that relieve boredom.
   o. Ensure that participation in alternative activities increases self-esteem and respect for others.
   p. Advocate for a healthy environment through political action and other efforts to change policies, laws, and community norms.
   q. Support measures that limit access to addictive substances.

r. Participate in activities that increase the access of poor and underserved groups to health care and other resources.

s. Participate in organizations that can influence national or statewide health care reform, such as the American Holistic Nurses' Association and the American Nurses Association.

t. Screen all clients and patients for actual or potential problems associated with addictive substances and behaviors.

 Pause for a moment . . .

❑ *I watch my belly rise and fall with the rhythm of my relaxed breathing.*
❑ *This balanced breathing helps me in my work and life.*

HOLISTIC NURSING PROCESS

Assessment

1. The frequency of problems associated with addiction makes it likely that every nurse will come in contact with people whose use of substances is problematic or dependent.

2. Because these problems may not be obvious and because it is essential to identify problems as early as possible, the nurse should routinely screen all patients or clients.

3. Screening involves a variety of activities:
   a. History taking, both in the adolescent (Exhibit 29–1) and in the adult (Exhibit 29–2).
   b. Observation of the client's presenting behavior: restlessness, impulsiveness, anxiety, selfishness, self-centeredness, lack of consideration, stubbornness, irritability on questioning, anger or rage, ill humor, physical evidence of inflicting violence on others, depression, isolation, self-destructiveness, low self-esteem, shame and guilt, reduced physical and mental functioning, excessive defensiveness and denial, projection of blame and responsibility onto others in the environment.[8]
   c. Physical examination and laboratory testing: systems review for indications of disease processes known to be associated with addiction; signs of traumatic injuries; results of drug screens from blood, urine, or hair samples; blood alcohol levels.

d. Use of screening tools (Exhibits 29–3 through 29–6).

4. For the client known to have problems associated with addiction, assessment should be based on multiple sources of information, including data from the client and the family, observations by health care professionals, reports from employer or school or legal representatives, and objective data from physical examination and laboratory testing.
   a. Present drug history should include the types of substances used, amount taken, frequency taken, patterns of use, and last use. Is there evidence of tolerance? Withdrawal symptoms? History of complications to withdrawal, such as seizures or hallucinations? Any chronic medical problems? Prior attempts at treatment?
   b. Other aspects of assessment include support systems and nature of relationships, work history, school performance, impact of addiction on family, degree of spiritual crisis, legal problems, financial needs, and coping strategies.

Nursing Diagnoses

1. The following nursing diagnoses compatible with strategies to overcome addictions are related to the human response patterns:
   a. Exchanging: Altered nutrition (more/less than body requirement)
   Potential for infection
   Potential for injury
   b. Communicating: Impaired verbal communication
   c. Relating: Social isolation
   Altered family process
   Sexual dysfunction
   d. Valuing: Spiritual distress
   e. Moving: Sleep pattern disturbance
   Self-care deficit
   f. Feeling: Altered comfort: pain
   Anxiety
   g. Knowing: Knowledge deficit
   Altered thought processes
   h. Choosing: Ineffective individual coping
   Noncompliance
   Altered self-concept
   i. Perceiving: Sensory-perceptual alteration
   Hopelessness
   Powerlessness

Exhibit 29-1 Clues to Adolescent Alcohol, Tobacco, and Other Drug Use

Social
- Complaints, jokes, remarks made by friends about alcohol and drug use
- Conflicts with boyfriend/girlfriend over alcohol/drug use
- Rejection by non-using peer group
- Peer group drift; increasing socialization with heavy users
- Binges with peers
- Risk-taking behavior
- Increased sexual activity, risky sexual practices
- Increased conflict with family

Physical
- Passing out (with or without injury)
- Blackouts
- Cigarette smoking
- Increasing sickness (colds, flu)
- Headaches, stomachaches
- Sweating, rapid pulse, chest tightness
- Hangovers
- Steady deterioration in personal appearance and hygiene

Legal
- Arrests for possession, driving while intoxicated, disorderly conduct
- On probation
- Arrested for stealing, breaking and entering, vandalism, truancy

Academic
- Declining grades
- Low achievement in middle/junior high
- Low expectations
- May appear to have learning difficulties
- Decreased attention and concentration
- Uninvolved in school activities
- Hyperactive
- Difficult to discipline
- May stop doing homework
- Increased absenteeism, tardiness
- Dropping out
- Rebellious, argumentative with authority figures
- No goals for life
- Increased aggressiveness, excessive fights

Psychological
- Lethargy, nonmotivation
- Agitation, restlessness
- Depression, suicidal thoughts
- Paranoia
- Defensiveness, secretiveness
- Euphoric, unusually self-confident
- Unwillingness to express real feelings
- Feelings of guilt, shame, rejection undermine self-esteem
- "Addict personality": Grandiose, defensive, self-absorbed, manipulative, arrogant

Sources: Dryloos, J. (1990). *Adolescents at risk: Prevalence and prevention.* New York: Oxford University Press. Goplerud, E. (1991). *Preventing adolescent drug use: From theory to practice.* Rockville, MD: Office for Substance Abuse Prevention. Kaminer, Y. (1991). Adolescent substance abuse. In R. Frances & S. Miller (eds.), *Clinical textbook of addictive disorders* (pp. 320–346). New York: The Guilford Press.

Client Outcomes

1. The patient hospitalized for detoxification will safely achieve a drug-free state without complication or injury. He or she will identify addiction as the source of problems and accept referral for further treatment.
2. The client in the early stage of recovery will demonstrate a willingness to participate actively in treatment to overcome problems associated with psychoactive substances. He or she will identify the connection between problems and use of psychoactive substances.
3. The client in recovery will demonstrate that he or she has integrated learning about addiction and begun lifestyle changes.
   a. The client will describe spiritual transformation.

   b. The client will identify triggers that might signal impending relapse and strategies for preventing that relapse.

Plan and Interventions

For the Client

1. Explain the process of detoxification and assist the client.
   a. All clients must go through detoxification if they have been physically dependent on psychoactive substances. Detoxification may be done with the client as an inpatient or as an outpatient; medication is used in gradually decreasing doses to replace the psychoactive substance until the person is drug-free.

Exhibit 29–2 Clues in Adult Client's History

Social
- Reclusive and isolated—withdrawal from social activities
- Social life revolves around drinking- or drug-related activities
- Change of friends
- Frequent conflicts and altercations with friends
- "Partying" a lot and would like to "cut down"
- Accidents, driving arrests
- Frequent alcohol/drug use among peers

Psychological
- Cares less about everything
- Mood disturbances/mood swings
- Suicidal thoughts
- Chronic or acute depression
- Lack of impulse control
- Thought disorders
- Sexual dysfunction
- Manipulative or evasive
- Frequent and/or chronic anxiety and stress
- Preoccupied with alcohol/drugs
- Low self-esteem
- History of physical or sexual abuse

Behavioral
- Drinking during pregnancy
- Changes in school performance
- Repeated intoxication
- Frequent requests for mood-altering substances, asking for increased dose and more refills
- Complains life is "a mess"
- Frequently cancels appointments
- Frequently blames others for problems
- Denial/minimization of problems
- Tolerance to pain medication, alcohol, anesthesia
- Tried to quit before but was unable to

Employment
- Frequent complaints about job, employer, coworkers
- Frequent absenteeism, tardiness, absent from workstation
- Frequent and unexplained job changes
- Job performance is diminished and productivity is low
- High incidence of on-the-job accidents and injuries

Family
- Family members complain about drinking or drug use
- Continued alcohol and drug use in spite of tension created in family
- Spouse or partner reports intimacy or sexual problems
- Unexplained alterations in family system, such as separation, divorce, abandonment
- Family members have been treated for alcoholism and/or drug addiction and/or depression
- Rejection or absence of involvement by family members
- High level of family conflict
- Decreased interaction with family members
- Secretive
- Less responsible at home
- Reports of financial problems

Medical
- More frequent trauma than would be expected
- Unexplained injuries and accidents
- Complaints of gastritis and/or heartburn with frequent use of antacids
- Signs of withdrawal syndrome such as tachycardia, hypertension, diaphoresis, muscle cramps, tremors, flu-like symptoms
- Malnourished with weight loss, decreased muscle mass, and/or ascites
- Unexplained burns on arms, hands, fingers, chest (from falling asleep with lit cigarette)
- Heavy smoker with harsh cough and hoarseness
- Complaints of tingling sensations in extremities
- Frequent infections, including cellulitis and abscesses
- History of treatment for hepatitis, cirrhosis, pancreatitis, subacute bacterial endocarditis, chronic pulmonary problems
- Seizures that first appear between ages 10–30
- Persistent fatigue or general debilitation
- Deterioration in personal hygiene
- Sleep disturbance
- Episodes of hyperactivity
- Disturbance in motor functions
- Confusion, disorientation, memory loss

b. Some programs use either acupuncture or transcutaneous electrical nerve stimulation to modulate central nervous system activity during drug withdrawal. This afferent nerve stimulation appears to relieve symptoms of withdrawal and also may significantly decrease subsequent craving for the substance.[9]

2. During the client's detoxification, perform thorough and frequent assessments, provide medication as ordered, provide comfort measures to assist patient to begin the process of healing, educate the client about the impact of addiction, collaborate with other members of the treatment team, intervene to resolve any medical complications of the client's ad-

Exhibit 29–3 The CAGE and CAGE-AID Questions (CAGE Adapted To Include Drugs)

1. In the last three months, have you felt you should **c**ut down or stop drinking or *using drugs*?
   ❑ Yes ❑ No

2. In the last three months, has anyone **a**nnoyed you or gotten on your nerves by telling you to cut down or stop drinking or *using drugs*?
   ❑ Yes ❑ No

3. In the last three months, have you felt **g**uilty or bad about how much you drink or *use*?
   ❑ Yes ❑ No

4. In the last three months, have you been waking up wanting to have an alcohol drunk or *use drugs?* (**E**ye-opener)
   ❑ Yes ❑ No

Each affirmative response earns one point. One point indicates a possible problem. Two points indicate a probable problem.

Note: CAGE = C, cut, A, annoyed, G, guilty, E, eye opener.

The original CAGE questions appear in plain type. The CAGE questions adapted to include drugs are the original CAGE questions *modified by the italicized text.*

The CAGE or CAGE-AID should be preceded by two questions:

1. Do you drink alcohol?
2. Have you ever experimented with drugs?

If the patient has experimented with drugs, ask the CAGE-AID questions. If the patient only drinks alcohol, ask the CAGE questions.

Source: The Society of Teachers of Family Medicine. Project SAEFP Workshop Materials, Screening and Assessment Module, p. 18. Funded by the Division of Health Professionals, HRSA, DHHS, Contract No. 240-89-0038.

diction, and make a referral or coordinate further treatment to ensure a strong beginning to the recovery process.

3. During recovery, continue to provide health education about addiction and its consequences, creating an interpersonal relationship with client that makes it safe to talk about issues and feelings.
   a. Teach new coping skills, providing opportunities to rehearse these skills.
   b. Have the client practice self-care measures that can be incorporated into newly achieved healthy lifestyle.

4. Explain that learning to overcome addictions involves recognizing the urge to use substances, associating that urge with particular situations or settings, identifying other options and evaluating them, choosing the best available strategies for managing the situation, and reaching spiritual transformation and acceptance.[10]

5. Teach the client general relaxation and imagery exercises with a focus on body-centered awareness of body responses to feelings.

6. Teach the client how to create specific imagery patterns, including the following:
   a. Active images that cleanse the body, like a waterfall, and create a protective shield to block out negative images.
   b. End-state images about the quality of life.
   c. Healing images to help the client connect with spiritual resources.
   d. Process images to overcome stressful situations.

7. Teach the client to reframe current situations and problems so that positive thoughts will produce positive actions.

8. Teach the client creative ways to recognize and express feelings, such as journal writing, painting or sculpting, music and dance, letter writing.

9. Have the client identify high-risk situations and triggers for relapse, and then develop strategies for dealing with them constructively.

10. Encourage the client to attend 12-step meetings.

11. Make a written contract for health, which includes healthy nutrition, regular exercise, regular practice of relaxation and imagery techniques, and healthy recreation.

12. Help the client to build a support system, including family, friends, sponsor, and therapist.

13. Deal with any resistance to spirituality that the client may display, because this resistance is likely to interfere with the client's attendance at 12-step meetings.

14. Advise the client to practice daily stress management techniques, such as deep muscle relaxation, guided imagery, massage, aromatherapy, rhythmic breathing, and cognitive restructuring.

15. Teach the client to complete daily affirmations, focusing on inner strengths and positive qualities. Help the client to forgive self and others and to move forward, learning to trust again.

Exhibit 29–4 Brief MAST

Short Michigan Alcohol Screening Test

1. Do you feel you are a normal drinker?
2. Do friends or relatives think you are a normal drinker?
3. Have you ever attended a meeting of Alcoholics Anonymous?
4. Have you ever lost friends or girlfriends/boyfriends because of drinking?
5. Have you ever gotten into trouble at work because of drinking?
6. Have you ever neglected your obligations, your family, or your work for 2 or more days in a row because you were drinking?
7. Have you ever had delirium tremens (DTs), severe shaking, heard voices, or seen things that weren't there after heavy drinking?
8. Have you ever gone to anyone for help about your drinking?
9. Have you ever been in a hospital because of drinking?
10. Have you ever been arrested for drunk driving or driving after drinking?

Brief MAST Scoring

Questions	Response Score Yes	Response Score No
1. Do you feel you are a normal drinker?	0	2
2. Do friends or relatives think you are a normal drinker?	0	2
3. Have you ever attended a meeting of Alcoholics Anonymous?	5	0
4. Have you ever lost friends or girlfriends/boyfriends because of drinking?	2	0
5. Have you ever gotten into trouble at work because of drinking?	2	0
6. Have you ever neglected your obligations, your family, or your work for 2 or more days in a row because you were drinking?	2	0
7. Have you ever had delirium tremens (DTs), severe shaking, heard voices, or seen things that weren't there after heavy drinking?	2	0
8. Have you ever gone to anyone for help about your drinking?	5	0
9. Have you ever been in a hospital because of drinking?	5	0
10. Have you ever been arrested for drunk driving or driving after drinking?	2	0

Total   _____ = _____

Score of 6 or more indicates probable diagnosis of alcoholism, except for questions 3, 8, or 9, which are diagnostic.

Source: Pokovny, A.D., Miller, B.A., Kaplan, H.B. (1972). The Brief MAST: A Shortened Version of the Michigan Alcohol Screening Test. *American Journal of Psychology* 129, 342–345.

For the Caregiver

1. Be a positive role model of health and respect for self.
2. Do a daily body scan to identify bodymind responses, and implement a daily program of healthy behavior, including nutrition, exercise, positive affirmations, recreation, balance, and effective stress management.
3. Help any colleague who may be experiencing problems with addiction.
   a. Talk to the colleague, and share your observations of the problems that addiction is creating for the colleague.
   b. Share information about treatment, and convey your sense of hope that the colleague can find help to resolve the current spiritual crisis.
   c. Demonstrate compassion and respect for the colleague.
   d. Show acceptance when the colleague returns to work and help provide support and reinforcement for efforts at healthy behaviors.

Evaluation

1. Determine if the client outcomes, such as sobriety and integration of healthy behaviors, have been achieved.

Exhibit 29–5 RAFFT

A relatively new screening instrument, particularly valuable because it focuses equally on alcohol and drug use. It was developed at Brown University for Project ADEPT.

- Do you drink or use drugs to *Relax*, feel better about yourself, or to fit in?
- Do you ever drink or use drugs while you are by yourself, *Alone*?
- Do you or any of your closest *Friends* drink or use drugs?
- Does a close *Family* member have a problem with alcohol or drug use?
- Have you ever gotten into *Trouble* from drinking or drug use?

Source: From "Adolescent Substance Abuse," by S.G. Riggs and A.J. Alario, 1989, in C.E. Dube, M.G. Goldstein, D.C. Lewis, E.R. Myers, and W.R. Zwick (eds.), *The Project ADEPT Curriculum for Primary Physician Training* (p. 27J), Providence, RI: Brown University. Copyright 1989 by Brown University. Reprinted by permission of National Training System, U.S. Office for Substance Abuse Prevention.

Exhibit 29–6 Trauma Scale Screening Tool

Five questions about history of trauma since 18th birthday.

1. Have you had any fractures or dislocations of your bones or joints?
2. Have you ever been injured in a traffic accident?
3. Have you ever injured your head?
4. Have you ever been in an assault or fight (excluding sports)?
5. Have you ever been injured while drinking?

More than one positive response would indicate a probable drinking problem.

Source: Skinner, H.A., Holt, S., Schuller, R., Roy, J., and Israel, Y. (1984). Identification of Alcohol Abuse Using Laboratory Tests and a History of Trauma. *Annals of Internal Medicine,* 101, 847–851.

2. Validate with the client the existence of the therapeutic relationship, and determine which specific interventions have been particularly helpful and which have been ineffective.

REFERENCES

1. L. Jack et al., *The Core Curriculum of Addictions Nursing* (Skokie, IL: Midwest Education Association, 1990), 8.
2. B.M. Dossey et al., *Holistic Nursing: A Handbook for Practice,* 2nd ed. (Gaithersburg, MD: Aspen Publishers, 1995), 519–520.
3. J. Lowinson et al., *Substance Abuse: A Comprehensive Textbook,* 2nd ed. (Baltimore: Williams & Wilkins, 1992), 575.
4. J. Kinney, *Clinical Manual of Substance Abuse,* 2nd ed. (St. Louis: Mosby–Year Book, 1996), 18.
5. Ibid.
6. M. Fleming et al., *Addictive Disorders* (St. Louis: Mosby–Year Book, 1992), 353.
7. D. Snow et al., *Prevention of Alcohol, Tobacco, and Other Drug Problems: An Independent Study for Nurses* (Raleigh, NC: National Nurses Society on Addictions, 1994), 23.
8. Dossey et al., *Holistic Nursing: A Handbook for Practice.*
9. Lowinson et al., *Substance Abuse: A Comprehensive Textbook.*
10. Dossey et al., *Holistic Nursing: A Handbook for Practice.*

CHAPTER 30

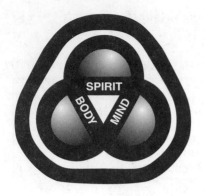

Incest/Child Sexual Abuse and Violence

E. Jane Martin

KNOWLEDGE COMPETENCIES

- Trace childhood sexual abuse from antiquity to the present.
- Identify the present incidence of incest/child sexual abuse.
- Discuss the repressed memories/false memories controversy.
- Describe the emotional and behavioral consequences of childhood sexual abuse for survivors.
- Describe the physical consequences of childhood sexual abuse for survivors.
- Explicate the application of the nursing process to care of the adult survivor.
- Discuss the specific nursing interventions of empowerment (including disclosure and teaching), grounding skills, relaxation, writing, anger expression and management, and imagery.

DEFINITIONS

Child Sexual Abuse: exploitative psychosexual activity that goes beyond the developmental level of the child, to which the child is unable to give informed consent, and that violates social taboos regarding roles and relationships (includes incest).[1]

Dissociation: a splitting off of dimensions of the personality into partial or whole alter personalities, each with a different degree of consciousness.[2]

Flashback: a nonpsychotic episode in the present in which the person actually relives the abuse as it originally happened.

Grounding: staying in or reorienting self to the present.

Incest: any type of exploitative sexual experience between relatives (or surrogate relatives) before the victim is 18 years old.[3]

Trigger: any sight, sound, smell, or other sensory experience that stimulates recall of a memory.

Violence: a component of all incest/child sexual abuse, regardless of the intent of the perpetrator.

 Pause for a moment . . .

❑ *My study of the **AHNA Core Curriculum** is satisfying.*
❑ *I am preparing for the successful completion of the holistic nursing certification (HNC) examination to prepare for my present and future role as a holistic nurse.*

THEORIES AND RESEARCH

History of Incest/Child Sexual Abuse

1. A universal taboo against incest is supported by cogent arguments: biologic (to prevent genetic defects), economic (to broaden the family base of power and wealth), sociologic (to solidify society through wider connections and relationships), and psychosocial (to prevent the collapse of the family because of sexual rivalries).[4]

2. In spite of the universal taboo against it, incest/child sexual abuse has existed since antiquity in every, or nearly every, known culture.[5]

a. In ancient Eastern cultures, the practice of pedophilia was common.
1) In India, children slept with adults, sexual activity began early, and child marriage was commonplace.
2) Historical data from ancient China support the institutionalization of practices of pederasty of boys, child concubinage, castration of young boys so they could be eunuchs, child marriage, boy and girl prostitution, and foot binding to break the bones of the foot and facilitate shaping it to become a penis substitute, a practice that continued into the twentieth century.

b. In Western cultures, incest/child sexual abuse is documented in poetry and on pottery from ancient Greece, in historical documents from early Roman times, in religious writings from the Egyptian–Hebrew culture, in educational treatises from Western European Christianity, in popular literature during the Enlightenment Period, in pornographic literature during the Victorian Period, and in Freud's early writings.

c. With Freud's retraction of his seduction theory and formulation of the Oedipal complex in its place, public knowledge of child sexual abuse by parental figures in the home was lost until the 1960s.

3. Since then, child abuse has been a subject of continued concern. Only since the 1980s, however, have sufficiently large samples been available for statistical analyses of the prevalence of child abuse. The present conservative estimates are truly alarming: 1:4 for girls and 1:7 for boys.[6]

4. National attention focused over the past decade on the rising incidence rate, the increase in public self-disclosure (often after the recall of repressed memories of childhood abuse), and the use of legal redress have elicited a backlash response.

a. When Miss America of 1958, Marilyn Van Derber Atler, broke years of silence and publicly told the story of her sexual abuse from age 5 until age 18 by her (then deceased) prominent, respected father, the prestigious audience was shocked and disbelieving, and the media attention was nationwide.[7]

b. Some accused parents, troubled and angered, have founded a support and advocacy organization called The False Memory Syndrome Foundation (FMSF). The targets of their anger are "New Age healers, self-help movement promoters, political activists, radical feminists, social service providers and mental health professionals."[8]

Consequences of Child Sexual Abuse

1. Adult survivors of incest/sexual abuse suffer a wide array of emotional disorders that manifest themselves in behavioral symptoms.[9]

a. Depression is the most common manifestation, occurring either intermittently or constantly throughout childhood into adolescence.
1) Associated with the depression are low self-esteem, feelings of worthlessness and hopelessness, inability to trust, passivity, lethargy, feelings of helplessness, inability to concentrate, inability to take control of one's life, confusion, and guilt.
2) Impulsive behavior is common and may include mood swings, rage, inappropriate spending, self-mutilation, "accidents," and suicide gestures and attempts.

b. Dissociation also occurs frequently and may be manifested by nightmares or night terrors, with resultant sleep disorders, amnesia (especially for segments of childhood), feelings of depersonalization, fainting spells, panic attacks, hyperventilation, flashbacks, denial of incest/abuse, and splitting or multiple personalities.

c. Relationships are frequently problematic; interpersonal skills are often impaired, and the survivor may seem to seek out those who revictimize him or her and to run from those who offer positive regard and nurturance.

2. Equally noteworthy is the wide range of physical symptoms that survivors suffer, many times affecting several organ systems and challenging precise medical diagnosis. Survivors rate their general health lower than non–sexually abused women rate their health, and survivors use health care more throughout their lives.[10,11]

a. Gastrointestinal symptoms are very common. They include nausea, gagging, vomiting, "nervous" stomach, stomach pains, ulcers, and irritable bowel.

b. Survivors often develop eating disorders, including anorexia nervosa, bulimia, and obesity. Some perceive food as the only area in which they feel in control; others hope to alter body appearance (very fat or painfully thin) in an attempt to appear unattractive and sexually unappealing.

c. Substance abuse is a pattern frequently found as survivors learned early that alcohol and drugs would temporarily numb the pain of their existence, a kind of chemical dissociation.

d. Sexual dysfunctions of all kinds commonly result from incest/sexual abuse.

   1) Manifestations include a range of behaviors from sexual promiscuity to the point of addiction all the way to sexual abstinence and phobia.

   2) Pain and discomfort, particularly in the anogenital and/or pelvic areas are frequently experienced, whether the person is sexually active or not.

   3) Intolerance or even fear of physical touch is another manifestation of sexual dysfunction and poor interpersonal skills.

e. Other general physical symptoms include headaches, insomnia, seizures, back pain, and chronic tension.

Pause for a moment . . .

❑ *I am practicing successful completion of the HNC examination.*

❑ *I am preparing for successful completion of the HNC examination as a mark of achievement and proficiency as defined by the AHNA Certification Board.*

HOLISTIC NURSING PROCESS

Assessment

1. In order to use therapeutic interventions effectively with adult survivors of incest/child sexual abuse, nurses must first
   a. Be personally comfortable with discussions of incest/child sexual abuse and aware of their attitudes toward it.
   b. Increase their knowledge about this serious problem.
2. Nurses then must
   a. Take the responsibility for asking about incest/child sexual abuse as part of their routine nursing history taking.

b. Initiate a discussion of the subject rather than wait for the client to offer information.
c. Use good communication techniques.
d. Allow sufficient time for the client to tell his or her story.
e. Provide psychologic support during the interview.

3. If more information is needed, nurses may ask a client to describe his or her perception of the effects of the incest/sexual abuse on eight life domains:
   a. Social (e.g., do you feel isolated, different from others, or unable to interact with others?).
   b. Psychologic/emotional (e.g., are you unable to feel anything, or do you have too many feelings?).
   c. Physical (e.g., do you have pain, headaches, or muscle tension, or do you feel sick when certain activities are mentioned?).
   d. Sexual (e.g., do you engage in sexual behavior or avoid it, do you have sexual fears?).
   e. Familial (e.g., has your family life changed, for example, through divorce, estrangement, increased closeness?).
   f. Sense of self (e.g., do you feel strong, powerless, worthwhile, ashamed?).
   g. Relation to men (e.g., do you trust them, feel hostile to them, avoid them?).
   h. Relation to women (e.g., do you trust them, feel hostile to them, avoid them?)[12]

Nursing Diagnoses

1. The following selected nursing diagnoses most common with incest/abuse survivors are related to the human response patterns:

   a. Relating: Social isolation
                Impaired social interaction
                Sexual dysfunction

   b. Valuing: Spiritual distress
                Spiritual well-being

   c. Choosing: Altered participation in family
                Impaired adjustment
                Ineffective coping

   d. Perceiving: Altered self-concept
                Disturbance in body concept
                Disturbance in self-esteem
                Disturbance in self-identity
                Powerlessness

   e. Feeling: Pain
                Grief
                Anxiety

Fear

Post-trauma response

f. Moving: Sleep disturbance

Client Outcomes

1. Outcomes should flow from the assessment data and problem list (nursing diagnoses) and be created with the client.
2. There should be one or more measurable outcome for each problem in each nursing diagnosis. For example, if the nursing diagnosis is relating and the problem is social isolation, the outcome can be that the client attends a scheduled social activity three times a week.

Plan and Interventions

1. Plan effectively by
   a. Using the assessment data, the nursing diagnoses, and the outcomes specific to each problem.
   b. Working with the client to develop a plan, including goals and interventions, that will facilitate the achievement of the identified outcomes.
      1) Part of the plan should focus on self-care, using the client's personal resources.
      2) Part of the plan should include the nursing interventions, including client education.
   c. Ensuring that the plan reflects both the client's priorities and the nurse's.
2. Provide a copy of the plan for the client, as well as for the client's record.
3. Implement the plan effectively by
   a. Promoting client participation in both self-care and nursing interventions.
   b. Providing a supportive environment.
   c. Providing safe care.
4. Document the care provided.

Empowerment

1. Support the client while empowering him or her, which enables the client to increase self-esteem and feel more in control of life events.
   a. Nurses need not be experts in working with survivors to be helpful.
   b. Many helping techniques decrease the guilt and shame associated with the long-kept, "dirty" secret.
2. Collaborate with the client in a true partnership.

a. Client goals and outcomes are the result of a joint planning effort.
b. The plan builds on the client's strengths.
c. With the nurse's support, the client comes to believe that he or she can and should make the decisions about his or her life.
3. Support the client and facilitate the disclosure whenever and however the client chooses.
   a. Disclosure is the first step for the survivor.
   b. The client must feel that he or she has the nurse's permission to "tell the story."
   c. The nurse should not express shock or horror at the details.
   d. The nurse should be comfortable with the client's silence if it occurs during the disclosure, should follow the client's lead, and help the client strategize when he or she is ready.
   e. The nurse can help the survivor realize that self-disclosure takes great courage and is a real strength.
4. Provide psychologic support if the client experiences flashbacks during the disclosure.
5. Teach basic principles of normal physiology and child development.
   a. Help the client forgive himself or herself for any sexual pleasure experienced during the abuse.
   b. Explain that current negative habits and traits can be linked to the incest/abuse and may have been adaptive when the survivor developed them, but they are no longer helpful and may even be destructive.
6. Explore new behaviors and teach those of interest to the survivor, such as assertiveness and anger control.

Grounding Skills

1. Help the survivor to stay grounded in or reorient self to the present.
   a. Clients have often developed their own ways of staying in the present.
   b. The nurse may observe this during the history taking (e.g., the client touching a piece of jewelry or holding a small object).
   c. The nurse should ask about or verify the grounding object rather than assume its existence.
2. Teach the client to assess and monitor his or her current level of awareness in order to stay grounded in the present.
   a. Grounding is especially helpful when a client experiences a flashback or dissociates.

b. The client should learn the signs of dissociation (e.g., losing track of thoughts, stopping in the midst of talking, staring into space, and flat affect).

c. Additional grounding skills to help the client stay oriented in the present include maintaining eye contact, stating aloud the day and date, or naming the people in the room.

3. Since survivors are often re-victimized or their children become victims, help the survivor become empowered to prevent either situation.

Relaxation

1. Teach the survivor relaxation exercises to reduce anxiety, promote grounding, and discourage dissociation.

a. Although survivors of abuse may be reluctant to take part in relaxation exercises, the skills can be very helpful to them.

b. Survivors may not feel "worthy" to take time away from their recovery to relax; they may equate relaxation with vulnerability and, in fact, may experience flashbacks when in a relaxed state.

c. Survivors may need to relearn the skill of relaxation, which can help them achieve more restful sleep, clearer thought processes, and more pleasant physical sensations.

2. Help the survivor use progressive relaxation, which uses the controlled tensing and relaxing of specific muscle groups.

a. It can allow the survivor to feel more fully in control of his or her body.

b. It can help alleviate feelings of helplessness and vulnerability.

c. If progressive relaxation is joined with systematic desensitization, the survivor could gain some comfort in regard to anxiety-inducing people or events.

Writing

1. Suggest that the survivor keep a journal, writing in it each day, and recording thoughts, feelings, dreams, nightmares, flashbacks, and memories.

a. Poetry and stories may be recorded as well as a detailed lifeline with its graphic portrayal of important family and life events.

b. The journal can help the client regain forgotten memories, see improvements in behaviors, and recall strategies that were useful in earlier difficult times. If a lifeline is included, it can reveal previously undetected patterns in the survivor's childhood, adolescence, and adulthood.

c. The journal can be brought into the treatment for the nurse's review and suggestions.

2. To facilitate full, uncensored expression of thoughts and feelings, encourage the survivor to write letters.

a. Initially, the letter is not intended to be sent.

1) It is written to a particular person (e.g., the abuser or the nonprotective parent) without regard for style, tone, emotional censorship, or guilt.

2) The survivor should freely express thoughts and feelings.

3) The letter can be brought into treatment and read aloud to facilitate verbal expression of feelings.

b. If the survivor decides to send the letter, he or she can rework it until satisfied with the form.

c. The value of this technique lies in the survivor's uncensored, full expression of feelings toward the person addressed.

d. If the survivor wants to send the letter and expects that the letter will "make a difference" (i.e., the person addressed will finally understand the survivor's pain and beg forgiveness), it is better that the survivor not send the letter, for that is almost never the outcome.

Anger Expression and Management

1. Teach the survivor to recognize and express his or her own anger.

a. Survivors have usually learned early that only the perpetrator is allowed to express anger in the home without punishment.

b. The survivor learns that anger equals power.

c. The survivor has usually internalized anger and may express it only in disguised form, such as passive–aggressive behavior, manipulativeness, depression, anxiety, and somatic complaints such as headaches, colitis, and ulcers.

d. It may also be expressed as self-blame, self-contempt, and self-defeating and self-abusive behaviors.

2. Explore appropriate anger management techniques as the survivor begins to get in touch with his or her anger.

a. The survivor must first learn that feelings of anger and rage are appropriate considering what happened; however, the survivor must also learn that indirect and aggressive expression of anger is not good.

b. The survivor must learn to "dose anger" (express it in small, manageable amounts). Using a 30-second to 3-minute timer to guide expression of anger for a safe amount of time can be helpful.

c. Use of an audiotape to record verbal expression of anger can be useful if the tape is played in the presence of a nurse or supportive friend who can help validate and justify the anger.

d. Physical exercise, such as running, can reduce anger.

e. Other techniques include throwing "soft" balls at a wall, hitting a punching bag with plastic pipe, and hitting sofa cushions or a bed with a tennis racket.

f. Anger workouts should be appropriate to the lifestyle and comfort level of the survivor.

Imagery

1. Assist the survivor in remembering experiences through imagery, which has not usually been punished in the past and is less likely to be censored by the survivor in the present. An effective guided imagery technique can help a survivor connect with the lost emotions associated with the abuse.

   a. The nurse assists the client to relax deeply.

   b. The nurse asks the client to close the eyes and imagine the face of the abuser (or some other significant person in the client's past). The nurse may suggest that the face appear on a TV screen to protect the client from overwhelming emotion.

   c. The client is asked to describe the facial expression and his or her somatic response to it (e.g., "knot in my stomach").

   d. Next the client is asked to interpret the image, to say what the face represents, and to identify the intensity of the somatic response.

   e. Then the client is asked what the face is saying and what the somatic response is. The nurse and client together determine how far to go with this exercise.

   f. Finally, the client is given an opportunity to respond to the abuser by releasing lost emotions.

2. Vary this technique to help clients connect with long-buried feelings of pain, anger, sadness, pleasure, etc. Also, if the client has never felt or cannot recall ever feeling safe or nurtured, for example, imagery can provide the means to present the possibility. Because acting "as if" produces the same biochemical response as the actual experience, the possibilities are limitless (see Chapter 24, Imagery).

Evaluation

1. In the process of evaluation, the nurse works to
   a. Evaluate outcomes based on the client's attainment of goals.
   b. Assess effectiveness of nursing and self-care measures in meeting outcomes.
   c. Revise the plan on an ongoing basis.
2. It is essential to document evaluation and outcomes in the client record.

REFERENCES

1. L.G. Kolkmeier, Sexual Abuse: Healing the Wounds, in *Holistic Nursing: A Handbook for Practice,* 2nd ed., B.M. Dossey et al. (Gaithersburg, MD: Aspen Publishers, 1995), 404.

2. C. Courtois, *Healing the Incest Wound: Adult Survivors in Therapy* (New York: W.W. Norton & Co., 1988), 154.

3. J.C. Urbancic, Intrafamilial Sexual Abuse, in *Nursing Care of Survivors of Family Violence,* ed. J. Campbell and J. Humphreys (St. Louis: Mosby, 1993), 133.

4. M. Lew, *Victims No Longer: Men Recovering from Incest and Other Sexual Abuse* (New York: Harper & Row, 1988), 19.

5. L. DeMause, The Universality of Incest, *Journal of Psychohistory* 19, no. 2 (1991): 123–164.

6. E.J. Martin, Incest/Child Sexual Abuse, *Journal of Holistic Nursing* 13, no. 1 (1995): 14.

7. L. Terr, *Unchained Memories: True Stories of Traumatic Memories Lost and Found* (New York: Basic Books, 1994), 123–126, 262.

8. M. Wylie, The Shadow of a Doubt, *Family Therapy Networker* 17, no. 5 (1993): 29.

9. Courtois, *Healing the Incest Wound,* 98–99.

10. J. Lesserman et al., Sexual and Physical Abuse History in Gastroenterology Practice: How Types of Abuse Impact Health Status, *Psychosomatic Medicine* 58, no. 4 (1996): 4–15.

11. Courtois, *Healing the Incest Wound,* 99–100.

12. Ibid., 368–369.

Practice Examinations

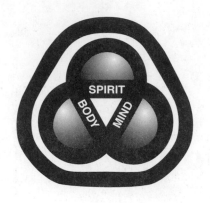

Taking the Practice Examinations

This section of the *AHNA Core Curriculum for Holistic Nursing* is designed to help you prepare for the HNC examination that is administered by the AHNA Certification Board under the direction of the National League for Nursing Testing Division. All of the sample test questions in this section are based on the information in the *AHNA Core Curriculum for Holistic Nursing* and follow the HNC examination blueprint. The HNC examination blueprint was compiled following the analysis of the IPAKHN Survey (Appendix B). You are encouraged to request a copy of the current HNC examination blueprint from the AHNA Certification Board.* The actual test is based upon the specific percentage for each part of the *AHNA Core Curriculum for Holistic Nursing.*

The practice examinations follow Section I of the *AHNA Core Curriculum for Holistic Nursing.* These sample questions provide examples of types of questions that will be found on the HNC examination. These sample test questions are to stimulate the general types of questions that are included in the HNC examination. None of these questions will be actual examination items. The questions are intended to teach and to prepare you for the HNC examination. They are designed for recall, comprehension, and situation level questions covering the basic knowledge of a holistic nurse in different practice environments.

_____

*For more information on the application for the HNC examination and the HNC Blueprint contact the AHNA: American Holistic Nurses' Association (AHNA), 4101 Lake Boone Trail, Suite #201, Raleigh, North Carolina 27607; (919) 787-5181 or toll free (800) 278-AHNA; Fax (919) 787-4916.

Prepare in advance for the HNC examination. Follow the study plan suggestions. As you prepare, use this knowledge in your practice settings. This reinforces retention of information and the improvement of your client skills. This is a valuable asset to your current clinical practice as well as a way to prepare for your future holistic nursing practice.

STUDY PLAN

The successful completion of the HNC examination requires careful planning and preparation. The process can be one of joy and excitement, because it allows you to sharpen your knowledge base in your holistic nursing practice. A systematic approach can increase your energy level as you assess your study needs, develop your study plan, use your study skills, and plan for the successful completion of the HNC examination (Exhibit II–1).

Assessing Study Needs

It is essential to determine which content areas you know well and which areas you need to review further. The following steps can help you assess your knowledge, skills, and abilities:

1. Review the contents of the *AHNA Core Curriculum.* Identify the areas that will need more of your time than the others. Reflect on your current education or practice environment. Because you are more familiar with these areas, they will require less of your time. Begin with the subjects that you find most difficult and about which you know the least. Take the practice examinations and determine the areas on

Exhibit II–1 Checklist for Developing a Study Plan

1. Prepare carefully for the HNC examination.
   - I will review the organization of the components of the AHNA Standards of Holistic Nursing (Appendix A). (The AHNA Standards of Holistic Nursing Practice provide the framework for the *AHNA Core Curriculum for Holistic Nursing* and the blueprint for the HNC examination.)
   - I will review the blueprint for the HNC examination.
   - I will study the *AHNA Core Curriculum* and then take the practice examinations.
   - I scored best on these practice examinations: _____ .
   - I am not satisfied with my scores on these practice examinations: _____ .
   - I need further study in these content areas: _____ .
2. Review your test-taking skills.
   - I can identify the components of a test question.
   - I read questions carefully before selecting an answer.
   - I can make reasonable "guesses" on questions when I am not certain of the correct answer.
   - Before I take the practice examinations, I will establish the conditions as if I were taking the actual examination (e.g., empty bladder, quiet environment without interruptions for _____ hours).
3. Make a study plan.
   - I will study in (quiet environment and location) _____ .
   - I will commit to study at these times and dates: _____ .
   - I will assemble all of the materials that I need to study: _____ .
4. Practice successful completion of the HNC examination.
   - I am preparing for the successful completion of the HNC examination as a mark of personal and professional achievement.
   - I am preparing for successful completion of the HNC examination because this indicates proficiency as defined by the AHNA Certification Board.
   - I am preparing for successful completion of the HNC examination to prepare for my present and future role as a holistic nurse.
   - I can do relaxation (primarily deep breathing) exercises to manage my test-taking anxiety and to be alert, relaxed, and calm while taking the HNC examination.
   - I can visualize complete success in this entire process.
   - I can give myself positive affirmations and feedback.

which you need to concentrate. Gaining confidence in these areas earlier in your study plan will give you great satisfaction.

2. Review your test-taking skills. How do you feel when you think about taking an examination? If you feel anxiety, you can change this pattern immediately; with your knowledge and skills, you can evoke deep relaxation to study the requirements and to take the test. Assess what has worked in the past to make you confident about taking a test. Like many, you may have some old, negative mind tapes about being a poor test-taker. These no longer serve you. Spend some time changing these "old worn-out mind tapes" into mind tapes of "achieving your goal of test success."

Some areas in the *AHNA Core Curriculum* are more difficult than others. As you learn these more difficult areas, however, you increase your ability to articulate your philosophy, mission, and work to your colleagues. You also become a better teacher with your clients.

Developing a Study Plan

Begin to develop your plan and prepare for the HNC examination as soon as you can. Having identified your strengths and weaknesses, you know where to start. It is best to study small sections of content over a long period of time. Avoid cramming, because it leads only to frustration and anxiety. Create a healing ritual as you begin to study. The following suggestions are offered:

- Find your special place to be quiet, focused, and relaxed. Place objects around you that remind you to be focused and relaxed while you study.
- Place your books, papers, and other resources near you.
- Highlight content with one or different colored markers.

- Tell your family or friends why you are preparing for the HNC examination so that they will support you in your endeavors. This will help them to better understand your need for quietness.
- Learn to use your time effectively. There are no rules in how you actually study. Find your own personal style.
- Make an audiocassette tape with your own voice covering the most difficult core content or all the core content. Then you can listen to it over and over again at your own pace.

Improving Your Study Skills

The *AHNA Core Curriculum* is designed to help you learn and refine your knowledge and skills base. Good study skills enable you to organize, acquire, remember, and use the information that you need to pass the HNC examination. Following are some further suggestions:

- Study to learn, not to memorize. Frequently, it is very useful to ask yourself, "How do I apply this in my clinical practice, education, or specific practice environment?" or "How can I apply this in order to more deeply understand the nurse as an instrument of healing?"
- Use study skills that have worked for you in the past (e.g., studying alone or in a group).
- While you study, formulate your own questions, and explain your answers. If studying in a group, each participant can add questions during the discussion process and discuss their rationale.
- Simulate a test-taking situation. Sit down to take the practice examinations without interruptions.
- Use relaxation and imagery strategies, as well as positive affirmations and positive feedback. Reward yourself in your own special way during and after a concentrated study session.
- Evaluate your progress. Keep a checklist as to specifics, such as practice examination scores, about certain content areas. Spend more time on those areas that you have not mastered and less time on the areas you know well.

TEST-TAKING STRATEGIES

The "test-wiseness," the "how-to" of test taking, is a skill that can be learned and practiced to improve test scores. Among the effective test-taking strategies are the following:

1. Understand the components of the multiple choice test item. A test item consists of background or situation information, a question, and four possible answers.
   a. The *background* (*situation*) is a nurse-based or a client-based situation. The content of the situation, such as presurgery, a client seeking help to learn relaxation and imagery skills, a client's health or family status, or ethnicity, is significant.
   b. The *question* (*stem*) poses the problem to be solved. The stem made be written as a direct question, "What would you do first?" or an incomplete sentence, "The nurse should. . . ."
   c. The *answers* are the possible responses to the stem. Of the four answers, only one is correct.
2. Each chapter also has situation questions. You will be asked to give basic responses (in any order) and optional responses (in any order) to the situation questions in each chapter. These questions assess the broad knowledge, clinical decision-making skills, and integration of holistic nursing practice. Your answers should be based on the core content within each chapter of the *AHNA Core Curriculum*.
3. Read each question with care. Do not rush. Do not read meaning into a question. If a word in a question is not familiar, try to figure out the meaning based on the context in which it appears in the question.
4. As you read the question, consider carefully what you are being asked, such as to set priorities, to select the best intervention, or to evaluate outcomes.
5. Look for key words, because these words give clues to the correct answer. These are such words as *except, not,* or *but.* Words such as *most, next,* or *first* indicate the order of steps or the priority.
6. On the multiple choice questions, try to answer the questions first before you look at your choices. Then look for the answer that is similar to the one that you generated.
7. If you do not know an answer, make a reasonable guess. "Intuition" and "hunches" often result in correct answers.

PREPARING FOR THE DAY OF THE HNC EXAMINATION

By the time you reach the day of the HNC examination, you have prepared as much as you can. This day involves physical and mental preparation. A few suggestions follow:

1. Get a good night's rest before the examination. Monitor your responsibilities the week of the

examination so that you do not arrive exhausted or worried about work or family.

2. Eat nourishing food before the examination. Complex carbohydrate foods provide the most energy. Avoid excess use of caffeine or sugar right before the examination.

3. Concentrate during the examination. Focus. Others may finish before you, but you will have plenty of time to finish. If you lose your concentration, just use your relaxation, deep breathing, imagery, affirmations, positive self-talk, and distraction to refocus.

4. Use your successful test-taking strategies prior to and during the examination to decrease any anxiety. Throughout the *AHNA Core Curriculum,* you will see the AHNA logo and some success strategies to remind you to use the following:

   a. Relaxation and deep breathing exercises to decrease anxiety and tension.

   b. Imagery rehearsal of preparing for the test, seeing yourself in the examination environment, feeling relaxed and confident, and successfully passing the examination.

   c. Affirmation and positive self-talk: "I am prepared for this exam," "I can pass this exam with flying colors," "I can see HNC after my name," "I can see the HNC certification recognition hanging in my office," "I am so proud that I made this commitment to take the HNC examination," etc.

   d. Distraction techniques: Any time worry or fear comes into your mind, let yourself take a deep breath, and with the next exhalation let the worry flow out.

Best wishes in your study preparation and in taking the HNC examination.

Sample Answer Sheet

Note: This sample answer sheet may be photocopied for your own use as you test yourself.

1. _____	6. _____	11. _____	16. _____
2. _____	7. _____	12. _____	17. _____
3. _____	8. _____	13. _____	18. _____
4. _____	9. _____	14. _____	19. _____
5. _____	10. _____	15. _____	20. _____

Situation 1:   Basic Responses   Optional Responses

Situation 2:   Basic Responses   Optional Responses

Situation3:   Basic Responses   Optional Responses

Situation 4:   Basic Responses   Optional Responses

PART I—DISCIPLINE OF HOLISTIC NURSING PRACTICE

CONCEPT I—HOLISTIC PHILOSOPHY

CHAPTER 1—HOLISTIC NURSING PRACTICE

 Pause for a moment . . .

❏ *I know my effective test-taking strategies.*
❏ *I understand the components of the test item.*

Test Questions 1–15

1. Holism is
   a. a theory that the function of human beings is accounted for by behavior of the constituent parts of the body—the atoms and electrons.
   b. a theory that the universe and living nature are seen correctly in terms of interactional wholes that are more than the mere sum of their parts.
   c. a theory of determinism.
   d. a theory of molecular dysfunction.

2. A bio-psycho-social-spiritual model
   a. combines spirituality with mind modulation of the autonomic nervous system.
   b. differentiates between psychologic and spiritual elements.
   c. integrates and recognizes the interrelationship of biologic, psychologic, sociologic, and spiritual dimensions.
   d. focuses on the physical and psychologic sequelae inherent in illness.

3. Holistic nursing emphasizes
   a. fragmentation of the client's problems into physiologic and psychologic problems.
   b. the organic or functional relationships between parts and wholes.
   c. the nuisance of the placebo effect.
   d. limited evidence for the domain of spirituality.

4. Era I medicine focuses on
   a. mind/body interactions of emotions and meanings.
   b. the combination of medical treatments and technology.
   c. nonlocal states of consciousness.
   d. mind/body therapies and outcomes.

5. Era II medicine focuses on
   a. the chemical reaction to medical treatments and technology.
   b. the limited effect of consciousness on the body.
   c. the interactions of emotions with behavior and mind/body responses.
   d. the molecular cause of disease and treatments.

6. In Era III medicine, consciousness is viewed as
   a. local in nature.
   b. nonlocal in nature.
   c. a brain-bound mind state.
   d. a body-bound mind state.

7. Complementary and alternative therapies targeted for evaluation by the Office of Complementary and Alternative Medicine (OCAM) include all but
   a. biobehavioral approaches.
   b. nutritional approaches.
   c. cardiovascular medications.
   d. manual healing methods.

8. Meaning can be viewed as
   a. unnecessary for the healthy function of individuals.
   b. not linked to mind modulation.
   c. having an influence on the outcome of illness.
   d. all physical or all mental.

9. The three *best* descriptions of relationship-centered care include all except
   a. patient–practitioner relationships.
   b. community–practitioner relationships.
   c. practitioner–practitioner relationships.
   d. medical records–hospital relationships.

10. Each component in relationship-centered care must address the following areas.
    a. knowledge, values, and skills.
    b. knowledge, values, and meaning.
    c. self-awareness.
    d. skills and self-awareness.

11. In a patient–practitioner relationship,
    a. the practitioner is the leader and tells the patient what is best.

b. the patient makes the decision and informs the practitioner.

c. the practitioner may include information about needed technology.

d. the patient and practitioner actively collaborate as often as needed.

12. In a community–practitioner relationship,
    a. a narrow view of cultural diversity and care exists.
    b. only a few significant relationships are addressed.
    c. harmful elements that block a person's healing are dismissed in healing.
    d. the multiple relationships, beliefs, and meanings are addressed.

13. To address practitioner–practitioner relationships, it is necessary to
    a. begin with a few practitioners interacting at a time.
    b. develop an understanding of the dynamics of groups, teams, and organizations.
    c. limit the number of alternative/complementary practitioners used by a patient.
    d. use only practitioners who follow scientifically proven therapies.

14. Strategies for creating relationship-centered care should include
    a. close autocratic supervision.
    b. competitive assessments of performance.
    c. emphasis on competencies of skills.
    d. mentorship and modeling of holistic behaviors.

15. To disseminate learning strategies for relationship-centered care, nurses
    a. discourage the sharing of personal stories.
    b. use only tested, computer-based programs.
    c. limit the use of support groups.
    d. assist individuals with the use of self-paced learning programs.

 Pause for a moment . . .

❑ *I know that the* background (situation) *is a nurse-based or a client-based situation.*

❑ *I pay attention to the content of the situation in each question.*

Situations 1–4

Situation 1:   You have been invited to be part of a team to draft a proposal to start a Mind/Body Center at the local community hospital. Your assigned task is to work with two other holistic nurse colleagues and to introduce holistic nursing into the hospital.

Question 1:   The American Holistic Nurses' Association (AHNA) is an excellent resource for you and your colleagues. What two basic AHNA documents can guide the introduction of holistic philosophy, holistic foundation, and holistic nursing standards? What optional topics can you introduce to clarify the discipline of holistic philosophy, holistic foundation, and holistic nursing standards?

Answer 1:   Basic Responses   Optional Responses

_____   _____

_____   _____

_____   _____

_____

Situation 2:   You have been asked to give a 1-hour talk to introduce the concepts of holistic nursing to the physicians in this community hospital. The allopathic model is the dominant model currently used.

Question 2:   What basic concepts will you introduce to these physicians so that they understand the discipline of holistic nursing practice? What optional steps can you take to help these physicians better understand the holistic framework and the discipline of holistic nursing practice?

Answer 2:   Basic Responses   Optional Responses

_____   _____
_____   _____
_____   _____

Situation 3:   The AHNA Description of Holistic Nursing and the AHNA Standards of Holistic Nursing Practice have been introduced to this community hospital. The nursing administration and the nursing staff have accepted the concepts that these documents address. You and your planning committee colleagues are now ready to introduce holistic caring–healing modalities for clinical practice to the community hospital nurses and the community hospital home health care nurses.

Question 3:   What are some basic steps to begin the teaching of these caring–healing modalities? What are some optional steps?

Answer 3:   Basic Responses   Optional Responses

_____   _____
_____   _____
_____   _____

Situation 4:   It is now 1 year since holistic nursing has been introduced into this community hospital. The nurses have begun to integrate caring–healing modalities into their clinical practices and personal lives. Several nurses have told you about nurse–patient healing interactions, as well as some aspects of their own personal healing journey. You recognize that a major part of holistic nursing practice is the nurse's self-care and the sharing of stories that illustrate exemplars of caring–healing nursing practice.

Question 4:   What basic steps can further advance the practice of holistic nursing in this hospital? What are some optional steps for greater implementation of relationship-centered care?

Answer 4:   Basic Responses   Optional Responses

_____   _____
_____   _____
_____   _____

CHAPTER 2—TRANSPERSONAL HUMAN CARING AND HEALING

 Pause for a moment . . .

❑ *I recognize that the question (stem) poses the problem to be solved.*

❑ *I know that the stem may be written as a direct question, What would you do first?, or an incomplete sentence, such as The nurse should. . . .*

Test Questions 1–15

1. The term *transpersonal* may mean:
   a. that which transcends the limits and boundaries of the individual ego.
   b. an experience of interconnectedness between two people.
   c. acknowledgment of something greater than the individual and personal.
   d. all of the above.

2. Transpersonal human caring
   a. is first and foremost a process of relationship.
   b. is a set of intervention strategies anyone can use.
   c. requires nurses to take more time with patients.
   d. cannot happen if the patient cannot communicate.
3. A "caring occasion" is
   a. an opportunity to celebrate with a patient's family.
   b. a healing encounter between nurse and patient where both are changed.
   c. any interaction between nurses and patients.
   d. the result of the performance of competent nursing care.
4. Healing is
   a. another way of talking about curing.
   b. an outcome of treatment given by the medical staff.
   c. measurable by standard tests and empirical observations.
   d. the emergence of "right relationship" at one or more levels.
5. To be whole means
   a. to be perfectly balanced at all levels—body, mind, and spirit.
   b. to have the use of all parts of the body.
   c. to be cured of all diseases.
   d. none of the above.
6. "Right relationship" in the context of healing
   a. maximizes free energy to do the work of the system.
   b. increases order and coherence in the system.
   c. maximizes freedom for creativity and change.
   d. all of the above.
7. The holistic nurse realizes that
   a. curing and healing are unrelated processes.
   b. curing is required for healing to begin.
   c. healing can occur with or without curing.
   d. once healing has begun, curing will follow.
8. Which of the following most accurately states the holistic nurse's understanding of the healing process?
   a. Healing emerges from within the body-mind-spirit of the patient, but cannot be manipulated or controlled.
   b. Healing is the result of the actions of health care providers.
   c. The outcome of a healing process can be determined at the outset by the patient and/or the health care team.

d. The patient is in control of the healing process, and the health care team must help the patient to achieve his or her goal.
9. Which way of being is usually *not* attributed to the "feminine principle"?
   a. A focus on the process rather than the outcome.
   b. Decisive intervention designed to fix the problem.
   c. An attitude of receptivity.
   d. Allowing space for the unfolding mystery.
10. When the nurse is with a patient, which of the following is most true within a holistic nursing perspective?
    a. The nurse is in the patient's environment.
    b. The nurse becomes the patient's environment.
    c. The nurse remains separate from the patient's environment.
    d. None of the above.
11. The holistic nurse can center and shift his or her consciousness in order to
    a. participate in the creation of a healing environment.
    b. keep herself or himself from experiencing burnout.
    c. facilitate rest and relaxation for the patient.
    d. all of the above.
12. The concept of the nurse as a "wounded healer" suggests that
    a. nurses who are wounded are the best healers.
    b. only nurses who have completed their own healing process can help others to heal.
    c. people who are actively involved in their own healing journey can accompany others on the path.
    d. once healed, the "wounded healer" nurse no longer needs to help others and is free to move into new soul work.
13. In holistic nursing, wholeness means that
    a. people are more than and different from the sum of their parts.
    b. people are body plus mind plus spirit.
    c. the mind can learn to control health, illness, and healing.
    d. when people grow spiritually, they can cure their own diseases.
14. The nurse may use which of the following in creating a healing environment with the patient?
    a. Eyes.
    b. Voice.
    c. Energy field.
    d. All of the above.

15. A true healing health care system will exist when
    a. only natural, nontoxic therapies are used.
    b. both curing medicine and caring/healing modalities can be accessed by all.
    c. nurses are the "gatekeepers" in the managed care system.
    d. all health care providers use complementary or alternative therapies.

Pause for a moment . . .

❑ *I can approach the situation questions as if I were in the situation.*

❑ *I can then think about my basic responses (in any order) and optional responses (in any order) for this situation.*

❑ *I understand that these situation questions assess my broad knowledge and integration of holistic nursing practice and are based on the AHNA Core Curriculum content.*

Situations 1–4

Situation 1: Mr. Smith, a 38-year-old man who has been newly diagnosed with HIV infection, comes to you for help in "winning the battle with HIV."

Question 1: How do you begin to work with him?

Answer 1: Basic Responses   Optional Responses

_____

_____

_____

_____

Situation 2: Ms. Jones, a 41-year-old woman with multiple sclerosis, wants to work with her condition "holistically" but is not sure what that means.

Question 2: How would you work with this client?

Answer 2: Basic Responses   Optional Responses

_____

_____

_____

_____

Situation 3: Ms. Lindsey, a 52-year-old women, has hypertension and reacts badly to medications that have been prescribed. She wants "energy work" to control her hypertension.

Question 3: Where do you begin with her?

Answer 3: Basic Responses   Optional Responses

_____

_____

_____

_____

Situation 4:   Mr. Hines, a 50-year-old man, has just received the results of his latest computed tomography (CT) scan, which shows widespread metastasis of his cancer. His doctors have told him that there is nothing else that the health care system can do.

Question 4:   How do you begin to help him?

Answer 4:   Basic Responses   Optional Responses

_____

_____

_____

_____

CHAPTER 3—THE NURSE AS AN INSTRUMENT OF HEALING

 Pause for a moment . . .

❑ *As I read the question, I understand that I am being asked to identify priorities, the best intervention, or to evaluate outcomes.*
❑ *I read each question carefully. I do not rush.*
❑ *I develop my skills to understand the question being asked.*

Test Questions 1–20

1. Presence is best defined as
   a. the accessing of the supernatural.
   b. a mode of communication.
   c. performing nursing functions for the patient.
   d. a mode of being with another with the wholeness of one's being.

2. A block to being present to another includes
   a. active listening.
   b. busyness.
   c. unconditional love.
   d. intentional touch.

3. To experience a sense of wholeness, a person needs to feel connected and in relationship with all the following except
   a. current affairs.
   b. himself or herself.
   c. creation.
   d. others.

4. One level of healing presence includes
   a. therapeutic presence.
   b. financial presence.
   c. business presence.
   d. technical presence.

5. Outcomes of presence include all but
   a. sense of well-being.
   b. increased vulnerability.
   c. increased coping strength.
   d. an enhanced sense of connection.

6. Characteristics of nurse healers include
   a. ego attachment to outcome.
   b. focus on particular results.
   c. awareness that self-healing is a continued process.
   d. ability to judge what is best for the client at any given moment in time.

7. Patterns of knowing include all of the following except
   a. personal knowledge.
   b. ethical knowledge.
   c. aesthetic knowledge.
   d. organizational knowledge.

8. A major tenet of nursing theories pertinent to healing is
   a. the patient's responsibility to comply with the plan of self-care as designed by the nurse healer.
   b. client dependence on the nurse as healer, teacher, and guide.
   c. placement of the person in an environment in which healing can occur naturally.
   d. focus on one part of the patient's healing at a time.

9. Creating sacred space includes all of the following except
   a. recognizing the nurse as environment.

b. using natural elements to create an environment.

c. unruffling the chaos in an environment.

d. asking the family to leave the room.

10. A whole person assessment includes all of the following except
    a. an assessment of body, mind, and spirit only.
    b. determining the impact of episodes and transitions upon a person's life.
    c. a disease-based history.
    d. genetic predispositions.

11. The essence of disease can be rooted in
    a. patterns of thought and beliefs.
    b. side effects of medication.
    c. the level of education.
    d. the diagnosis of the patient.

12. The nurse facilitates a healing intervention by doing all of the following except
    a. aligning with the highest intention.
    b. determining outcomes in advance.
    c. assessing the client's energy fields.
    d. helping the client to achieve balance at the end of the session.

13. The capacity to hold another is enhanced by
    a. self-care and presence to personal process.
    b. imagining self as a big container.
    c. freedom from fear of hugging.
    d. set boundaries for client interaction.

14. Healing can be defined as
    a. a conscious procedure done to the client.
    b. the consistent return of the integrity and wholeness of the natural state of the individual.
    c. the nurse's power to help the client.
    d. the removal of symptoms.

15. Outcomes of a healing intervention include all but
    a. a sense of peace and integration.
    b. a deeper understanding of the meaning of life's events.
    c. a total remission of the disease process.
    d. pain relief.

16. Co-creating a plan of conscious living includes which one of the following?
    a. Detoxing from alcohol.
    b. Following doctor's orders.
    c. Taking medications as prescribed.
    d. Using a spectrum of interventions to promote a balanced approach to living.

17. Designing a system of support involves
    a. identification of people to help the individual in self-care strategies.
    b. third-party reimbursement.
    c. referral to the family physician.
    d. client dependence on the nurse's plan of care.

18. Nursing theory helps to better define the dynamics of healing through all but the following concepts:
    a. creating environments that support the client's process.
    b. facilitating the client's access to inner wisdom, healing, and guidance.
    c. recognizing that health is consistent with the openness or closure of a system.
    d. designing a plan of care based on physician's orders.

19. System closure would imply
    a. a disease in progress.
    b. the decrease of healthy interchange between an individual and the environment.
    c. wound healing.
    d. a therapeutic way to solve problems.

20. The concept of the wounded healer is important in that
    a. it helps us determine whether or not we are capable of caring for another.
    b. it shows us that we are prone to burnout.
    c. it creates a connection based on the common human experience of suffering.
    d. it demonstrates the reason for a high rate of substance abuse in caregivers.

 Pause for a moment . . .

❑ *I do not read meaning into a question.*

❑ *I understand all the words in the question.*

❑ *I recognize when a word in a question is not familiar, and I try to figure out the meaning based on the context in which it appears in the question.*

Situations 1–5

Situation 1:   Marty J., a four year-old boy, has parents who are verbally abusive. The home environment is violent. Both parents are chain smokers, and Marty is prone to multiple upper respiratory infections and asthmatic symptoms. Marty is considered hyperactive and wets the bed every night. Because of the hyperactivity and the diagnosis of possible attention deficit disorder, the mother has sought out the support of a nurse friend.

Question 1:   What would you do to help Marty?

Answer 1:   Basic Responses   Optional Responses

_____

_____

_____

_____

Situation 2:   Helen K., a 15-year-old girl, is interested in finding a boyfriend. She is a pretty girl with many friends, is a cheerleader, plays piano, is a member of several clubs, and follows a self-imposed regimen of jogging, swimming, and biking. Her mother noticed her looking thinner and found her vomiting after dinner one night. When confronted, Helen said she was getting too fat and was just trying to keep in good shape so that boys would find her attractive.

Question 2:   What would be your focus for intervening with Helen?

Answer 2:   Basic Responses   Optional Responses

_____

_____

_____

_____

Situation 3:   Ms. Raines, a successful, 35-year-old attorney, has been happily married for the past 10 years. Her schedule is very demanding, and she follows a daily program of exercise and nutrition that helps her relax and keep healthy. The couple has been attempting to have children for the past 5 years, with the help of an infertility specialist. Their first GIFT procedure having been unsuccessful, the couple is open to other approaches as they perceive the clock to be ticking away.

Question 3:   What recommendations would you have for the couple?

Answer 3:   Basic Responses   Optional Responses

_____

_____

_____

_____

Situation 4:   Ms. Frankin, a 60-year-old executive, has been recently diagnosed with a localized tumor of the colon. To date, she has enjoyed perfect health and seeks the nurse healer to help guide her through this episode. Ms. Frankin opts for surgery with a plan of healing to follow after recuperation.

Question 4:   What would you encourage in the plan of healing?

Answer 4:   Basic Responses   Optional Responses

_____

_____

_____

_____

Situation 5:   Ms. Neil, a 68-year-old wife and mother of two, has advanced cancer of the liver, ovary, and bones. The family is wealthy and asks the nurse healer to help them find a cure for her cancer from around the world. The nurse healer researches the possibilities and presents the family with options, but in her intimate conversations with Ms. Neil, she discovers that she is spiritually aligned and at peace with death.

Question 5:   What would you recommend to the family?

Answer 5:   Basic Responses   Optional Responses

_____

_____

_____

_____

CONCEPT II—HOLISTIC FOUNDATION

CHAPTER 4—CONCEPTS OF HEALTH-WELLNESS-DISEASE-ILLNESS

 Pause for a moment . . .

❑ *I look for key words in questions because these words give me clues to the correct answer.*
   — These are such words as "except," "not," or "but."
   — Words such as "most," "next," or "first" indicate the order of steps or the priority.

Test Questions 1–20

Match the following terms with the best definition:

1. Engagement
2. Self-responsibility
3. Dialectic
4. Health
5. Wellness
6. Disease
7. Illness

a. integrated, congruent functioning aimed at reaching one's highest potential
b. a subjective experience of suffering and symptoms
c. harmony/unity, a process of becoming, expanding consciousness
d. the process of commitment, involvement, and performance of value-consistent health behavior
e. a relationship in which there is synthesis of subjective and objective perspectives
f. the desire, will, and ability to choose and act on one's own behalf
g. a discrete entity causing specific symptoms or a deviation from a normal state, imbalance

8. Mr. Brown collaborates in his care and willingly chooses value-consistent healthy behaviors. Which of the following terms best describes this behavior?
   a. Noncompliance.
   b. Compliance.
   c. Engagement.
   d. Lack of engagement.

9. Which of the following statements best describes the central idea of the health belief model?
   a. Individual health behaviors are chosen based on past experiences.
   b. Individual perceptions of the seriousness of and personal susceptibility to a disease, moderated by demographic and social factors, and the perceived threat of the disease can predict the likelihood of the individual's taking a preventive health action.
   c. Individual beliefs about the outcomes of prevention and treatment, moderated by the perception of care providers of the seriousness of the disease, indicate individual potential for lack of engagement.

10. Ms. Coombs, a 34-year-old woman, has recently learned that she has breast cancer. She has a strong social support network and a positive attitude. Nurses are most likely to facilitate engagement if they
    a. develop a simple, basic care regimen for Ms. Coombs.
    b. focus on clarifying values and strengthening social networks.
    c. focus on teaching and matching teaching style to coping style and locus of control.
    d. focus on consciousness raising and involvement in community agencies.

11. Mr. Waters, a 65-year-old retiree, has recently lost his wife of 40 years. It seems that most of his family and friends have either died or moved away. He has developed chronic obstructive lung disease. He believes the condition cannot improve and continues to smoke two packs of cigarettes per day as he has for 35 years. The nursing intervention most likely to facilitate engagement is
    a. collaboration with Mr. Waters to develop a simple care regimen.
    b. referrals to several self-help groups.
    c. focus on values clarification.
    d. focus on cognitive strengthening.

12. The stage of change that is characterized by awareness of the need for change, but no commitment to action is termed the
    a. precontemplation stage.
    b. maintenance stage.
    c. contemplation stage.
    d. realization stage.

13. Movement through the stage of change is characterized by
    a. linear progress forward.
    b. a circular pattern of relapse.
    c. a spiral pattern of progress, some relapse, and further progress.

14. Which of the following is true about the integration of change processes and the stages of change?
    a. All of the processes of change can be used in any stage.
    b. For each stage, there are some processes more appropriate than others.

15. Mr. Roberts has had an alcohol problem for about 5 years. He is beginning to realize that this problem is interfering with his work and his relationships, but he is not committed to making a significant change in his behavior. Which of the following change processes might be useful to him?
    a. Counterconditioning.
    b. Stimulus control.
    c. Consciousness raising.
    d. Logotherapy.

16. Which of the following statements is true about the dialectic relationship of health-wellness-disease-illness?
    a. Health and illness are opposite ends of a continuum.
    b. The phenomenon of health-wellness-disease-illness is best understood by breaking it down into its component parts.

    c. This phenomenon has cognitive and affective dimensions through which individuals ascribe meaning and significance to their experience.
    d. A major component of health is wellness, and a major component of illness is disease. These phenomena represent totally different dimensions of human experience.

17. Which of the following statements best characterizes values?
    a. Values are affective subsets of attitudes.
    b. Values have inherent right and wrong properties.
    c. Values are dynamic and motivational because they possess cognitive, affective, and behavioral dimensions.
    d. Values indicate faith in a person, idea, or object.

18. To determine the dominant values of a culture, which of the following questions would be the most useful?
    a. What are the traditional beliefs about illness causation?
    b. Who are the traditional healers?
    c. What is the relationship of human beings to nature?
    d. What are the major health practices?

19. Which of the following statements best describes the process of values clarification?
    a. Values clarification is a strategy of discovery that involves choosing, prizing, and acting for the purpose of becoming more authentic and genuine.
    b. Values clarification is somewhat useful, but usually takes too much time to be practical in a clinical setting.
    c. Values clarification increases anxiety in situations involving personal risk.
    d. Values clarification may be helpful in identifying moral conflicts, but not useful in solving these conflicts because it does not change behavior.

20. Which of the following is true regarding workplace wellness programs?
    a. Workplace wellness programs do not reduce health costs to employers.
    b. The most effective workplace wellness programs incorporate worker families and significant others.
    c. Using needs assessment data from successful programs ensures the effectiveness of a new workplace wellness program.

d. Research and program evaluation increase the cost:benefit ratio of workplace wellness programs and are, therefore, not integral to success.

Pause for a moment . . .

❑ *I answer the question before I look at the choices.*
❑ *I then look for the answer that is similar to the one that I generated.*

Situations 1–4

Situation 1:   Mr. Jones, a 45-year-old man, is a new home care client. He is homebound following the open reduction of a spiral fracture of the tibia and fibula. The surgery took place 5 days ago. Because he has a history of deep vein thrombosis, he is on anticoagulant therapy. He lives alone in a two-story house, is used to a fast food diet, and has a sedentary job. For the best wound and bone healing results, you realize that some exercise, good nutrition, and safe mobility are care priorities. You are also aware that Mr. Jones needs a vitamin K–restricted diet. You will be visiting twice each week to draw blood to determine anticoagulant status.

Question 1:   What will you assess in order to determine which strategies will facilitate the engagement process?

Answer 1:   Basic Responses   Optional Responses

Situation 2:   In the course of your home visiting, you notice that Mr. Jones smokes about two packs of cigarettes per day. He tells you that he really has thought about quitting. He mentions that he quit once 5 years ago, but started smoking again during his divorce last year. He states that his company has smoking cessation classes, but he quit "cold turkey." He asks for your advice.

Question 2:   Describe the stage of change Mr. Jones is experiencing.

Answer 2:   Basic Responses   Optional Responses

Situation 3:   In spite of his current disability and lifestyle, Mr. Jones describes himself as healthy. In discussing this, he mentions that he has always been able to work and make a good living. He describes himself as a "self-made man," determined and powerful. He has never had a serious disease. He states, "When I feel good, I'm healthy. Even if I'm laid up, I can still feel OK. The better I feel, the healthier I am." He believes that being healthy is within his control. "I can manage OK even if I can't walk right now." He recognizes the dangers of smoking because his father, who was the picture of health, died at age 56 of lung cancer. Despite his description of himself as healthy, he is worried about the cough that he has developed over the last few months.

Question 3:   Discuss the meaning and significance of health in Mr. Jones' experience of health-wellness-disease-illness.

Answer 3:   Basic Responses   Optional Responses

_____   _____

_____   _____

_____   _____

_____   _____

Situation 4:   You are an occupational health nurse in a large manufacturing company. Your employer has asked you to develop a wellness program for the employees.

Question 4:   What do you need to know to develop an effective program?

Answer 4:   Basic Responses   Optional Responses

_____   _____

_____   _____

_____   _____

_____   _____

Chapter 5—Psychophysiology of Bodymind Healing

 Pause for a moment . . .

❏ *If I do not know an answer, I make a reasonable guess. "Intuition" and "hunches" are often correct answers.*

❏ *I understand that the HNC examination is based on the* **AHNA Core Curriculum.**

Test Questions 1–20

1. Bodymind best refers to
   a. a state of integration among body, mind, and spirit.
   b. the interaction between body and mind.
   c. the effect the body has on the mind.
   d. a combined state of body and mind.

2. Which of the following changes in our understanding of our bodymind system can be attributed to Einstein's theory of relativity?
   a. All bodymind events have an identifiable cause and effect.
   b. Symptoms indicate a breakdown in our bodymind system.
   c. The world and bodyminds are an interconnected dynamic system.
   d. All things and events connect and are relative to the others.

3. The knowledge that our immunity cannot be explained in terms of a single set of rules operating in one world comes from which of the following theories?
   a. Bohr's complementarity.
   b. Prigogine's dissipative structures.
   c. Plank's quantum mechanics.
   d. Heisenberg's uncertainty principle.

4. Which of the following underlies our current understanding of immune functioning?
   a. Novelty in evolution is the result of random mutation and natural selection of the most fit.
   b. Novelty in evolution is akin to creative problem solving in humans.
   c. Evolution is the steady and uniform development of organisms from the simple to the complex.
   d. Organisms exhibit a fundamental self-organizing force that can be explained by physical principles.

5. Which of the following statements best describes the principle underlying bodymind healing?
   a. Interventions are directed to the mind to heal the body and the spirit.
   b. Physical and psychologic factors influence the body and mind equally.
   c. The direction of causality and mechanisms of the associations of the mind and body are not known.

d. The body is under the direction of the mind and the spirit.

6. Which of the following best describes how perceptions are processed by our brains?
   a. Perceptions registered in the cerebral cortex are first processed along a complex series of cortical pathways that are connected with the affect system by way of the bidirectional corticolimbic system. The perceptions are stored in both areas of the brain.
   b. Perceptions are stored in the cerebral cortex, where they acquire meaning, and are later processed along the corticolimbic system, where they are stored and may be recalled in the presence of similar stimuli.
   c. Perceptions are first processed in the limbic system where they acquire meaning and attach emotion. They are then sent to the cerebral cortex where they are stored and available for recall in the presence of new stimuli.
   d. Perceptions are simultaneously processed in the anterior frontal lobe of the cerebral cortex and the hypothalamic area of the midbrain. Images are stored in the anterior frontal lobe, and the associated emotions are stored in the hypothalamus. New stimuli will release the image and the stimuli instantaneously.

7. Self-regulation theory is based on which of the following principles?
   a. Imagery patterns become blueprints that can be reinforced or reframed with focused attention into patterns that may modulate positive changes at the biochemical levels within cells.
   b. Imagery patterns can be used to create new blueprints that can be used to retrieve stored information and their associated emotional and biochemical responses.
   c. Imagery patterns generate biochemical responses that can be modified with concentration through a cybernetic feedback loop and, thus, effect positive healing outcomes.
   d. Imagery patterns can be modified by helping a client gain access to the raw material of inner memories and re-experience the attached emotion.

8. Which of the following interventions effectively modulates ultradian stress syndrome?
   a. Following a regular pattern of 120 minutes of activity alternated with 30 minutes of rest.
   b. Following a regular schedule that allows for a 20-minute nap in the morning and afternoon.
   c. Integrating the ultradian healing response in your schedule throughout the day.

d. Following a schedule that synchronizes your infradian rhythms with your ultradian and circadian rhythms.

9. The therapeutic benefit of holistic nursing interventions such as imagery, touch, and relaxation with patients who are experiencing chronic pain may be best explained as follows:
   a. They simply distract from the pain.
   b. They bring about changes in one part of the system, which leads to changes in the whole system.
   c. They work primarily on the cortico-limbic-thalamic system.
   d. They basically exert a placebo effect.

10. The peripheral nervous system is divided into the somatic and autonomic nervous systems. Identify which secrete acetylcholine at the synapse.
    a. The somatic and the parasympathetic nervous systems.
    b. Both branches of the autonomic nervous system.
    c. The parasympathetic branch of the autonomic nervous system.
    d. All nerves originating in the brain.

11. From the following, choose the correct sentence:
    a. The sympathetic nervous system secretes acetylcholine at the pre- and postganglionic synapses.
    b. The parasympathetic nervous system secretes epinephrine at the postganglionic synapses.
    c. Stimulation of the sympathetic nervous system aids digestion by increasing motility.
    d. The enteric nervous system connects the gastrointestinal tract with the central and autonomic nervous systems.

12. Psychophysiology explains how thinking and feeling influence the body. A lesion in which of the following would interfere with one's ability to process feelings?
    a. Parasympathetic or sympathetic nervous system.
    b. Limbic structures or motor fibers of the somatic nervous system.
    c. Prefrontal cortical region or hypothalamus.
    d. Enteric intrinsic nerve plexus or limbic structures.

13. Identify the gut-brain neuropeptides.
    a. Substance P and somatostatin.
    b. Somatostatin and cholecystokinin.
    c. Cholecystokinin and growth hormone.
    d. Substance P and cholecystokinin.

14. Your patient has a low sodium level, a high potassium level, and low blood pressure. Identify

the source and name of the hormone secreted to return the body to dynamic equilibrium.

   a. The adrenal cortex mineralocorticoid named hydrocortisone.

   b. The adrenal medulla mineralocorticoid named aldosterone.

   c. The adrenal cortex glucocorticoid named hydrocortisone.

   d. The adrenal medulla glucocorticoid named aldosterone.

15. Which axis is responsible for the secretion of epinephrine during times of stress?

   a. The sympathetic-adrenal-medulla axis.

   b. The hypothalamus-pituitary-adrenal axis.

   c. The sympathetic-adrenal-cortex axis.

   d. The cortico-hypothalamus-adrenal-cortex axis.

16. Identify the statement that best illustrates the influence of the psychophysiologic state.

   a. "A bone marrow biopsy is a routine part of treatment."

   b. "Bone marrow biopsies are done to evaluate treatment."

   c. "I do not think that I can bear to have another bone marrow biopsy."

   d. "The bone marrow biopsy will be done in the morning at the doctor's office."

17. The gate control theory of pain supports which of the following statements?

   a. Past pain experiences, plus interpretation of the meaning of the pain, determine whether the gate is open or closed.

   b. Most people experience the same amount of pain with the same type and severity of injury.

   c. Whether the gate is open or closed is dependent solely on the type of messages sent to the substantia gelatinosa.

   d. Serotonin, histamine, and bradykinin, released when there is tissue damage, determine the interpretation of the injury and open or close the gates.

18. Patients who are experiencing stressful and painful events have difficulty learning. The best concept to explain this statement is

   a. Psychophysiology.

   b. State-dependent memory.

   c. Psychoneuroimmunology.

   d. Mind modulation.

19. What serum changes can be expected in persons experiencing a stress situation?

   a. High levels of fatty acids and glucose.

   b. Low levels of protein with muscle buildup.

   c. High levels of albumin and enhanced tissue healing.

   d. Low blood pressure, heart rate, and respiratory rate.

20. Your patient asks if his illness is caused by stress. Your best answer is

   a. "Yes. Your illness is caused by stress."

   b. "No. Stress has no effect on diagnosis or course of illness."

   c. "Although the research is inconclusive, there is evidence that high levels of stress may have an effect."

   d. "What makes you ask such a question?"

 Pause for a moment . . .

❑ *I can imagine that today is the day of the HNC examination.*

❑ *I am arriving for the HNC examination physically and mentally prepared.*

❑ *I am proud of my accomplishments!*

Situations 1–4

Situation 1: Mr. Judge, a 46-year-old computer programmer, was told by his doctor that he has "high blood pressure" and needs to learn how to relax. He asks for your help because he feels that he cannot relax and still keep his job.

Question 1: How can you help Mr. Judge lower his blood pressure while meeting the demands of his job?

Answer 1: Basic Responses   Optional Responses

Situation 2:   Ms. Parris, a 30-year-old woman, is having difficulty sleeping. As a result, she has been feeling tired for the past 3 months. She realizes that her daily living patterns are contributing to her difficulties.

Question 2:   How can you help Ms. Parris get more restful sleep?

Answer 2:   Basic Responses   Optional Responses

_____

_____

_____

_____

Situation 3:   Ms. Jones, a 65-year-old woman, is complaining that her pain medication is not working. She is demanding large amounts of pain medication at frequent intervals. She has just learned that her cancer is no longer in remission.

Question 3:   What interventions are appropriate to help her with her pain?

Answer 3:   Basic Responses   Optional Responses

_____

_____

_____

_____

Situation 4:   Jimmy J., a 16-year-old automobile accident victim, is in traction with a broken, infected right leg that is not improving in spite of high doses of powerful antibiotics. The physician has just informed Jimmy's parents that Jimmy may lose his leg. When you see Jimmy, he is angry and crying with pain.

Question 4:   How can you help Jimmy with his problem?

Answer 4:   Basic Responses   Optional Responses

_____

_____

_____

_____

CHAPTER 6—SPIRITUALITY AND HEALING

 Pause for a moment . . .

❑ *I am eating nourishing food and will do so before the HNC examination. Complex carbohydrate foods will provide me with the most energy.*

❑ *I am avoiding excess use of caffeine or sugar right now and will continue this before the HNC examination.*

❑ *I am relaxed and at ease and will arrive at the HNC examination in this same relaxed state.*

Test Questions 1–14

1. Which of the following does not harmonize with a description of spirituality?
   a. Spirituality permeates all of life.
   b. Spirituality is an organized system of beliefs and practices.
   c. Spirituality is an interconnectedness with the Absolute, others, nature.
   d. Spirituality shapes and gives meaning to life.
2. Which of the following statements may provide openers for exploring a person's spirituality?

1. "My injury has kept me from gardening this year."
2. "My daughter comes to visit every day."
3. "I'm not able to go to church like I used to."
4. "I feel most at peace when I am outside."
    a. 2, 3, 4
    b. 3 only
    c. 1, 2, 3, 4
    d. 1, 2, 4

3. All of the following are true about forgiveness, except that
    a. it is a conscious choice.
    b. it is a deep human hunger and need.
    c. there may be difficulties in forgiving others.
    d. it is generally easy to forgive oneself.

4. Your patient, who is scheduled for surgery tomorrow, asks you out of the blue to stay and pray with her. The most appropriate nursing response to her request would be to
    a. ask her how she usually prays.
    b. tell her that you will call the chaplain for her.
    c. begin to pray aloud that she will trust in the Lord and be healed.
    d. tell her that you know she is afraid, but that everything will be OK.

5. Which of the following is the true statement?
    a. All people express spirituality in the same way.
    b. Belief in God is fundamental to spirituality.
    c. Spirituality is related to meaning and a source of purpose, strength, and guidance.
    d. A person who is not religious is not spiritual.

6. In assessing spirituality, which of the following questions would be most appropriate?
    a. What gives your life meaning?
    b. What is your religious preference?
    c. Do you want the chaplain to visit?
    d. Can we arrange for you to attend services in the chapel?

7. When you enter your patient's hospital room to give him morning care, you notice that he is standing at the east-facing window with his hands above his head, chanting something in a language you do not understand. You should
    a. call the doctor and say that the patient is acting strange and may need a psychiatric consult.
    b. ask him to get back in bed so you can proceed with his care.
    c. interrupt and ask him what he is doing.
    d. note that he is not in distress and quietly leave and return later to give morning care.

8. When you are talking to the patient later that day, what would be the least appropriate approach to exploring his behavior?
    a. Tell him you noticed that he was facing the east window this morning and wondered if he could tell you about what he was doing.
    b. Assume that he was praying and not say anything about it so as not to embarrass him.
    c. Ask him about how and when he prays.
    d. Ask him how he expresses his spirituality and if there are things you can do to help him have the time and space he needs.

9. Which of the following is true regarding spiritual care?
    a. It is important to provide answers to the questions clients raise.
    b. It is important to call a minister, priest, rabbi, or the hospital chaplain as soon as persons raise spiritual concerns.
    c. It is important to know one's own spiritual perspective and wellness.
    d. It is important to encourage clients to pray.

10. Which of the following statements are true about the role of religious faith?
    a. Religious faith can affect the course and outcome of illness.
    b. There is a role for prayer in the course of illness.
    c. Faith helps in dealing with death.
    d. All of the above.
    e. None of the above.

11. To understand others' spirituality, it is more important to
    a. read up on their religion or faith expression.
    b. listen to their story.
    c. ascertain who is significant to them and what is of value to them at the present time.
    d. a and b.
    e. b and c.

12. Which is the most true regarding the place of story in spiritual care?
    a. Stories are useful only in working with children or the elderly.
    b. The nurse should try to clarify all the details of the person's story.
    c. Stories provide understandings not revealed in traditional history taking.
    d. The nurse's goal is to finish the patient's story.

13. Mr. Ricardo lists "atheist" on his information form. The nurse
    a. should avoid any comments or questions concerning spirituality.

b. should ask him what he means by "atheist."

c. should recognize him as a spiritual being and listen for spiritual issues he may express.

d. should tell him that there are no such things as atheists and ask him what he really believes.

14. Which of the following are involved in being present with another?

1. Intentionality.
2. Active listening.
3. A desire to listen and to hear.
4. An ability to center and focus.
   a. 1, 2, 3, 4
   b. 1, 2, 4

c. 1, 3, 4
d. 2, 3, 4

 Pause for a moment . . .

❑ *I will be physically rested by getting a good night's sleep before the HNC examination.*

❑ *I am going to monitor my responsibilities the week of the HNC examination so that I arrive rested and free of worry.*

Situations 1–4

Situation 1:   Ms. George, a 72-year-old grandmother, has been hospitalized with complications of a fractured hip for the past month. For the past few days, she has seemed depressed and frequently questions aloud if she will ever see her grandchildren (who live out of state) again. She has also expressed worry about her cat, wondering if anyone has been taking care of it.

Question 1:   How can you explore and address the spiritual concerns evident here?

Answer 1:   Basic Responses   Optional Responses

_____

_____

_____

_____

Situation 2:   Ms. Jones, a 29-year-old mother of four, comes for a routine examination and mentions that she feels frazzled, stays busy all the time, and never has any time for herself. She loves her kids, but would sometimes like them all to go away; then she feels guilty for thinking that. She notes that the only time she gets to herself is at church when they are in the children's program.

Question 2:   How can you help Ms. Jones further explore her spiritual concerns?

Answer 2:   Basic Responses   Optional Responses

_____

_____

_____

_____

Situation 3:   Mr. Sosa, a 33-year-old man, is scheduled for surgical removal of a pituitary tumor. During your routine check of his vital signs, he tells you that he is not religious and does not know if he remembers how to pray, but this has got him worried. Although he thinks everything will be OK, he asks that you pray for him if you believe in God. He adds that he wishes that he had not had an argument with his brother before entering the hospital.

Question 3:   How do you respond to Mr. Sosa?

Answer 3:   Basic Responses   Optional Responses

_____

_____

_____

_____

Situation 4:   Joe P., a 15-year-old boy, is in serious condition in the intensive care unit after a motorcycle accident. His father said that he will stay the night in the room because Joe needs him; then he began to put crystals and other objects around the room and to hang some pouches and feathers over the bed. It is after visiting hours.

Question 4:   How do you deal with this situation?

Answer 4:   Basic Responses   Optional Responses

_____

_____

_____

_____

CHAPTER 7—ENERGETIC HEALING

 Pause for a moment . . .

❑ *I have plenty of time to finish the HNC examination.*
❑ *If I lose my concentration, I will use my relaxation, deep breathing, imagery, affirmations, positive self-talk, and distraction.*

Test Questions 1–10

1. Like an electromagnet, the human being
   a. has parallel circuits and boosters.
   b. is surrounded by a field of varying densities.
   c. analyzes frequencies in an environment.
   d. transmits information.
2. A Fourier analyzer detects
   a. a specific frequency of energy.
   b. the amperage of direct current.
   c. a magnetic field.
   d. a wave, separating it into its frequencies.
3. Acupuncture points act like
   a. a flow of alternating current.
   b. electrical boosters.
   c. parallel electrical lines.
   d. off and on switches.

4. "Energetic healing" implies that
   a. healing occurs through electrical energy.
   b. healing occurs through the use of the electromagnetic and other energy.
   c. healing energizes a person.
   d. exercise energizes a person and leads to healing.
5. A person's aura is most like
   a. a smoke screen.
   b. a halo such as is seen in paintings of Jesus.
   c. a person's charisma.
   d. an information-filled electromagnetic field.
6. Quantum physics suggests that
   a. events happen in definable space at a specific time.
   b. matter is solid.
   c. nature is a complicated set of structures.
   d. dynamic energy packets are the fundamental aspect of the universe.
7. What is the content of the three levels of the unconscious in Assagioli's psychosynthesis model of the dimensions of the psyche?
   a. Drives, ego, conscience.
   b. Survival, love and belonging, achievement.
   c. Immature self, on-call skills, aspirations.
   d. Self, family, community.

8. If the lowest level of the unconscious as described by Assagioli's psychosynthesis model were to observe a quantum waveform and collapse it into an actuality, what might that actuality look like?
   a. Anger at childhood experiences.
   b. Ability to cook a meal.
   c. Concern for the environment.
   d. Love for a child.

9. The quantum theory of consciousness-created reality proposes that
   a. a photograph will cause particles to collapse into actualities from quantum waveforms.
   b. consciousness is the primary element.
   c. events are objective, but are interpreted differently by each person.
   d. we make our own beds so we have to lie in them.

10. If you had a wound on your chest, which one of the following would not be an appropriate self-healing measure?
    a. Wear green.
    b. Listen to music in the key of F.
    c. Touch the wound.
    d. Keep your emotions to yourself.

Pause for a moment . . .

❏ *I can concentrate during my studying so that I can concentrate during the HNC examination.*
❏ *I focus while I study, and I will focus during the HNC examination.*
❏ *I will finish at my own pace even when others finish before me.*

Situations 1–4

Situation 1:   You are healthy but want to be healthier.

Question 1:   Using the Energetic Healing Modalities Model, describe one action that you can take from each circle.

Answer 1:   Basic Responses   Optional Responses

_____

_____

_____

_____

Situation 2:   You have clients who scorn holistic approaches.

Question 2:   How can you treat them holistically without violating either your principles or theirs?

Answer 2:   Basic Responses   Optional Responses

_____

_____

_____

Situation 3:   You are in charge of all things on your unit in a hospital.

Question 3:   How can you change the environment to assist the patients in their efforts to maximize their own healing?

Answer 3:   Basic Responses   Optional Responses

_____

_____

_____

_____

Situation 4:   Your nursing colleagues are at war with each other. Each complains that the others are not finishing their work, are not communicating, etc.

Question 4:   How can you use the Energetic Healing Modalities model to help your colleagues heal?

Answer 4:   Basic Responses   Optional Responses

_____

_____

_____

_____

Concept III—Holistic Ethics

Chapter 8—Holistic Ethics

 Pause for a moment . . .

❑ *I have plenty of time to finish the HNC examination.*
❑ *If I lose my concentration, I will use my relaxation, deep breathing, imagery, affirmations, positive self-talk, and distraction.*

Test Questions 1–10

1. In general, ethics is concerned with
   a. judgments of approval or disapproval.
   b. rightness or wrongness.
   c. disciplined reflection on the moral choices that people make.
   d. all of the above.
2. Within the framework of holistic ethics, acts are not performed for the sake of law, precedent, or social norms, but rather from the desire to
   a. satisfy the needs of the whole.
   b. behave in a caring way.
   c. do good freely in order to witness, identify, and contribute to unity.
   d. pave the way for others as a role model of ethical decision making.
3. Holistic ethics provides guidelines for
   a. behaviors befitting healers.
   b. a caring nursing-based practice.
   c. others who use their presence to heal.
   d. the development of spirit in the healer.

4. Awareness of ethical issues is accelerating because of
   a. case management and managed care.
   b. advances in technology and scarcity of resources.
   c. redesign of job descriptions and reengineering of the workplace.
   d. increased interest in cognitive issues on the part of the profession of nursing.
5. The development of holistic ethics comes from a philosophy that couples
   a. the two traditional forms of ethics: deontologic and teleologic.
   b. the evolving concepts of holism and ethics.
   c. religion and spirituality.
   d. meaning and consciousness.
6. The underlying principle in a holistic ethical view is being, and its corollary is
   a. consciousness.
   b. action.
   c. spirituality.
   d. precedent.
7. In order to make ethical decisions appropriately, it is necessary to
   a. operate from a set of principles.
   b. have some sort of analytic method to sort out and classify the elements of the problem.
   c. work within a framework of being and consciousness.
   d. do all of the above.
8. The Patient Self-Determination Act requires that all individuals receiving medical care

a. also receive written information about their right to accept or refuse care.
b. have a chaplain present to witness their signature.
c. also be informed about the option of euthanasia.
d. understand the new restrictions about length of stay.

9. Ethically knowledgeable nurses can
a. make decisions for their patients or clients.
b. direct the physician in the proper way to deliver care.
c. lobby for experimental treatments.
d. ask to participate in their agency's ethics committees.

10. Nurses have been politically active in ethical issues that concern nursing since

a. the Health Care Reform Act of 1990.
b. the inception of nursing.
c. becoming involved in public health issues during the Industrial Revolution.
d. the formation of institutional ethics committees in the 1980s.

 Pause for a moment . . .

❑ *I can concentrate during my studying so that I can concentrate during the HNC examination.*
❑ *I focus while I study, and I will focus during the HNC examination.*
❑ *I will finish at my own pace even when others finish before me.*

Situations 1–3

Situation 1: Don H., an 8-year-old boy, was committed to a psychiatric hospital by his stepfather after his mother died (the boy's father was unable to be reached). Don had been hospitalized in the past for psychiatric disorders; this time the diagnosis was schizophrenia. There were standing orders to restrain him and place him in solitary confinement if his behavior was uncontrollable. When his admitting sedation wore off, Don became hostile, screaming, and angry, voicing dismay that he had been abandoned. As ordered, he was placed in an empty, locked room for a 2-hour "cooling off" period. After repeated periods of confinement over a period of time, his condition worsened. Eventually, Don was transferred to a state mental hospital for permanent institutionalization.

Question 1: (Basic) Identify some of the ethical considerations in this case. (Optional) What are some of the ethical issues that may be discussed regarding this situation?

Answer 1: Basic Responses   Optional Responses

_____

_____

_____

Situation 2: Ms. Smith, an 88-year-old grandmother, suffered an acute myocardial infarction, was admitted to the hospital, and went into respiratory and cardiac arrest the day after admission. She was resuscitated and placed on a respirator, but after 3 days of no response, she was taken off the respirator and pronounced dead.

Question 2: (Basic) Identify some of the ethical considerations in this case. (Optional) What are some of the ethical issues that may be discussed regarding this situation?

Answer 2: Basic Responses   Optional Responses

_____

_____

_____

Situation 3:   Tom A. was born prematurely with multiple anomalies. His young mother was unprepared to deal with the decisions that suddenly faced her. During the team conference, the mother was told that the baby's condition was grave, that immediate surgical intervention might save the child's life, but that the child would most likely be severely retarded. The mother decided not to sign the consent and opted for palliative care only. After 4 days, however, the mother changed her mind and called for life support measures and surgery. Following major surgery, Tom was transferred to an institution for the rest of his life.

Question 3:   (Basic) Identify some of the ethical considerations in this case. (Optional) What are some of the ethical issues that may be discussed regarding this situation?

Answer 3:   Basic Responses   Optional Responses

_____

_____

_____

_____

CONCEPT IV—HOLISTIC NURSING THEORIES

CHAPTER 9—NURSING THEORIES

 Pause for a moment . . .

❑ *I know my strongest test-taking skills.*
❑ *My effective test-taking skills will contribute to my HNC examination success.*

Test Questions 1–13

1. A theory is
   a. a proven set of facts.
   b. a set of concepts.
   c. a concrete description of reality.
   d. a framework for interpreting the world.
2. Phenomena of concern to nursing include
   a. person, health, nursing.
   b. concepts of care and cure.
   c. relationships between internal and external environments.
   d. health, illness, and treatment.
3. Use of nursing theory in practice
   a. guides the nurse in technical skills.
   b. creates presence.
   c. facilitates communication between nurses and other health care professionals.
   d. encourages nurses to reflect on their work.

4. Theories develop over time. Which of the following is true for a theory developed to the level of explanation?
   a. A nurse can use concepts of the theory to predict patient outcomes.
   b. A nurse can use concepts of the theory to prescribe specific nursing interventions.
   c. A nurse can use the theory to understand client behaviors.
   d. A nurse can use the theory to promote cost containments.
5. Nursing diagnoses can be used with theory by
   a. rewriting diagnoses in theory language.
   b. writing the diagnoses to reflect the theory used in the etiology part of the diagnostic statements.
   c. researching and validating the theory concepts.
   d. establishing the nursing interventions needed for best client outcomes.
6. According to Nightingale, health is achieved by
   a. the healing powers of nature.
   b. the nursing treatments given.
   c. the herbs and medications taken.
   d. the presence of another.
7. A young mother in active labor is having her first baby. The pregnancy has been uncompli-

cated, and she is looking forward to becoming a mother with great delight. According to Roy's theory, the labor is considered
   a. a focal stimuli.
   b. a contextual stimuli.
   c. a residual stimuli.
   d. an adaptation response.
8. In the Modeling and Role-Modeling Theory, modeling a client's world means
   a. drawing a picture of the client's environment.
   b. behaving in such a way that the client can imitate your behaviors.
   c. assessing the client's relationships.
   d. understanding the world from the client's perspective.
9. Watson and Leininger both believe that caring is the essence of nursing. From the perspective of these theories, caring is
   a. a significant human-to-human experience.
   b. the process of giving nursing care.
   c. the exchange between the nurse and client energy fields.
   d. a subjective state.
10. To describe the person as a unified whole means that
   a. the person has component parts that can be understood in the context of the whole.
   b. the person has several dimensions.
   c. the person is complete after going through stages of development.
   d. the person is seen as a complete, whole being.

11. According to Rogers, persons evolve
   a. through various stages of psychosocial development.
   b. in one direction only, through space and time.
   c. in several directions over time.
   d. according to their own genetic drive.
12. According to Newman, disease is
   a. an indication of pathology needing treatment.
   b. a reflection of the whole.
   c. an imbalance.
   d. an adaptation response.
13. Parse emphasizes the nurse's role as a
   a. guide.
   b. caretaker.
   c. professional.
   d. primary care provider.

 Pause for a moment . . .

❑ *I am using my distraction techniques.*
   — *Any time that worry or fear comes into my mind, I will let go of the anxiety.*
   — *If a thought of failure comes to my mind . . . I take a deep breath, and with the next exhalation, I let the worry flow out.*
❑ *I will successfully pass the HNC examination.*

Situation 1

Situation 1: Describe a client situation and your nursing care, based on the nursing theory of your choice.

Question 1: Explain how your assessment of the client situation is grounded in a specific theory, and how your interventions were guided by your choice of theory.

Answer 1: Basic Responses   Optional Responses

_____   _____

_____   _____

_____   _____

_____   _____

Concept V—Holistic Nursing and Related Research

Chapter 10—Holistic Nursing and Related Research

Pause for a moment . . .

❏ *My affirmations and positive self-talk are*
—*I am prepared for the HNC examination.*
—*I can pass the HNC examination with flying colors.*
—*I can see HNC after my name.*
—*I can see the certification for holistic nursing hanging in my office.*
❏ *I am so proud that I set this goal and made this commitment to take the HNC examination.*

Test Questions 1–8

1. An example of quantitative research is
   a. correlational research.
   b. phenomenologic research.
   c. ethnographic research.
   d. philosophic research.
2. An example of qualitative research is
   a. descriptive research.
   b. grounded theory research.
   c. quasi-experimental research.
   d. experimental research.
3. Experimental research methods evaluate
   a. the response of the whole human being to variables.
   b. life experiences and their meanings.
   c. cause-and-effect interactions between variables.
   d. all of the above.
4. Grounded theory research is used to
   a. study a culture and the people in the culture.
   b. analyze meanings, identify values and ethics, and study the nature of knowledge.
   c. uncover what problems exist in a social situation and how the persons involved handle them.
   d. explain how people communicate with one another and how symbolic meanings in society develop.
5. When studying the effects of holistic interventions on the bodymind, what type of research should be used?

a. Qualitative research methods.
b. Quantitative research methods.
c. The biomedical scientific process.
d. Both qualitative and quantitative research methods.
6. The placebo response occurs in what percentage of people?
   a. 10 to 25 percent.
   b. 35 to 70 percent.
   c. 25 to 30 percent.
   d. 60 to 100 percent.
7. The Office of Alternative Medicine at the National Institutes of Health was established to
   a. develop educational curricula on alternative therapies for nursing and medical schools across the United States.
   b. certify legitimate practitioners of alternative therapies.
   c. endorse books and products related to alternative therapies.
   d. support investigations evaluating the effects of alternative healing practices.
8. Alternative therapies are used
   a. instead of traditional medical therapies.
   b. in most hospital institutions.
   c. to control the mind.
   d. in a complementary approach with conventional medical practices.

Pause for a moment . . .

❏ *I am practicing my successful test-taking strategies prior to the HNC examination so that I can remember to use them during the HNC examination.*
❏ *Relaxation and deep breathing exercises decrease my anxiety and tension.*
❏ *Imagery rehearsal of preparing for, seeing myself in the HNC examination environment, feeling relaxed and confident, and successfully passing the HNC examination is exciting.*

Situations 1–2

Situation 1: As a radiology nurse, you notice that many magnetic resonance imaging (MRI) procedures have been canceled recently related to patients' anxiety while they are in the machine. You believe that a music therapy program in the radiology department may reduce the number of canceled MRIs.

Question 1: How can you evaluate the effectiveness of a music therapy program in reducing the number of canceled MRI procedures?

Answer 1: Basic Responses   Optional Responses

_____

_____

_____

_____

Situation 2: As a coronary care nurse, you believe that a music therapy program may help in the psycho-physiologic recovery of patients admitted to your coronary care unit (CCU) with acute myocardial infarction (AMI).

Question 2: How can you determine the effectiveness of a music therapy program in the CCU for AMI patients?

Answer 2: Basic Responses   Optional Responses

_____

_____

_____

_____

CONCEPT VI—HOLISTIC NURSING PROCESS

CHAPTER 11—HOLISTIC NURSING PROCESS

 Pause for a moment . . .

❑ *I am using my distraction techniques.*

— *Any time that worry or fear comes into my mind, I will let go of the anxiety.*

— *If a thought of failure comes to my mind . . . I take a deep breath, and with the next exhalation I let the worry flow out.*

❑ *I will successfully pass the HNC examination.*

Test Questions 1–14

1. The idea of a nursing process composed of distinct steps was first mentioned by
   a. Krieger in 1972.
   b. Kreuter in 1957.
   c. Nightingale in 1845.
   d. Peplau in 1952.
2. The essence of the nursing process as defined in the holistic nursing standard of care is
   a. using primarily holistic nursing interventions, such as therapeutic touch, herbal remedies, and humor.

b. the client's experiencing the presence of the nurse as a shared humanness.

c. making certain the client is following all the recommended practices for nutrition, exercise, and stress reduction.

d. carrying out all physician orders exactly as prescribed.

3. Nurses should choose a theoretical model for their practice that is

a. realistic, useful, consistent with personal religious preferences.

b. realistic, abstract, consistent with professional values and philosophy.

c. idealistic, useful, consistent with professional values and philosophy.

d. realistic, useful, consistent with professional values and philosophy.

4. The ethical pattern of knowing used in the nurse–client interaction is focused on

a. objective information measurable by the senses.

b. intuitive perception of meaning.

c. sense of form, structure, and creativity.

d. underlying concept of integral wholeness of all people and nature.

5. The primary role of the client in the assessment aspect of the nursing process is to

a. participate actively in the process.

b. answer the nurse's questions concisely.

c. avoid expressing personal perceptions of health care.

d. refrain from offering unsolicited information.

6. Some of the human response patterns identified as forming the foundation for nursing diagnoses are

a. exchanging, valuing, choosing, knowing.

b. exchanging, valuing, choosing, eliminating.

c. metabolizing, valuing, choosing, knowing.

d. valuing, choosing, exchanging, protecting.

7. An actual nursing diagnosis is defined as

a. a human response that may develop in a vulnerable client.

b. a description of an individual's existing health concerns.

c. a human response that has a potential for enhancement.

d. an interpretation of medical diagnoses from a nursing perspective.

8. In using personal knowledge in the outcome phase of the nursing process, the nurse

a. intuits the client's degree of enthusiasm for possible outcomes.

b. chooses outcomes that are personally appealing to the client.

c. uses scientific principles to determine reasonable outcomes.

d. decides what outcomes are in the best interest of the client.

9. The nurse impedes creation of appropriate client outcomes by

a. discussing possible ways to achieve desired outcomes with the client.

b. helping the client to identify concrete milestones for observing desired changes.

c. encouraging the client's expression of life hopes and dreams.

d. making final decisions about the desired outcome.

10. The knowledge base used by the nurse in advocating for the client's desired quality of life is the

a. scientific.

b. ethical.

c. esthetic.

d. personal.

11. Finding nursing interventions that will enhance outcome achievement involves helping the client

a. ask the physician which ones are best.

b. ask significant others to make the decision.

c. state values, beliefs, and resources affecting selection of interventions.

d. choose the intervention practiced by the nurse.

12. Which of the four patterns of knowing is the nurse using when responding reflectively to the client's reaction to interventions?

a. Scientific.

b. Ethical.

c. Esthetic.

d. Personal.

13. One aspect of the nurse's role in the implementation phase of the holistic nursing process involves

a. controlling all elements of the intervention.

b. focusing attention on procedural steps.

c. giving decision-making power to the client.

d. avoiding being distracted by client feedback.

14. To apply the scientific pattern of knowing in the evaluation step of the nursing process, the nurse

a. follows intuitive insights into the client's experience.

b. observes and reflects changes in patterns to the client.

c. bases conclusions on client perceptions.

d. looks for valid indicators of health enhancement.

Pause for a moment . . .

❑ *My special words, a prayer, or a phrase to bring me into the present moment are* _____.
❑ *As I repeat my special words, prayer, or phrase silently to myself for a few minutes, I feel* _____.
❑ *I combine these with my rhythmic, relaxed breathing and relaxation.*
❑ *I repeat this 10 times to deepen being in this present moment.*
❑ *Then I return to my important studying.*

Situations 1–4

Situation 1:   Mr. Brown, a 79-year-old retired office worker, comes to the Holistic Nursing Center because, he says, "at this time in my life I want to know how I am with God." He not only attends church services, but also reads and studies scriptures daily. Mr. Brown has regular medical care for diabetes mellitus of 45 years' duration and gastroesophageal reflux; he also describes difficulty with sleeping. Mr. Brown says he has come to the Center because he believes "in your kind of healing work."

Question 1:   What would be your focus and actions in proceeding with nursing assessment?

Answer 1:   Basic Responses   Optional Responses

_____

_____

_____

_____

Situation 2:   Ms. Sullivan is a 41-year-old unemployed former court reporter who has been on the adult psychiatric unit for 2 days for the treatment of cocaine withdrawal. She and her 15-year-old daughter reside with her mother in a mobile home. She is attractive, dresses stylishly, and has been pleasant and sociable with all patients and staff on the unit. You have previously determined with her that some nursing diagnoses with high priority are anxiety related to possible resuming of drug use, situational low self-esteem related to job loss and absence of financial resources, and social isolation related to avoidance of drug-using acquaintances.

Question 2:   How can you proceed to develop appropriate, specific outcomes related to each nursing diagnosis?

Answer 2:   Basic Responses   Optional Responses

_____

_____

_____

_____

Situation 3.   Ms. Gibson is a 61-year-old former nun and retired secretary. She has come to the Holistic Nursing Center for relief of a stiff neck that has bothered her for many years. Acupuncture and massage provided temporary relief. Ms. Gibson works as a volunteer at an emergency shelter for children. She also helps her 85-year-old mother with transportation and house cleaning.

Question 3:   How will you proceed to identify nursing interventions to achieve defined client outcomes?

Answer 3:   Basic Responses   Optional Responses

_____

_____

_____

_____

Situation 4:   Ms. Robinson, a 26-year-old woman, has just completed her second semester of an associate degree nursing program. A classmate brought her to the Holistic Nursing Center because she had been dismissed from the program and was very angry and depressed. She has returned for her third appointment. On previous appointments, you used healing touch with counseling and discussion of journaling.

Question 4:   How will you proceed to implement the ongoing plan of care?

Answer 4:   Basic Responses   Optional Responses

_____

_____

_____

_____

PART II—CARING AND HEALING OF CLIENTS AND SIGNIFICANT OTHERS

CONCEPT VII—MEANING AND WHOLENESS

CHAPTER 12—THERAPEUTIC COMMUNICATION: THE ART OF HELPING

 Pause for a moment . . .

❑ *I am aware of my test-taking skills.*
—*I can identify the components of a test question.*
—*I can read questions carefully before selecting an answer.*

Test Questions 1–15

1. Communication is best described as
   a. linear from sender to receiver.
   b. serendipitous.
   c. constant.
   d. intentional.

2. Communication occurs when
   a. sender launches message.
   b. receiver intakes message.
   c. message is determined to be meaningful.
   d. all of the above.

3. Helping communications
   a. focus on client's problems.
   b. occur naturally.
   c. invest the helper actively.
   d. facilitate self-discovery by the client.

4. Holistic nurses need to
   a. use accurate helping skills.
   b. counsel most patients.
   c. teach clients how to communicate effectively.
   d. provide psychotherapy.

5. Select the false statement.
   a. Helping communications can occur in 5-minute exchanges.
   b. Core helping skills facilitate deep exploration.
   c. Active listening is helpful in building positive affect.
   d. Change can most easily occur with client goals.

6. Focused exploration helps the client to
   a. make changes in his or her patterns.
   b. see the bigger picture.
   c. solve problems.
   d. feel rapport with the nurse.

7. Many nurses tend to use only the first and third stages of a helping relationship.
   a. True.
   b. False.

8. Core helping skills include
   a. empathy, self-disclosure, concreteness.
   b. empathy, respect, concreteness.
   c. empathy, genuineness, feedback.
   d. respect, genuineness, rapport.

9. The second stage of the helping model
   a. is critical to identify the underlying problem.
   b. involves the nurse's perceptions.
   c. clarifies deeper issues.
   d. is all of the above.

10. Deeper exploration uses the skills of
   a. empathy, feedback, confrontation.
   b. self-disclosure, brainstorming, additive empathy.
   c. goal setting, alternative ways to cope.
   d. confrontation, immediacy, and troubleshooting.

11. Confrontation
   a. points out dysfunction.
   b. challenges the client to see own weaknesses.
   c. highlights discrepancies in client's presentation.
   d. blames client.

12. The highest risk skill is
   a. feedback.
   b. self-disclosure.
   c. immediacy.
   d. additive empathy.

13. Communication is the context in which all of nursing is fulfilled.
   a. True.
   b. False.

14. Perception is affected by
   a. filters.
   b. beliefs.
   c. sensory limitations.
   d. all of the above.

15. Communication needs to be
   a. purposive to fulfill the goals of nursing.
   b. spontaneous and natural to comfort client.
   c. focused on client's needs and goals.
   d. incisive to assist client clarify and self discover.

 Pause for a moment . . .

❏ *I know my strongest test-taking skills.*
❏ *My effective test-taking skills will contribute to my HNC examination success.*

Situations 1–4

Situation 1: Ms. King came late to a session because she had a car accident on the way. You note that she is shaking, crying, muscularly tense, and obsessing about the fact that she did not see the other car.

Question 1: Your basic response would be to say:

   a. You shouldn't blame yourself for this accident.
   b. You are tense and shaken because you had an unexpected accident.
   c. You came late because you were delayed by the accident.
   d. You seem depressed because you didn't see the other car.

What would you then do to assist Ms. King?

Answer 1:   Basic Responses   Optional Responses

_____

_____

_____

_____

Situation 2:   You meet a new client, Billy N., and he begins to explain that he was sent by his principal to work with you on learning to handle his stress levels better.

Question 2:   Your initial basic response to him is?

    a. You are here because you need to learn to deal with stress.
    b. You were made to come by your principal.
    c. You feel upset because others think you have a problem handling stress.
    d. You handle stress badly, and others want you to get help.

What would be your next approach to begin work with Billy?

Answer 2:   Basic Responses   Optional Responses

_____

_____

_____

_____

Situation 3:   Ms. Parry has come to you for nutritional counseling, but she continues to overeat and rarely does the homework you assign. She asks you to sign a note to her employer that she is making progress on her eating problem, since her job is in jeopardy if she does not lose weight.

Question 3:   Your best basic response is?

    a. I need to share some feedback with you. When I am asked to write a note indicating that you are making progress when you fail to follow through on your agreements, I feel used and angry.
    b. You want me to rescue you by lying to your boss. I will not write the note, but I will support you in making the needed changes.
    c. On one hand, you come for nutritional counseling to deal with your obesity; yet on the other hand, you do nothing to reduce your eating or fulfill your homework.
    d. All of the above.

How would you handle Ms. Parry for the next step?

Answer 3:   Basic Responses   Optional Responses

_____

_____

_____

_____

Situation 4:   Ms. Becker indicates that she is having trouble making life pattern changes, yet she is quite insistent that she wants to continue working with you.

Question 4:   As a troubleshooter, you decide the first basic response is

  a. Review the main goals that Ms. Becker has set for herself.
  b. Review the steps that she is struggling with.
  c. Clarify what she is afraid of.
  d. Reassure her that change is hard.

Explain the process you would use to deal with this problem.

Answer 4:   Basic Responses   Optional Responses

_____

_____

_____

_____

CHAPTER 13—CULTURAL DIVERSITY AND CARE

Pause for a moment . . .

❑ *I am aware of my test-taking skills.*
— *I can identify the components of a test question.*
— *I can read questions carefully before selecting an answer.*

Test Questions 1–15

1. Cultural competence is demonstrated by all except
   a. recognizing the dynamics of one's own beliefs and values.
   b. reading about other cultures.
   c. avoiding any controversial discussion with people of another culture so as not to offend.
   d. attempting to articulate issues from another's perspective.
2. Ms. James is of Haitian heritage; the best approach to understanding her is to
   a. avoid using the term *Black*.
   b. read about foods commonly eaten by Haitians and change her menu plan accordingly.
   c. research the voodoo religion so as to be able to understand her spiritual beliefs.
   d. ask about the history of her family.
3. Members of the Hispanic culture may include
   a. persons born in Central and South America.
   b. persons of the Caucasian race.
   c. persons of the Mongolian race.
   d. persons of the Negroid race.
   e. all of the above.
   f. only two of the above.
4. The theory of orthogonal cultural identification holds that
   a. the longer a family has been in the United States, the more they adopt U.S. culture.
   b. groups with strong heritage consistency acculturate faster.
   c. adaptation is a complex process wherein acculturation interacts with heritage consistency.
   d. children always adapt faster than their parents.
5. Mr. Thompson, an elderly African-American, is always late for his clinic appointment. He arrives 45 minutes late. The best interpretation (incorporating cultural understanding) of his behavior is
   a. he is lazy and disorganized.
   b. he does not respect others or value their time.
   c. this is a way of acting out anger and aggression at the establishment and the White race.
   d. his view of time may be present oriented.
6. The Hong family is from China. Hui, age 27, has polycystic kidney disease and his medical team has suggested a transplant. He nods in approval, but will not discuss the issue or sign any papers without a family discussion. Understanding of cultural relationships to others may help interpret this behavior. Chinese culture often has which approach to relationships with others?

a. Lineal.
b. Collateral.
c. Individual.
d. Institutional.

7. Ms. Hu, of Southeast Asian background, is 25 weeks pregnant. She speaks broken English. In teaching her about nutritional requirements, she frequently nods in agreement. The nurse should interpret this as
   a. an indication that she understands the nutritional instructions and plans to follow them.
   b. a sign that she is afraid to displease you and fears punishment.
   c. a sign of respect for you and your position of authority and her desire to keep you from "losing face."
   d. a negative response of disagreement.

8. Which of the following are true of a culture that is organized around written communication?
   a. Visual and auditory images are persuasive in presenting information.
   b. Books with essential truths presented as parables and proverbs are printed.
   c. Communication is based on the fastest transmission of facts.
   d. Scientific information is presented in precise, often quantitative format.

9. The Mexican tradition of eating specific foods for their "hot" or "cold" properties is an example of which major cultural paradigm regarding health?
   a. Magicoreligious health paradigm.
   b. Holistic health paradigm of balance.
   c. Scientific paradigm.
   d. Biomedical paradigm.

10. A hallmark of the Western Judeo-Christian-Islamic religious tradition is
    a. polytheism.
    b. pantheism.
    c. essential unity of all.
    d. monotheism.

11. Ms. Davis is a healer who prays with her clients and is determined to convert them to her beliefs by helping them heal. She views all who do not believe in God as heathens who need to be saved, and she feels her healing abilities are to be used to convert others. From a cultural competence perspective, she is making which common error?
    a. Cultural imposition.
    b. Cultural blindness.
    c. Confusion of race and ethnicity.
    d. Underestimation of the importance of socioeconomic status.

12. One of the fundamental tasks that a nurse needs to undertake to develop cultural competency is to
    a. understand that biomedicine is a cultural system in which both she and the patient must interact.
    b. read original ethnographies from the anthropologic literature to get accurate information.
    c. be well informed about every culture to be able to understand that culture.
    d. treat all Whites alike, as they belong to the same culture.

13. Ms. Hernandez, a Central American immigrant who speaks English, returns to a clinic and has not adhered to dietary instructions to eat fruits and vegetables as they are "cold." The best nursing diagnosis would be
    a. impaired communication related to lack of understanding.
    b. lack of engagement in recommended health behaviors related to noncoherent explanatory systems between provider–client.
    c. noncompliance related to language differences.
    d. lack of knowledge related to low educational level.

14. Ms. White, age 78, is a devout Christian and is skeptical about new ideas. She is troubled with high blood pressure and claims to be nervous. The nurse uses touch in the form of a backrub and prays with her. She is using which mode of cultural intervention?
    a. Cultural preservation.
    b. Cultural accommodation.
    c. Cultural repatterning.
    d. Cultural stereotyping.

15. Traditional health practices of Native Americans include
    a. attention to the sins of one's ancestors.
    b. "root healers."
    c. mistrust of any healing that is not supported by scientific research.
    d. use of ceremonies like the "vision quest."

 Pause for a moment . . .

❑ *I know my strongest test-taking skills.*
❑ *My effective test-taking skills will contribute to my HNC examination success.*

Situations 1–4

Situation 1:   Ms. Smith is a nurse who has practiced in a small town hospital for 20 years. She has recently moved to a larger city with more cultural diversity. She is learning about developing more healing interventions to use with patients.

Question 1:   What is the best approach for her to develop cultural competence?

Answer 1:   Basic Responses   Optional Responses

_____

_____

_____

_____

Situation 2:   Mr. Taylor, a 46-year-old African-American, has been diagnosed with cancer. He is interested in using methods other than pills for pain relief.

Question 2:   What approach can you use to help design the best plan of care for him?

Answer 2:   Basic Responses   Optional Responses

_____

_____

_____

_____

Situation 3:   Ms. Lopez, a 23-year-old first-generation Mexican-American, is five months pregnant. Her husband comes to the clinic with her. She is using herbal teas, avoids certain foods, eats clay, prays every day, and likes to get massages for her backache.

Question 3:   What approaches to her prenatal care would best incorporate her cultural beliefs?

Answer 3:   Basic Responses   Optional Responses

_____

_____

_____

Situation 4:   Ms. Wilson, a 40-year-old White computer analyst, has been involved with "New Age" ideas for the past 5 years. Her company is reorganizing, and she is under a lot of stress. She was raised as a Methodist, but now meets with a small group of women who are exploring Buddhist ideas. She is seeking help for her tension headaches; she has been to the doctor, and she prefers not to use pharmaceuticals.

Question 4:   What is the best approach to helping her, demonstrating cultural competence?

Answer 4:   Basic Responses   Optional Responses

_____

_____

_____

_____

Chapter 14—Relationships

Pause for a moment . . .

❑ *I am aware of my test-taking skills.*
— *I can identify the components of a test question.*
— *I can read questions carefully before selecting an answer.*

Test Questions 1–15

1. Nurses need skills in communicating the value of their work to others because
   a. cost cutting is vital in the 1990s.
   b. managed care does not understand person-centered caring.
   c. patients often cannot speak up for their needs.
   d. of all of the above.
2. Effective communication consists of
   a. listening and being kind.
   b. valuing ourselves above others.
   c. a quality of mutual self-respect.
   d. getting approval.
3. Maslow contributed to holistic philosophy by
   a. emphasizing the development of healthy personalities.
   b. suggesting we all have needs.
   c. studying school children.
   d. founding several organizations.
4. Jung believed that everyone, including nurses, patients, and administrators,
   a. ought to get along.
   b. shares a collective human awareness.
   c. plays psychologic games.
   d. needs to be more assertive.
5. The Parent, Adult, and Child states are held
   a. in the conscious mind.
   b. in the unconscious mind.
   c. in the superego.
   d. firm in negotiations.
6. A psychologic game is
   a. fun for all the participants.
   b. a series of crossed transactions.
   c. a game in which everyone wins.
   d. uncomplementary interactions resulting in a payoff.
7. Better relationships are possible when the nurse
   a. expresses her anger.
   b. tells her boss the truth.
   c. can identify her ego states.
   d. tells her co-workers about her problems.
8. When confronted with a powerful authority, most nurses are likely to invoke
   a. the Healer archetype.
   b. their sense of self-worth.
   c. the Adaptive Child.
   d. a sense of trust in a Higher Power.
9. The archetype that helps the nurse to communicate effectively in difficult situations is the
   a. Wounded Healer.
   b. Nurturing Parent.
   c. Free Child.
   d. Warrior.
10. One of the principles of negotiation is that
    a. some compromises are made by both parties.
    b. once agreements are reached, there can be trust.
    c. someone has to feel left out.
    d. there is no way of enforcing an agreement.
11. A holistic nursing diagnosis of relationships includes
    a. consideration of the client's unspoken ego state
    b. awareness of the nurse's interaction patterns
    c. ways of holding firm to one's convictions
    d. plenty of options
12. Centering is useful
    a. before any relationship interaction.
    b. after an unpleasant encounter.
    c. whenever needed.
    d. for all of the above.
13. Reframing means
    a. being hard on people while protecting the ideas behind the issues.
    b. being hard on the issues while maintaining rapport with the individuals concerned.
    c. seeing everything from a framework of caring and kindness.
    d. being centered at all times to ensure understanding.
14. Being centered, grounded, and factual is most representative of the
    a. Nurturing Parent.
    b. Healer archetype.
    c. Warrior.
    d. Collective Unconscious.
15. The following best exemplifies an "I" statement:
    a. "I resent the supervisor's attitude. We have enough problems getting along already."

b. "I blame you for this patient's confusion."
c. "I think we have some real problems in health care."
d. "I'm uncomfortable with your choices and wish you would reconsider."

Pause for a moment . . .

❑ *I can make reasonable "guesses" on questions when I am not certain of the correct answer.*
❑ *Before I take the practice examination, I will set the conditions as if I were taking the actual examination (empty bladder, quiet environment without interruptions for _____ hours).*

Situations 1–4

Situation 1: Nurse Norris is told by his supervisor that he is sloppy and much too flippant with his patients. He resents the criticism and shows the supervisor that he is strong by telling others what a "bitch" she is. To her face, he is friendly and tells her off-color jokes.

Question 1: Using the transactional model, describe the ego states involved in the situation. How should you respond to him if he told you his feelings? How can the relationship between the supervisor and Mr. Norris be improved? Is there a psychologic game going on?

Answer 1:   Basic Responses   Optional Responses

_____

_____

_____

_____

Situation 2: The nurses in home care agency X are having difficulty getting their paychecks on time. They are told via a memo that the agency needs their trust, and things will work out gradually if they are patient.

Question 2: What ego state is likely to be evoked in the nurses by the memo? Which archetype is likely to be activated? What adult decisions need to be made? How can the relationships in this agency be healed?

Answer 2:   Basic Responses   Optional Responses

_____

_____

_____

_____

Situation 3: Nurse Eastman is commandeering with her patient who is noncompliant with the medical protocol.

Question 3: What other options does she have?

Answer 3:   Basic Responses   Optional Responses

_____

_____

_____

Situation 4:   Nurse Greene wants to introduce holistic ideas to her unit. She assumes people will be interested.

Question 4:   What would be the best way for her to proceed in creating curiosity and interest in her project? What would limit her effectiveness? How may staff feel threatened by her proposal?

Answer 4:   Basic Responses   Optional Responses

_____

_____

_____

_____

Chapter 15—Death and Grief

Pause for a moment . . .

❏ *I know my strongest test-taking skills.*
❏ *My effective test-taking skills will contribute to my HNC examination success.*

Test Questions 1–15

1. Grief, which follows the death of a loved one, is
   a. pervasive, affecting all aspects of life.
   b. a set of well-defined stages people go through in order.
   c. a precursor to clinical depression in most people.
   d. a diagnosis requiring intervention.

2. The difference between life review and reminiscence is
   a. length of interview.
   b. degree of structure in the format.
   c. number of participants in the group.
   d. written vs. oral techniques.

3. Assessment of pain most importantly depends on
   a. the patient's description of pain.
   b. past history of pain management patterns for that patient.
   c. characteristics of the medications proposed.
   d. use of a standard, pain assessment scale.

4. According to the gate control theory of pain, painful sensory impulses can be inhibited (the gate closed) by stimulation of related nerve fibers using
   a. distraction or heat.
   b. imagery or hypnosis.
   c. touch or cold.
   d. medication or immobility.

5. One's perception of pain is influenced by
   a. emotion and caffeine.
   b. age and severity of injury.
   c. intelligence and exercise tolerance.
   d. memory and learning.

6. Assessment of spiritual concerns most importantly requires assessment of one's
   a. concept of God or deity.
   b. religious denominational affiliation.
   c. attendance at religious events or services.
   d. method of prayer or meditation.

7. Environmental characteristics that predispose hospital nurses who care for the dying to experience signs of stress include
   a. professional competition, lack of equipment.
   b. inflexible visiting hours, poor temperature control.
   c. lack of collaboration, inexperience.
   d. poor staff communications patterns, role-overload, and ambiguity.

8. Which of the following statements about near-death experiences (NDEs) is true?
   a. NDEs are proof of life after death.
   b. NDEs are a form of hallucination.
   c. NDEs are often comforting to a client and family.
   d. NDEs are always dramatic.

9. A widow who celebrates her wedding anniversary each year for 5 years after her husband's death should be
   a. assessed for suicide risk.
   b. encouraged to do so if it helps her acknowledge her feelings.

c. distracted by good friends to help her move beyond her grief.

d. taught to use a variety of coping skills.

10. A professional nurse evaluates care for a dying client to determine if it has met the client's goals for comfort and

a. communication with the doctor.

b. increased wisdom during the dying process.

c. participation in care for as long as possible.

d. progress toward cure.

11. A prerequisite professional skill for the nurse to be able to provide comfort to the client who is dying is

a. love.

b. presence.

c. compassion.

d. self-discipline.

12. A major use of support groups for people who love someone who is dying is to

a. tell people what will happen during death.

b. encourage completion of the grieving process.

c. develop spiritual resources.

d. provide a safe place to express feelings.

13. Potential outcomes for the self-transcendent person generally include

a. less depression, increased hope.

b. new connections to people, introspection.

c. ability to meditate deeply, less fear of death.

d. increased church attendance, increased verbalization.

14. Knowledge that a family must have in order to be comfortable and achieve some kind of peace during the death of a loved one is

a. the nature of the afterlife.

b. what others think should be done.

c. how to complete funeral arrangements.

d. changes in the body during the death process.

15. Self-care for the nurse before caring for the dying individual most importantly begins with

a. exercising daily for good health.

b. setting limits for involvement with people.

c. centering, to be in a focused and caring state.

d. prioritizing care according to the nursing process.

 Pause for a moment . . .

❑ *The test taking skills that have worked best for me in the past to make me confident about taking a test are* _____ .

❑ *I am changing some old, negative mind tapes about being a poor test taker. These no longer serve me.*

❑ *I am spending time developing my plan to change these "old worn-out mind tapes" and to create new success mind tapes of "achieving my goal of test success."*

Situations 1–3

Situation 1:   Mr. Pearson, a 23-year-old student nurse, asks you what it means to help someone have "a peaceful death." The ideas of peace and death seem contradictory to him.

Question 1:   How do you describe a "peaceful death"?

Answer 1:   Basic Responses   Optional Responses

_____   _____

_____   _____

_____   _____

_____

Situation 2:   Ms. Riordan, another student nurse in the conference group, wants to know how to support the family during the grief process.

Question 2:   List at least five interventions that help to support the family during the grief process.

Answer 2:   Basic Responses   Optional Responses

_____   _____

_____   _____

_____   _____

Situation 3:   Ms. McMullough, RN, is a home health nurse who is helping her terminally ill client with pain control. She has just increased the dose of pain medication and would like to add a nonpharmacologic technique other than cognitive or behavioral (because of the patient's impaired state of consciousness).

Question 3:   List at least four other nonpharmacologic pain reduction strategies that she may try.

Answer 3:   Basic Responses   Optional Responses

_____   _____

_____   _____

_____   _____

CONCEPT VIII—CLIENT SELF-CARE

CHAPTER 16—SELF-ASSESSMENTS

 Pause for a moment . . .

❏ _I simulate a test-taking situation._
❏ _I sit down to take the practice examination without interruptions for a 1- or 2-hour period._
❏ _I am doing a great job!_

Test Questions 1–10

1. The major distinguishing factor of holistic self-assessment is
   a. assessment of the environment.
   b. assessment of the energy system/field.
   c. assessment of the nutritional status.
   d. assessment of the spiritual well-being.
2. The purpose of learning self-assessment skills is
   a. to become aware of our innate healing potential.
   b. to learn how to be spiritual.
   c. to assess others.
   d. to teach nutrition.
3. The purpose of physical self-assessment is
   a. to identify risk factors.
   b. to increase optimum level of health.
   c. to seek wholeness of physical potential.
   d. all of the above.
4. The goal of emotional self-assessment is to
   a. become emotionally balanced.
   b. practice self-counseling techniques.
   c. become aware of one's feelings.
   d. know when to seek help.
   e. follow both b and c.
5. The goal of spiritual self-assessment is to
   a. develop a relationship to a higher power.
   b. choose one religion over another.
   c. learn how to meditate properly.
   d. explore one's spiritual potential.
6. The goal of social self-assessment is to
   a. be more friendly to one's neighbors.
   b. know one's relationship to the community and to the world at large.
   c. alleviate fears of social interaction.
   d. compare one's social standing to others in the community.

7. Self-responsibility is vital to self-assessment because
   a. the individual no longer needs professional help.
   b. there is less chance that the individual will blame others for illness.
   c. the individual acknowledges his or her own role in establishing and maintaining wellness.
   d. it prevents the individual from becoming ill.
8. The individual can strengthen his or her self-assessment skills by practicing the following:
   a. philosophy.
   b. relaxation and imagery processes.
   c. aerobic exercise.
   d. nutritional cooking habits.
9. Before giving the client any physical self-assessment tools, a nurse should
   a. assess the client/patient.
   b. obtain the results of the client's most recent physical examination.

c. provide the client with the necessary information.
d. teach the client about risk factors and ways to identify them.
10. Which of the following patients/clients are poor candidates for self-asessment interventions?
   a. People with low self-esteem.
   b. People with no kinesthetic awareness.
   c. People with no social skills.
   d. None of the above.

 Pause for a moment . . .

❏ *I identify my test-taking skills.*
❏ *The "test-wiseness," the "how-to" take a test, is a skill that I am learning.*
❏ *I practice taking the practice examinations so that I can retain the information and improve my test scores.*

Situations 1–4

Situation 1: Ms. Parker, a 42-year-old woman, seeks your help to learn how to assess her general well-being. She wants to start by learning about healthful nutrition.

Question 1: How would you introduce her to the general principles of nutrition?

Answer 1: Basic Responses

_____

_____

_____

_____

Situation 2: Ms. Smith, a 25-year-old woman, has been suffering from depression intermittently. She has been feeling good lately and has come to you to learn how to remain aware of her emotions and to avoid falling into a depression again.

Question 2: How can you help her assess her emotional status?

Answer 2: Basic Responses

_____

_____

_____

Situation 3: Mr. Rogers, a 60-year-old man, was recently discharged from a medical center after a triple bypass operation. He has gone through a cardiac rehabilitation program and is now ready to maintain a moderate exercise routine on his own. He comes to you to learn guidelines for self-assessment in this area.

Question 3:   What would you tell him?

Answer 3:   Basic Responses

_____

_____

_____

_____

Situation 4:   Ms. Black, a 35-year-old woman, is interested in holistic health care. She comes to see you to discuss what she can do to participate in the process.

Question 4:   How would you proceed?

Answer 4:   Basic Responses

_____

_____

_____

_____

CHAPTER 17—COGNITIVE THERAPY

 Pause for a moment . . .

❑ *I am aware of my test-taking skills.*
❑ *I can identify the components of a test question.*
❑ *I can read questions carefully before selecting an answer.*

Test Questions 1–15

1. Which of the following is true of cognitive therapy?
   a. Stress and suffering are caused by our perception(s), and these perceptions (thoughts) are often distorted and unrealistic.
   b. By changing negative (distorted) thoughts, we can change the way we feel physically.
   c. By changing negative (distorted) thoughts, we can change the way we feel emotionally.
   d. All of the above.
   e. None of the above.
2. Physiology can be affected by
   a. depression.
   b. anxiety.
   c. anger.
   d. hostility.
   e. all of the above.
3. In response to stress, individuals often engage in health-risking behaviors, such as
   a. increased smoking, alcohol and fatty food consumption.
   b. relaxation response.
   c. increased exercise.
   d. social support.
   e. all of the above.
   f. none of the above.
4. Cognitive therapy was introduced by
   a. Hans Selye.
   b. Walter Cannon.
   c. Aaron Beck.
5. Symptoms of depression and anxiety respond favorably to:
   a. a high-fat diet.
   b. decreased exercise.
   c. cognitive therapy.
6. Hypertension has been shown to be caused by:
   a. stress.
   b. vigorous exercise.
   c. a low-fat diet.
7. In order to deal effectively with stress, it is more important to

a. change external events.
b. change the way we think about things.
c. isolate oneself socially.

8. In the health contract, goals should be
   a. detailed.
   b. comprehensive.
   c. unstructured.
   d. achievable.

9. The following may be symptoms or signals of stress:
   a. crying.
   b. smoking.
   c. back pain.
   d. tight neck and shoulders.
   e. being critical of others.
   f. none of the above.
   g. all of the above.

10. Automatic thoughts:
    a. are not in our control.
    b. can be challenged and reframed.
    c. include neither of the above.

11. Irrational beliefs
    a. are bad.
    b. are always in our conscious awareness.
    c. can lead to negative mood states.

12. Automatic thoughts are
    a. quick, fleeting.
    b. usually not in our conscious awareness.
    c. frequently unrealistic, illogical, and distorted.
    d. all of the above.
    e. none of the above.

13. In preparing for a cognitive therapy session, it is important for the nurse to take time to

a. center himself or herself before beginning.
b. be hypervigilant and on guard.
c. do neither of the above.

14. Cognitive therapy is more applicable in
    a. the outpatient setting.
    b. the inpatient setting.
    c. both of the above.

15. Which of the following is a realistic achievable outcome of cognitive therapy? The patient will be able to
    a. self-monitor negative automatic thoughts and silent assumptions.
    b. identify the distortions in these automatic thoughts.
    c. identify the assumptions that underlie these automatic thoughts.
    d. substitute more realistic, self-enhancing thoughts.
    e. replace self-defeating silent assumptions with more effective coping skills.
    f. communicate more effectively.
    g. do all of the above.
    h. do none of the above.

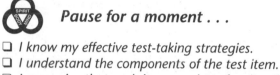 *Pause for a moment . . .*

❏ *I know my effective test-taking strategies.*
❏ *I understand the components of the test item.*
❏ *I recognize that each item consists of a situation or background information, a question, and several possible answers.*

Situations 1–4

Situation 1:   Mr. Foster, a 56-year-old man, has had coronary artery disease for 5 years and experiences stable exertional angina. He has done well with exercise, healthy nutrition, relaxation, and stress management. Recently, he was admitted to the hospital because of an increase in his anginal pain, and he is awaiting cardiac catheterization. On the morning of the procedure, he experiences chest pain.

Question 1:   What is the stress? What physical response, thoughts, feelings, and behaviors can Mr. Foster be having? What cognitive distortions? How can he contribute to his symptom reduction? What can you do?

Answer 1:   Basic Responses   Optional Responses

Situation 2:   Ms. Havior, a 36-year-old woman, has had fibromyalgia for 3 years. Recently, she has been feeling much better thanks to her swim therapy program and new medications. Now, however, she relates that she has lost all momentum because of a flare-up of symptoms last week.

Question 2:   What physical response, thoughts, feelings, and behaviors can Ms. Havior be having related to her recent flare-up? What cognitive distortions? How can she reframe them? What can you do?

Answer 2:   Basic Responses   Optional Responses

_____

_____

_____

_____

Situation 3:   Mr. Cross, a 25-year-old man, has had problems with insomnia for the last 2 years. After establishing that there is no biologic reason for his sleep disturbance, you ask him to describe his physical response and thoughts, feelings, and behaviors when he cannot fall asleep.

Question 3:   What physical response, thoughts, feelings, and behaviors can Mr. Cross be having related to his insomnia? What cognitive distortions? How can he reframe them and change his behavior? What can you do?

Answer 3:   Basic Responses   Optional Responses

_____

_____

_____

_____

Situation 4:   Ms. Kennedy, a 60-year-old woman, was recently admitted to the hospital with chest pain. Although her physician ruled out a myocardial infarction, she diagnosed coronary artery disease, angina, hypertension, and dyslipidemia. Ms. Kennedy also is overweight, sedentary, and under a great deal of stress. She has never been in the hospital before, nor had any serious illness. She appears very anxious and depressed, and it is difficult to do discharge teaching or planning.

Question 4:   What physical response, thoughts, feelings, and behaviors can Ms. Kennedy be having? What cognitive distortions? How can she reframe them and change her behavior? What can you do?

Answer 4:   Basic Responses   Optional Responses

_____

_____

_____

_____

CHAPTER 18—NUTRITION

Pause for a moment . . .

❏ *I recognize that the question (stem) poses the problem to be solved.*
❏ *I know that the stem may be written as a direct question, What would you do first?, or an incomplete sentence, such as The nurse should. . . .*
❏ *I understand that the answers (options) are the possible responses to the stem. There is one correct answer and three incorrect answers.*

Test Questions 1–17

1. Good nutrition is best defined as
   a. feeling satiated at the end of a meal.
   b. taking vitamin supplements.
   c. receiving adequate nutrients to prevent disease.
   d. receiving optimal nutrition for wellness.
2. Recommended daily allowances (RDAs) are guidelines for
   a. prevention of nutritional deficiency diseases.
   b. high-level wellness.
   c. interventions for people with chronic disease.
   d. prenatal care.
3. Factors that lower cholesterol levels include
   a. smoking and alcohol.
   b. soluble fibers.
   c. insoluble fibers.
   d. margarine.
4. Antioxidant vitamins protect the body from
   a. free radical damage.
   b. anemia.
   c. osteoporosis.
   d. migraine headaches.
5. Essential fatty acid deficiency is associated with
   a. cardiovascular disease.
   b. immune system dysfunction.
   c. skin problems.
   d. all of the above.
6. Women can reduce their risk of osteoporosis by
   a. reducing caffeine and alcohol in the diet.
   b. increasing weight-bearing exercise.
   c. taking calcium supplements daily.
   d. doing all of the above.

7. Which drug(s) increase the need for certain vitamins and minerals?
   a. Antibiotics.
   b. Aspirin.
   c. Birth control pills.
   d. All of the above.
8. Foods that contain soluble fiber include
   a. whole grain cereals.
   b. celery.
   c. oranges.
   d. cabbage.
9. When is the best time to take nutritional supplements?
   a. With meals.
   b. On an empty stomach.
   c. In the morning.
   d. Before bedtime.
10. The level of saturated fats is high in
    a. fish.
    b. meat.
    c. olive oil.
    d. almonds.
11. Margarine is
    a. an essential fatty acid.
    b. a transfatty acid.
    c. a polyunsaturated fat.
    d. a monosaturated fat.
12. Neurotransmitter production is dependent on
    a. antioxidants.
    b. vitamin B_6.
    c. iodine.
    d. selenium.
13. Environmental exposure to DDT and other pesticides and their metabolites
    a. is not a health risk factor in humans.
    b. increases estrogen levels in women.
    c. is easily resolved by the liver.
    d. is neutralized by stomach acids.
14. The use of sulphites as a preservative is associated with increased risk of
    a. migraine headaches.
    b. constipation.
    c. asthma.
    d. diverticulitis.
15. Efforts to promote immune system function in HIV-infected patients may include
    a. increasing caloric intake in the form of fats.
    b. increasing dairy products in the diet.

    c. consuming 60 percent of the diet in the form
      of animal protein.

    d. decreasing saturated fats and simple sugars in
      the diet.

16. Vitamin B_{12} deficiency and low hydrochloric
    acid levels are common in

    a. children.

    b. athletes.

    c. elderly persons.

    d. adolescents.

17. When assessing nutritional needs, include

    a. cultural factors.

    b. emotional factors.

    c. activity level.

    d. all of the above.

Pause for a moment . . .

❑ *I can approach the situation questions as if I were in the situation.*

❑ *I can then think about my basic responses (in any order) and optional responses (in any order) for this situation.*

❑ *I understand that these situation questions assess my broad knowledge and integration of holistic nursing practice and are based on the **AHNA Core Curriculum** content.*

Situations 1–4

Situation 1: Mr. Love, a 45-year-old man whose father died of heart disease at a young age, is seeking assistance with dietary changes. His own attempts to make changes have been unsuccessful. He is overweight, has a high-stress job, and is fearful that he will die prematurely like his father.

Question 1: What lifestyle changes can Mr. Love make to lower his risk of cardiovascular disease?

Answer 1:   Basic Responses   Optional Responses

Situation 2: Mr. Young, a 38-year-old man, was diagnosed with HIV infection in 1992. He recently experienced his first opportunistic infection, an intestinal parasite. He has heard that nutrition can strengthen the immune system and is seeking information and guidance.

Question 2: What interventions would you suggest to Mr. Young to strengthen his immune system?

Answer 2:   Basic Responses   Optional Responses

Situation 3: Ms. Poe, a 45-year-old premenopausal woman, has a yearly mammogram because both her mother and aunt had breast cancer. She is interested in changing her diet to promote health and prevent disease.

Question 3: What dietary and lifestyle guidelines would you encourage her to adopt to promote health and decrease her risk of cancer?

Answer 3:   Basic Responses   Optional Responses

_____

_____

_____

_____

Situation 4:   Ms. Mead, a 22-year-old obese woman, is seeking counseling for weight loss. She has tried various diet programs, including diet pills. She states that she eats compulsively when anxious.

Question 4:   How would you help Ms. Mead make changes in her eating patterns and well-being?

Answer 4:   Basic Responses   Optional Responses

_____

_____

_____

_____

CHAPTER 19—MOVEMENT AND EXERCISE

 Pause for a moment . . .

❑ *I do not read meaning into a question.*
❑ *I understand all the words in the question.*
❑ *I recognize when a word in a question is not familiar, and I try to figure out the meaning based on the context in which it appears in the question.*

Test Questions 1–15

1. Exercise is best defined as
   a. rigorous physical activity.
   b. a conscious act of movement.
   c. an aerobic expression of the physical body.
   d. an unconscious act of movement.
2. Which of the following least identifies movement/exercise as a universal process?
   a. All beings are expressions of the earth and move in accordance with their own rhythmic patterns.
   b. A universal perspective of movement/exercise respects self-knowledge.
   c. Movement/exercise is solely a human experience.

   d. The caring process is a mutual opportunity for self-reflection/pattern recognition for both the nurse and client.
3. Which of the following is an energy principle related to movement/exercise?
   a. Energy and matter are the same thing.
   b. Consciousness is a form of energy.
   c. The human is a pandimensional being within a universe of dynamic energy in many different frequencies and forms.
   d. All of the above.
4. Which of the following statements about the body-mind-spirit relationship effect of movement/exercise is false?
   a. It decreases memory.
   b. It elevates mood.
   c. It improves self-esteem.
   d. It strengthens the immune system.
5. Which of the following is not a possible physiologic effect of movement/exercise?
   a. It can raise the level of high-density lipoproteins and lower that of triglycerides.
   b. It can increase lung ventilation and lung diffusion capacity.
   c. It can increase blood clot formation.
   d. It can increase insulin sensitivity and glucose tolerance.

6. Conscious participation in movement/exercise can involve
   a. intention.
   b. self-awareness.
   c. motivation.
   d. all of the above.
7. Vehicles for recognizing patterns include
   a. body scan.
   b. inner advisor.
   c. meditation.
   d. all of the above.
8. A patient is interested in increasing her energy. Which of the following exercise benefits can you point out?
   a. Exercise increases the number of small blood vessels to muscles, thereby supplying them with more oxygen and blood.
   b. Exercise increases lung ventilation and lung diffusion capacity.
   c. Exercise increases ability to metabolize fat for energy.
   d. All of the above.
9. Pattern is best defined as
   a. a set perspective of characteristics.
   b. a determined way of being.
   c. an evolving energetic profile with distinguishing characteristics.
   d. clearly defined parameters or characteristics.
10. Subtle energy is
    a. not commonly visible.
    b. represented solely in material mass.
    c. extremely low frequencies.
    d. easily detected auditorially.
11. Which of the following is true?
    a. The pre-access phase involves goal setting.
    b. The pre-access phase involves pattern recognition.

c. The pre-access phase involves intention and centering.
d. The pre-access phase involves evaluation of goals.
12. Examples of holographic models are
    a. Ayurvedic.
    b. Rayid.
    c. Chinese Five Element/Phase.
    d. all of the above.
13. Moshe Feldenkrais is known for his work in
    a. physiologic norms.
    b. body awareness.
    c. quantum physics.
    d. establishment of vital signs.
14. Expressions of subtle movement do not include
    a. touch.
    b. low impact aerobics.
    c. breath work.
    d. imagery.
15. Holistic nursing process for movement/exercise
    a. is focused on physical intervention.
    b. is mutual and co-participative.
    c. is based on the nurse's identifying patient goals.
    d. concludes with an evaluation by the nurse.

 Pause for a moment . . .

❑ *As I read the question, I understand that I am being asked to identify priorities, to determine the best intervention, or to evaluate outcomes.*
❑ *I read each question carefully. I do not rush.*
❑ *I develop my skills to understand the question being asked.*

Situations 1–4

Situation 1: As a registered nurse, you are working with Mr. Pulaski, a 32-year-old construction worker who has requested your assistance in developing a movement/exercise program. He has a history of a right shoulder injury and occasional low back pain. X-rays are normal, and he is asymptomatic at this time. His goal is to strengthen his body and prevent further injury.

Question 1: How would you apply the holistic nursing process in caring for Mr. Pulaski?

Answer 1: Basic Responses   Optional Responses

_____

_____

_____

_____

Situation 2:   Ms. Schuster, a 47-year-old woman and single parent of three, comes to you to explore how her movement/exercise patterns relate to a larger picture of how she moves/relates to her life. She desires an expanded self-awareness for herself and her role as a mother.

Question 2:   How can an awareness of her way of moving/exercising—gained through the emerging paradigm of holistic movement/exercise—serve as a holographic representation of her/your life patterns?

Answer 2:   Basic Responses   Optional Responses

_____

_____

_____

_____

Situation 3:   Mr. Chuen, a 76-year-old man, moved to the United States from China in 1994. He had a cerebrovascular accident in 1989 and currently uses a wheelchair. He shares that he is most familiar with traditional Chinese medicine and has practiced tai chi for many years. He seeks assistance with movement/exercise.

Question 3:   What special considerations would you have in your care for Mr. Chuen?

Answer 3:   Basic Responses   Optional Responses

_____

_____

_____

_____

Situation 4:   As a holistic nurse, you are aware of movement/exercise as a universal process. You have an opportunity to share a perspective of this emerging paradigm with nursing colleagues.

Question 4:   Identify three energetic principles relevant to movement/exercise. Include one principle related to the human/earth community.

Answer 4:   Basic Responses   Optional Responses

_____

_____

_____

_____

CHAPTER 20—ENVIRONMENT

 Pause for a moment . . .

❑ *I answer the question before I look at the choices.*
❑ *I then look for the answer that is similar to the one that I generated.*

Test Questions 1–15

1. Earth ethics is *best* described as
    a. a field of study in philosophy.
    b. a set of guidelines to sustain a viable life support system.
    c. a way of viewing the world.

   d. a concept of recent development among scientists and other scholars.

2. Ecology is the study of
   a. the earth.
   b. living things.
   c. the universe.
   d. interrelationships.

3. Of the four key elements of sustainable economic development, which of the following is incorrect?
   a. Stabilizing world population.
   b. Reversing tide of deforestation.
   c. Managing and cleaning up the world's water supply.
   d. Increasing use of nuclear energy.

4. Of four specific measures to prevent infection and disease, which of these is most important?
   a. Buildup of immunity.
   b. Vaccination.
   c. Public education.
   d. Local stewardship.

5. By-products of health care processes and services are the responsibility of the
   a. state.
   b. municipality.
   c. health care organization.
   d. county.

6. All of the following are waste management goals, except
   a. consistent waste management systems.
   b. contract with local waste disposal company.
   c. guidelines for establishing mergers.
   d. maximization of cost effectiveness.

7. The CERES principles address
   a. cost/risk management.
   b. relationships of business with environment.
   c. guidelines for establishing mergers.
   d. standards of practice.

8. The following are ecologic hazards, as identified by the Environmental Protection Agency, except
   a. global climate change.
   b. stratospheric ozone depletion.
   c. interruption of migratory patterns of birds.
   d. indoor air pollution.

9. The systems approach to world order is
   a. a passing fad.
   b. not scientifically based.
   c. a recent invention.
   d. a paradigm shift.

10. The view of "environment as client" is
   a. a new paradigm in nursing.
   b. taught in schools of nursing.
   c. widely endorsed by nurses.
   d. a distortion of nursing.

11. The ecocentric world view means that
   a. human beings and the world are not separate.
   b. human beings and the world are separate.
   c. humans have dominion over the earth.
   d. humankind is the reason earth exists.

12. Clients who suffer from environmental exposures experience all but
   a. acceptance and understanding of employers and family.
   b. an assault on their immune system.
   c. a lengthy time in diagnosis and treatment.
   d. employers concerned with legal issues.

13. Assessment for environmental exposure is
   a. limited to allergists.
   b. vital for diagnosis.
   c. part of every physical examination.
   d. simple and straightforward.

14. Which of the following is not true?
   a. The chemical industry spends less on prevention of side effects than on product development.
   b. Many substances cause subtle damage to the body's systems.
   c. Protection against cancer is protection against other toxic outcomes.
   d. Many of the toxic linkages of chemicals to human health are known.

15. Which of these foods is more likely to be chemical-free?
   a. Fresh frozen.
   b. Local organic.
   c. Sun-dried.
   d. Imported.

 Pause for a moment . . .

❑ I look for key words in questions, because these words give me clues to the correct answer.
   — These are such words as except, not, or but.
   — Words such as most, next, or first indicate the order of steps or the priority.

❑ I move on to the next question if I am not sure, remembering to come back before concluding the examination.

Situations 1–4

Situation 1: Ms. Marks, a 36-year-old woman, seeks your help regarding her workplace. Since her building was renovated, she has had recurring headaches and loss of appetite. Her symptoms diminish when she returns home and over the weekend. Her employer and family tell her that she is exaggerating.

Question 1: What would your initial response be to her?

Answer 1:   Basic Responses   Optional Responses

_____

_____

_____

_____

Situation 2: You are employed in a hospital surgical intensive care unit and notice that aseptically wrapped supplies and equipment are being discarded as infectious rather than as solid waste.

Question 2: What steps would you take to investigate and change this situation?

Answer 2:   Basic Responses   Optional Responses

_____

_____

_____

_____

Situation 3: You are in a community health practice and are becoming increasingly overwhelmed by the enormity of environment-related illnesses among your clients. There are some obvious toxic sources and signs of environmental degradation in your geographic area.

Question 3: How would you begin to address this situation?

Answer 3:   Basic Responses   Optional Responses

_____

_____

_____

_____

Situation 4: You are invited to speak to a class of 30 middle school boys and girls on the topic of relating health to environment.

Question 4: What aspects would you want to be sure to include in your presentation?

Answer 4:   Basic Responses   Optional Responses

_____

_____

_____

_____

CHAPTER 21—LAUGHTER, PLAY, AND HUMOR

 Pause for a moment . . .

❏ *If I do not know an answer, I make a reasonable guess. "Intuition" and "hunches" are often correct answers.*
❏ *I understand that the holistic nursing certification (HNC) examination is based on the* **AHNA Core Curriculum.**

Test Questions 1–12

1. Humor is best defined as
   a. an ability to make people laugh.
   b. a willingness to laugh.
   c. an ability to recognize and appreciate the absurdity of a situation.
   d. an ability to remember and tell good jokes.
2. The difference between hoping humor and coping humor is that
   a. coping humor is used during stress and hoping humor is used any time.
   b. hoping humor accepts life and gives courage while coping humor gives detachment and releases tension.
   c. hoping humor makes others feel good and coping humor makes you feel good.
   d. there is no difference between hoping and coping humor.
3. Humor can help the nurse cope with stress by
   a. releasing endorphins that create relaxation and well-being.
   b. giving the nurse the ability to "bounce back" into a positive attitude.
   c. helping the nurse to maintain a psychologic distance from the pain and suffering.
   d. changing negative feelings into positive feelings.
4. Research has proven that
   a. people who like gallows humor are not compassionate caregivers.
   b. the person who creates humor under stress is denying the seriousness of the situation.
   c. people with a strong sense of humor are less emotionally distraught under stress.
   d. humor and laughter during stress have no significant benefits.

5. Measurements of neurologic changes during laughter reveal that humor
   a. stimulates primarily the left side of the brain.
   b. is experienced entirely in the right or creative side of the brain.
   c. is experienced on both sides of the brain simultaneously.
   d. is experienced at first on the left side and then moves to the right side.
6. Cancer patients benefit from laughter therapy because
   a. natural killer cells increase their reproduction rate.
   b. serum cortisol levels will rise and stimulate the immune system.
   c. it will relieve the pain and suffering.
   d. the activity of the natural killer cells will increase.
7. To assess a patient's responsiveness to humor, a nurse must
   a. observe the kind of humor that the patient creates.
   b. see the patient laugh in response to a cartoon that most patients find funny.
   c. laugh at the same things the patient does.
   d. understand the values of the patient's culture, gender, and generation.
8. People are most uncomfortable by humor that
   a. is scatological or bathroom oriented.
   b. is racist or sexual.
   c. is simplistic or nonsensical.
   d. makes fun of their profession.
9. Therapeutic humor programs are
   a. usually limited to the pediatric department.
   b. helpful to patients, family, and staff.
   c. inappropriate for seriously ill or terminal patients.
   d. most effective when created by one or two enthusiastic staff members.
10. When designing a comedy cart or laughter library, the selection of books and tapes should
    a. be evaluated for appropriateness and funniness by several people.
    b. include any donation that a staff or patient believes to be funny.
    c. be made based primarily on cost and availability.
    d. include only the most recent and popular releases.

11. Clowns who wish to bring humor to the hospital bedside should
    a. show up in makeup and costume and offer to entertain.
    b. engage the patient in playful, interactive activities to stimulate laughter.
    c. ask each patient for permission to enter the room.
    d. bring their own music and large comical props for a dramatic impact.
12. Guidelines for appropriate use of humor with patients include the following:
    a. Use a humorous intervention within the first 20 minutes of meeting a patient to establish the connection of shared laughter.
    b. If a patient seems offended by your humor, keep trying a different joke or prop until you get a laugh.

c. Use humorous interventions after you have attended to the physical or emotional pain that the patient may be experiencing.
d. If the patient does not respond with observable laughter, he or she is unable to appreciate the humor you shared.

Pause for a moment . . .

❑ *I can imagine that today is the HNC examination.*
❑ *I am arriving for the HNC examination physically and mentally prepared.*
❑ *I am proud of my accomplishments!*

Situations 1–4

Situation 1: Mr. Jones, a 49-year-old man, is anxious about his exploratory surgery scheduled for the next morning. You have assessed his knowledge, completed his preoperative teaching, and allowed time for him to express his concerns and questions. He tells you he cannot stop thinking about all the things that could possibly go wrong tomorrow.

Question 1: How would you introduce Mr. Jones to a therapeutic humor intervention?

Answer 1: Basic Responses   Optional Responses

Situation 2: Ms. Floyd, a 32-year-old woman, has recurrent breast cancer. After two mastectomies, each followed by chemotherapy and radiation therapy, she has now returned to the hospital for a bone marrow transplant and 3 weeks of intensive chemotherapy. She is angry, hopeless, and depressed about being in the hospital for many weeks.

Question 2: How would you assess Ms. Floyd's sense of humor and then integrate humorous modalities into the plan of care?

Answer 2: Basic Responses   Optional Responses

Situation 3: Mr. Cornwall, a 26-year-old man, has severe kidney disease and requires dialysis four times each week in the outpatient unit. He is angry and frustrated about his debilitated condition. He is resentful of the dietary restrictions and occasionally ignores all limits and eats exactly what he wants.

Question 3:   How would you use humor to help Mr. Cornwall resolve his frustration and release his feelings of animosity?

Answer 3:   Basic Responses   Optional Responses

_____

_____

_____

_____

Situation 4:   Jennifer L., a 7-year-old girl, has suffered a spinal cord transection from a motor vehicle accident, which left her paralyzed from the waist down. She has been in the hospital and rehabilitation unit for more than 1 month and will probably remain for another month. Jennifer is lonely and depressed. Her mother, who was driving the car when the accident occurred, is reluctant to visit because she feels she has ruined her child's life.

Question 4:   How would you create a humor intervention to lift Jennifer's spirit and help to reunite mother and daughter?

Answer 4:   Basic Responses   Optional Responses

_____

_____

_____

_____

CHAPTER 22—SELF-REFLECTION

 Pause for a moment . . .

❑ *I am eating nourishing food and will do so before the holistic nursing certification (HNC) examination. Complex carbohydrate foods will provide me with the most energy.*

❑ *I am avoiding excessive use of caffeine or sugar right now and will continue to do so before the HNC examination.*

❑ *I am relaxed and at ease and will arrive at the HNC examination in this same relaxed state.*

Test Questions 1–12

1. Self-reflection skills are best defined as those that
   a. guide healing.
   b. connect the individual with inner wisdom.
   c. expand healing awareness.
   d. connect the person with the universe at large.

2. Intuitive awareness is
   a. a type of cognition.
   b. instinctive knowing.
   c. immediately known without reasoning.
   d. an unconscious experience.

3. Events that are external to the individual
   a. have variable physiological effects on functioning.
   b. alter one's physiology.
   c. determine the individual's perception of the events.
   d. lead to adaptive coping responses.

4. Self-reflection nursing interventions are based on
   a. concepts of assertiveness and empowerment.
   b. the nurse as an authority on health.
   c. past experiences of the nurse and client.
   d. predictable outcomes.

5. The focus of self-reflection nursing interventions is
   a. connection with past successes and failures.
   b. awareness of barriers to current healing.

c. understanding one's personal inner wisdom.

d. all of the above.

6. Self-care knowledge, a major concept in the nursing theory of Modeling and Role-Modeling,

   a. means that nursing clients know how to care for themselves.

   b. means that nursing clients know what will be helpful to them.

   c. means that nursing clients may be deficient in important health-enhancing knowledge.

   d. means all of the above.

7. In Newman's theory, Health as Expanding Consciousness, clients gain freedom to act in new ways

   a. by taking responsibility for themselves.

   b. by experiencing chaos and disequilibrium.

   c. as consciousness expands.

   d. as nurses coach them in learning new skills.

8. Health as expanding consciousness is

   a. based on a model of disease prevention.

   b. based on understanding patterns of the whole.

   c. based on identifying and solving problems.

   d. based on eradicating disease and promoting health.

9. As a person's consciousness expands through relationships,

   a. there is a gain in freedom of action.

   b. there is a decrease in energy expended.

   c. there is resolution of pain and suffering.

   d. there is awareness of maladaptive patterns.

10. Self-reflection interventions

   a. are prescribed by the nurse for specific, measurable outcomes.

   b. focus on deficits within the person's behavioral repertoire.

   c. can be used only with individuals, not with groups.

   d. emphasize a person's inner strengths and wisdom.

11. Self-reflection interventions are most effective when the nurse

   a. is aware of his or her own inner resources.

   b. recognizes the chaos in the client's person-environment pattern.

   c. accurately diagnoses the client's deficits.

   d. understands the meaning of health and disease to the client.

12. Interventions that promote self-awareness and self-reflection

   a. focus on an expansion of consciousness.

   b. enhance creativity.

   c. facilitate authentic dialogue between and within persons.

   d. involve all of the above.

Situations 1–4

Situation 1: Ms. James, a 31-year-old mother of three young children, visits the community health clinic and is concerned about her increasing feelings of fatigue. She expresses frustration because she spends all her time trying to meet the demands of her husband and children.

Question 1: Following Margaret Newman's conceptual nursing model (health as expanding consciousness), what nursing interventions might best help Ms. James to feel more at ease?

Answer 1:   Basic Responses   Optional Responses

_____

_____

_____

_____

Situation 2: Billy M., a 15-year-old boy, has recently landed on the street after an intense argument with his father over Billy's sexual orientation. (Billy thinks he might be gay or bisexual.)

Question 2: As the nurse at a drop-in clinic for homeless youth, what are some barriers to self-reflection that Billy may experience?

Answer 2:   Basic Responses   Optional Responses

_____   _____
_____   _____
_____   _____

Situation 3:   As a clinician in an outpatient psychiatric unit, you have been assigned to develop an intervention to aid a group of older women who have a history of depression.

Question 3:   What are some nursing interventions that would be appropriate for this group?

Answer 3:   Basic Responses   Optional Responses

_____   _____
_____   _____
_____   _____

Situation 4:   Mr. Smith, a 54-year-old man, is receiving chemotherapy for lung cancer. As his nurse, you listen carefully to what he says about his treatment and his hopes for the future. He confides in you that he is afraid of dying from the treatment more than from the disease. He continually questions the reason for these treatments when "they probably won't do me any good anyway!" Through your continuous assessment, you learn that Mr. Smith has very little knowledge about the physiology of his body, cancer, or chemotherapy.

Question 4:   What *initial* nursing interventions would help Mr. Smith?

Answer 4:   Basic Responses   Optional Responses

_____   _____
_____   _____
_____   _____
_____   _____

Concept IX—Health Promotion

Chapter 23—Relaxation

 Pause for a moment . . .

❑ *I have plenty of time to finish the holistic nursing certification (HNC) examination.*

❑ *If I lose my concentration, I will use my relaxation, deep breathing, imagery, affirmations, positive self-talk, and distraction.*

Test Questions 1–16

1. Relaxation is best defined as
   a. the ability to think in sensory images.
   b. a psychophysiologic state characterized by parasympathetic dominance.
   c. Cannon's "fight or flight" response.
   d. a time for cooling out.

2. Benefits of relaxation training include
   a. easing muscle tension pain from skeletal muscle contractions.
   b. being able to fall asleep while performing relaxation exercises.
   c. dulling the senses.
   d. decreasing stamina for participation in athletic activities.
3. Which of the following is not a major route to the meditative state?
   a. Through the intellect.
   b. Through the emotions.
   c. Through the body.
   d. Through inaction.
4. Autogenics is defined as
   a. the increased muscle tension with which the body responds to stress.
   b. brief phrases used to focus attention on areas of the body for the purpose of inducing change in those areas from within.
   c. a homeostatic mechanism in the brain.
   d. progressive muscle relaxation.
5. Hypnosis
   a. is effective with disorders of the medulla.
   b. does not alter one's state of consciousness.
   c. is the process whereby muscles are quieted so that mental attention can be directed to positive statements.
   d. is rarely used for specific purposes such as altering physiologic functioning.
6. Biofeedback
   a. opens doors to sources of feedback that are ordinarily out of awareness.
   b. does not require any special equipment.
   c. prepares a person to deal with the actual or imagined threat of an emergency.
   d. increases heart rate and respiratory rate.
7. In addition to changes in the autonomic nervous system, changes in which of the following systems accompany the relaxation response?
   a. Endocrine.
   b. Immune.
   c. Neuropeptide.
   d. All of the above.
8. Mindfulness
   a. can be easily learned and requires little practice.
   b. activates the sympathetic nervous system.
   c. is an attitude of remaining fully awake and aware.
   d. requires the ability to dwell on each thought that comes to mind.

9. The sense of timelessness
   a. has healing properties.
   b. requires a repetitive focus on one particular word or phrase.
   c. requires losing control of oneself.
   d. is a stressor to people who claim to have too little time.
10. Choices of relaxation interventions
    a. are best determined by the nurse or other health care provider.
    b. require consideration of the person's condition, time available, and personal preferences.
    c. are almost always initially resisted by clients.
    d. are expected to be changed from week to week.
11. The most effective way to establish the efficacy of relaxation methods is through
    a. trial and error.
    b. clinical practice.
    c. scientific research.
    d. biofeedback.
12. Although used for centuries, it was not endorsed as part of medical education by the American Medical Association until the 1950s.
    a. Progressive muscle relaxation.
    b. Meditation.
    c. Biofeedback.
    d. Hypnosis.
13. Which of the following is *not* characteristic of changes evoked by the relaxation response?
    a. Decrease in peripheral blood flow.
    b. Increase in production of alpha waves.
    c. Decrease in oxygen consumption.
    d. Increase in activity of natural killer cells.
14. Which relaxation method is being used successfully for treating addictions and attention deficit–hyperactivity disorders?
    a. Electroencephalographic biofeedback.
    b. Hypnosis.
    c. Body scan.
    d. Meditation.
15. Which intervention is an introduction that can be used prior to using interventions to promote deeper relaxation?
    a. Self-hypnosis.
    b. Breath awareness.
    c. Tension awareness.
    d. Imagery.
16. The deepening stage of hypnosis is primarily characterized by
    a. suggestions for positive change.

b. spiral images, such as moving down a staircase or elevator.
c. repeat of the induction stage.
d. deepening of a state of relaxed alertness.

Pause for a moment . . .

❑ I can concentrate during my studying so that I can concentrate during the HNC examination.
❑ I focus while I study, and I will focus during the HNC examination.
❑ I will finish at my own pace, even when others finish before me.

Situations 1–4

Situation 1:   Ms. Hampton, a 39-year-old woman, has recently had surgery, chemotherapy, and radiation for breast cancer. She has read several books dealing with alternative therapies and is eager to use holistic approaches to enhance her own healing.

Question 1:   How would you introduce Ms. Hampton to breath awareness as a beginning approach?

Answer 1:   Basic Responses   Optional Responses

_____

_____

_____

_____

Situation 2:   Mr. Adams, a 47-year-old advertising executive, has had several sessions with you. He has found relaxation and imagery work useful in dealing with job burnout. Today, he is upset because his boss told him in his recent annual evaluation conference that his job performance is unsatisfactory and requires improvement. He says that he is "uptight" and feels "like an accident waiting to happen."

Question 2:   How can you facilitate Mr. Adams' relaxation?

Answer 2:   Basic Responses   Optional Responses

_____

_____

_____

_____

Situation 3:   Ms. Rush, a 65-year-old woman, has hypertension. Before beginning to teach her biofeedback techniques, you are helping her to understand the relaxation process by leading her through several breathing exercises. This is her first session.

Question 3:   To determine the client outcomes of the relaxation interventions, what questions will you ask her in order to evaluate her subjective experiences.

Answer 3:   Basic Responses   Optional Responses

_____

_____

_____

_____

Situation 4:   Mr. Stratman, a 53-year-old man, has decided to incorporate meditation as a relaxation modality into his cardiac fitness program. He is asking you to explain how this will help him, as this is his first attempt at meditation.

Question 4:   What information will you give him?

Answer 4:   Basic Responses   Optional Responses

_____

_____

_____

_____

CHAPTER 24—IMAGERY

 Pause for a moment . . .

❑ *My affirmations and positive self-talk are*
  — *I am prepared for the holistic nursing certification (HNC) examination.*
  — *I can pass the HNC examination with flying colors.*
  — *I can see HNC after my name.*
  — *I can see the HNC certificate hanging in my office.*
❑ *I am so proud that I set this goal and commitment to take the HNC examination.*

Test Questions 1–19

1. Imagery is best defined as
   a. thoughts that arise from our senses.
   b. the attainment of a paranormal state of mind.
   c. a natural means of communication.
   d. an interaction with a higher power.
2. In which area of the brain are images formed?
   a. Hypothalamus.
   b. Limbic system.
   c. Anterior frontal lobe.
   d. Medulla.
3. In which area of the brain are emotions processed?
   a. Hypothalamus.
   b. Cerebral cortex.
   c. Limbic system.
   d. Anterior frontal lobe.
4. The goal of imagery is to
   a. provide a focus for organizing an individual's body-mind-spirit energy toward healing and inner peace.

   b. keep a person's mind busy so as not to concentrate on the problem or event.
   c. increase logical hemispheric functioning that is intense and repetitive.
   d. replace biotechnology that is not effective in the acute care setting.
5. Correct biologic imagery
   a. bubbles up into the imagination, particularly with concentration.
   b. involves general images of various steps and procedures.
   c. implies images as they might appear under a microscope.
   d. is common in daydreaming and deep dream states.
6. Symbolic imagery is
   a. ineffective in stabilizing or reversing a problem/disease.
   b. a metamorphosis of personal images that cannot be forced.
   c. the step-by-step rehearsal of images away from desired outcomes.
   d. the imagery process of interpreting another person's experience.
7. When conducting an imagery session, keep in mind that
   a. it can be dangerous to allow a client to create his or her own images.
   b. imagery generally increases the client's respiratory rate.
   c. it is necessary to obtain specifics about the client's images during a session.
   d. no one can predict what images will occur in the client's imagination.

8. The most powerful images are usually
   a. concrete.
   b. symbolic.
   c. end-state.
   d. general healing.
9. In order to "speak to a body part," the client must use
   a. symbolic imagery.
   b. active imagery.
   c. general healing imagery.
   d. end-state imagery.
10. Which of the following statements about receptive imagery is true?
   a. It is common in hypnagogic sleep.
   b. It can be experienced only in your dreams.
   c. It usually takes the form of an inner guide.
   d. It is the conscious formation of an image.
11. Which of the following statements is true about concrete imagery?
   a. It is unique to each patient.
   b. It is seldom used in guided imagery.
   c. It is usually a precursor to symbolic imagery.
   d. It tends to block the patient's inner healing resources.
12. Mr. Smith, age 42, is anxious about a scheduled computed tomography scan of the head. Which of the following types of imagery would you suggest?
   a. Process imagery.
   b. End-state imagery.
   c. General healing imagery.
   d. Receptive imagery.
13. General healing imagery
   a. focuses on an event, person, or thing of special significance.
   b. usually takes the form of biologically correct images.
   c. helps clients move step by step toward a final, healed state.
   d. allows the client to rehearse being in a final, healed state.
14. Which of the following patients are poor candidates for imagery interventions?
   a. Those with organic brain syndrome.
   b. Those who cannot work with their eyes closed.
   c. Those with no experience using imagery.
   d. Those who are dominantly analytic.
15. Which of the following best describes the most important function of a client's baseline images?

   a. They serve as a standard against which the nurse can assess his or her later images.
   b. They help the nurse evaluate his or her imagery potential.
   c. They indicate which brain hemisphere is dominant.
   d. They tell the nurse what parts of the client are in need of healing.
16. If the client is troubled by distracting thoughts during imagery sessions,
   a. shorten the length of the imagery sessions.
   b. analyze the distracting thoughts.
   c. lengthen the relaxation time before sessions.
   d. obtain orders for an anxiolytic agent.
17. Before beginning an imagery session, the nurse should
   a. make sure the client understands that a deep sleep is the ultimate goal.
   b. tell the client to analyze all images that emerge.
   c. tell the client that uncomfortable images are sometimes the most revealing.
   d. have the client develop a positive expectation of the end result.
18. When intervening with imagery,
   a. limit the sessions to 10 minutes.
   b. continuously assess the patient's state of relaxation.
   c. use the same exercise daily without variation.
   d. focus on the analysis of images.
19. Skilled imagery guides
   a. use long phrases.
   b. avoid the use of metaphors.
   c. offer the client choices.
   d. focus on one sensory modality at a time.

 Pause for a moment . . .

❑ *I am practicing my successful test-taking strategies prior to the HNC examination so that I can remember to use them during the examination.*
❑ *Relaxation and deep breathing exercises decrease my anxiety and tension.*
❑ *Imagery rehearsal of preparing for, seeing myself in the HNC examination environment, feeling relaxed and confident, and successfully passing the HNC examination is exciting.*

Situations 1-4

Situation 1:   Ms. Smith, a 45-year-old woman, seeks your help to learn how to manage her tension head-aches. She returns to you after 1 week of practice with relaxation exercises. She has kept a diary and reports successfully integrating relaxation skill into her daily routine. Today, however, she describes having a very stressful day at the office and being unable to relax. She says that her head feels "like a firecracker getting ready to explode."

Question 1:   How would you introduce Ms. Smith to general imagery and then to receptive and active imagery to decrease her tension headaches?

Answer 1:   Basic Responses   Optional Responses

_____

_____

_____

Situation 2:   Mr. Jones, a 52-year-old man, has known about his cancer for 1 month. He wants to strengthen his imagery skills. He was introduced to relaxation and breathing exercises at a weekend workshop 3 months ago and enjoyed it very much. He has read two books on imagery and is enthusiastic about how he can enhance his own healing.

Question 2:   How can you help him assess his imagery process?

Answer 2:   Basic Responses   Optional Responses

_____

_____

_____

Situation 3:   Mr. Long, a 55-year-old man, had a myocardial infarction 1 month ago and is anxious that he will be a cardiac cripple.

Question 3:   How can you help him with process imagery?

Answer 3:   Basic Responses   Optional Responses

_____

_____

_____

Situation 4:   Jane W., a 16-year-old girl, has been in a full leg cast for 6 weeks and is scheduled for removal of the cast from her left leg. She has moderate anxiety in regard to the cast removal.

Question 4:   Using concrete objective information, how can you help Jane decrease her anxiety?

Answer 4:   Basic Responses   Optional Responses

_____

_____

_____

CHAPTER 25—MUSIC THERAPY

 Pause for a moment . . .

❑ *I am using my distraction techniques.*
  — *Any time worry or fear comes into my mind, I will let go of the anxiety.*
  — *If a thought of failure comes to my mind . . . I take a deep breath, and with the next exhalation I let the worry flow out.*
❑ *I will successfully pass the HNC examination.*

Test Questions 1–15

1. Sound is heard by the human ear when it vibrates between
   a. 16 to 20 cycles/sec.
   b. 16 to 25,000 cycles/sec.
   c. 200 to 50,000 cycles/sec.
   d. 200 to 5,000 cycles/sec.
2. Cymatics refers to the
   a. study of patterns of shapes evoked by sound.
   b. advancing impulses set up by a vibration or impulse.
   c. waves that resonate.
   d. tuning forks designed to vibrate at the same pitch.
3. The following is true about sound as it relates to the human body:
   a. Arterial vessels resonate with all outside stimuli.
   b. Atoms are the only body structures that do not vibrate.
   c. The body is a vibratory transformer.
   d. The body can take in sound but does not emit it.
4. Music therapy is a vehicle for achieving the relaxation response because it
   a. quiets ceaseless thinking.
   b. produces a hypermetabolic response.
   c. is similar to therapeutic touch.
   d. reduces electromagnetic resonance.
5. Music therapy can be used to reach nonordinary states of consciousness by
   a. shortening perception of time.
   b. lengthening perception of time.
   c. stimulating perception of time.
   d. acknowledging perception of time.

6. Because music is nonverbal in nature, it appeals to the
   a. left hemisphere of the brain.
   b. frontal lobe.
   c. cerebral cortex.
   d. right hemisphere of the brain.
7. The following is advisable when helping clients choose appropriate music for a session:
   a. Choose only music with words.
   b. Choose music that is 5 to 7 minutes in length.
   c. Allow the client to choose music of his or her choice.
   d. All of the above.
8. A mingling of the senses during relaxation and music therapy is called
   a. synesthesia.
   b. iso-principle.
   c. resonance.
   d. chakras.
9. Music therapy is used for individuals with a critical illness for the purpose of
   a. entertainment.
   b. communicative music making.
   c. musical enrichment.
   d. psychophysiologic relaxation.
10. To achieve therapeutic outcomes, music therapy should be practiced by patients
    a. 5 minutes every hour.
    b. once a day for 45 minutes.
    c. every other day for 10 minutes.
    d. 20 minutes twice a day.
11. During music therapy sessions, patients are instructed to
    a. concentrate on the music's words, their messages, and their meanings.
    b. analyze the music's rhythm, instruments, and meter.
    c. let the music suggest what to think and what to feel.
    d. become aware of how long, in terms of minutes and seconds, the session lasts.
12. The iso-principle in music therapy refers to
    a. the number of vibrations or cycles per unit of time.
    b. the fluctuation or variation between minimum and maximum values.
    c. a match of the music with the client's physiology, mood, and mind state.

d. an intervention to establish the body's fundamental frequency at 8 cycles/sec.

13. In preparing for a music therapy session, the client should be instructed to
    a. find a comfortable position.
    b. participate in sessions at night before bedtime.
    c. refrain from changing positions.
    d. keep eyeglasses on or contact lenses in.

14. Physiologic outcomes of a relaxed music therapy session include
    a. increased peripheral temperature.
    b. increased respiratory rate.
    c. increased heart rate.
    d. all of the above.

15. The beneficial effects of music therapy usually become apparent to clients

a. immediately during the first session.
b. after 1 year of therapy.
c. after two to three sessions.
d. none of the above.

Pause for a moment . . .

❏ *My special words, a prayer, or a phrase to bring me into the present moment are* _____ .
❏ *As I repeat my special words, prayer, or phrase silently to myself for a few minutes, I feel* _____ .
❏ *I combine these with my rhythmic, relaxed breathing and relaxation.*
❏ *I repeat this for 10 times to deepen being in this present moment.*
❏ *Then I return to my important studying.*

Situations 1–4

Situation 1: Mr. McGee, a 55-year-old man, became claustrophobic during a magnetic resonance imaging (MRI) procedure for visualization of a right parotid mass. Highly anxious, he demanded to be removed from the machine. The MRI was cancelled and rescheduled in a week.

Question 1: How would you help Mr. McGee reduce his fear of the upcoming test and cope with the procedure?

Answer 1: Basic Responses Optional Responses

_____

_____

Situation 2: Mr. Meiers, a 62-year-old chief of military police, was recently admitted to the coronary care unit for an acute myocardial infarction. On the first day of his admission, he continued to have mild chest pain and was diaphoretic, hyperventilating, and highly anxious. He was introduced to music therapy as an intervention to help reduce his stress. Following the second music therapy session, he stated that he was "not doing it right" and did not want to participate in any more music therapy sessions.

Question 2: How might you encourage him to continue his participation in music relaxation during his recovery in the coronary care unit?

Answer 2: Basic Responses Optional Responses

_____

_____

Situation 3:   Ms. O'Brien, a 32-year-old woman, recently learned that she has mild hypertension. She has just taken a job as a nursing unit manager in the emergency department of a large county hospital. She is working long hours because of the demands of the job and admits to overwhelming stress related to her workload. When she returns home from the hospital in the evening, she finds she is unable to unwind and relax following the stress of the day.

Question 3:   How might you help Mrs. O'Brien in findings ways to relax at home following her stressful day at work?

Answer 3:   Basic Responses   Optional Responses

_____   _____

_____   _____

_____   _____

_____   _____

Situation 4:   In the day surgery recovery room, many patients are agitated, vomiting, and anxious upon awakening from their anesthesia. You believe that some form of relaxation might be beneficial for patients in the immediate postoperative period.

Question 4:   How might you set up a postoperative music therapy program in the recovery room?

Answer 4:   Basic Responses   Optional Responses

_____   _____

_____   _____

_____   _____

_____   _____

CHAPTER 26—TOUCH

Pause for a moment . . .

☐ *I have plenty of time to finish the HNC examination.*
☐ *If I lose my concentration, I will use my relaxation, deep breathing, imagery, affirmations, positive self-talk, and distraction.*

Test Questions 1–12

1. Touch therapy is best defined as
   a. a method for curing disease.
   b. a process of working with the emotions and the mind.
   c. specific healing techniques that work with energy.
   d. hand techniques used on or near the body to support a client's movement toward optimal function.

2. Acupressure is a technique that
   a. uses hand motions away from the body.
   b. uses thumb and finger pressure along meridians.
   c. does not require the hands to touch the body.
   d. uses small needles to stimulate energy flow.

3. Intention is best defined as
   a. attention to the situation before you.
   b. attention directed to another time and place.
   c. an outward flow of energy.
   d. motivation for touch established when working with a client.

4. Which is not a common response to therapeutic touch?
   a. Flushed skin.
   b. Deep sighs.
   c. Increased respiration.
   d. Verbalized relaxation.

5. Harlow's studies in the 1950s demonstrated the significance of

a. nutritional therapies with institutionalized babies.

b. effluerage in the growth of premature babies.

c. touch in the development of monkeys.

d. energy healing working with barley seeds.

6. Oskar Estebany was a

a. social scientist working with children who failed to thrive.

b. touch theorist who studied mammal development.

c. healer used in many studies to demonstrate the relationship between touch and maturation.

d. German scientist who discovered a unique healing modality.

7. Nursing studies have confirmed that touch therapies

a. increase heart rate.

b. increase client verbalizations.

c. physically strengthen muscles and joints.

d. decrease systolic blood pressure.

8. Which of the following statements is most accurate?

a. Nurses touch older patients as often as younger ones.

b. Nurses frequently use touch as a nursing comfort measure, especially in critical care units.

c. Less mobile patients responded less positively to touch.

d. Poverty of touch is acute among the elderly.

9. In preparation for an initial touch therapy session, a nurse may be advised to pay attention to

a. centering himself or herself.

b. preparing the environment with soft lighting, proper equipment, and quietude.

c. communicating clearly with the client during the procedure.

d. all of the above.

10. Techniques of therapeutic massage are similar, involving the use of effleurage, petrosauge, and tapotement, which are:

a. hand movements that apply direct pressure to the skin.

b. classic nursing back rub strokes designed to enhance circulation of blood and lymph.

c. techniques to increase heart rate.

d. products that can be used to increase relaxation.

11. In a therapeutic touch session, the nurse stops when

a. there are no noticeable differences in temperature or density.

b. the client falls asleep.

c. the session has lasted 1 hour.

d. there is a physical change in the client's field.

12. Which nursing diagnosis is compatible with touch intervention and relates to the category of perceiving?

a. Altered circulation.

b. Impairment in skin integrity.

c. Altered meaningfulness.

d. Physical mobility impaired.

 Pause for a moment . . .

❑ *I can concentrate during my studying so that I can concentrate during the HNC examination.*

❑ *I focus while I study, and I will focus during the HNC examination.*

❑ *I will finish at my own pace, even when others finish before me.*

Situations 1–2

Situation 1: Ms. Quigley, a 48-year-old woman, had come to the wellness center where you work for therapeutic massage several times prior to the unexpected death of her husband, a prominent leader in the community. She had developed a strong bond with you as you provided therapeutic touch, acupressure, guided imagery, and music therapy. Her major loss, however, has caused her to feel suddenly overwhelmed with demands and decisions. Her friends have tried to cheer her up, but they are uncomfortable with expressions of grief. She has come to see you 1 week after the funeral. Now, rather than physical release alone, her need for emotional release is very strong. She seeks spiritual answers through the modality of touch.

Question 1: How can touch therapies help Ms. Quigley to heal?

Answer 1:   Basic Responses   Optional Responses

_____

_____

_____

_____

Situation 2:   You are working as a school nurse; a teacher brings in a 7-year-old second-grade student who is coughing and apprehensive. Bronchial wheezing is evident. You sit the child upright while providing a few minutes of therapeutic touch. Within minutes, the child's condition dramatically improves. You call the mother, who is amazed at the child's quick recovery, given previous history and multiple visits to the local emergency room. She asks you to teach her what to do in the future when this occurs.

Question 2:   How can you support this mother and child and help them to minimize the number of future emergency room visits?

Answer 2:   Basic Responses   Optional Responses

_____

_____

_____

_____

CHAPTER 27—WEIGHT MANAGEMENT

 Pause for a moment . . .

❑ *I am eating nourishing food and will do so before the HNC examination. Complex carbohydrate foods will provide me with the most energy.*

❑ *I am avoiding excessive use of caffeine or sugar right now and will continue to do so before the HNC examination.*

❑ *I am relaxed and at ease and will arrive at the HNC examination in this same relaxed state.*

Test Questions 1–15

1. What is the difference between being overweight and being overfat?
   a. Fat and muscle weigh approximately the same, so there is no real difference.
   b. Overweight is a body weight 10 to 20 percent above ideal or body mass index ranging from 25 to 29, while overfat is a percentage of body fat more than 28 percent for women and 20 percent for men.
   c. People who are overfat will also be overweight.
   d. Overweight is a body weight more than 20 percent above ideal or body mass index ranging from 20 to 25, while overfat is a percentage of body fat more than 25 for women and 15 for men.
2. Weight cycling is
   a. progressive difficulty maintaining weight loss from multiple dieting attempts.
   b. continuous weight gain and loss for unknown reasons.
   c. vacillation within a 10-pound weight range below and above ideal weight for height.
   d. cycles of weight gain and loss in the past year.
3. Set point theory, a biologic theory of obesity, states that
   a. hypermetabolic drugs can permanently reset metabolic rate.
   b. a set amount of weight is determined by the number of fat cells at birth.
   c. weight gain is caused by caloric intake greater than work expended.

d. body weight returns to about the same weight no matter how many diets a person attempts.

4. Cognitive theories of obesity focus on
   a. overeating behaviors as totally determined by learned responses.
   b. negative self-talk that triggers the desire to eat and overeat.
   c. self-monitoring and response control that can correct most overeating.
   d. negative body images that can contaminate the self-concept to drive overeating behaviors.

5. Reversal theory, a phenomenologic theory of arousal, motivation, and action, states that
   a. individuals' behaviors are determined by eight ways of being, all in effect at any given time.
   b. individuals' behaviors are determined by a chain reaction of first being aroused, which causes them to be motivated, and finally causes them to act.
   c. individuals' behaviors are inconsistent because they view life choices from two different perspectives.
   d. individuals' behaviors are caused by whether they believe that they can perform a certain action or not.

6. Reversal theory states that
   a. Motivations can be determined by removing the metalevel state associated with each state.
   b. Motivations are experienced from the degree to which individuals are aroused.
   c. Motivations are experienced in four pairs of opposing states.
   d. Motivations are determined by the cognitions in effect at the time.

7. Name the metamotivational opposing states associated with being strong and tough versus being tender and nurturing.
   a. Mastery and sympathy.
   b. Alloic and autic.
   c. Telic and paratelic.
   d. Conformist and negativistic.

8. Tension stress is
   a. the stress response of epinephrine release followed by muscular rigidity.
   b. the multiple daily hassles that irritate individuals.
   c. the suppression or enhancement of motivation by stressors.
   d. the unpleasant feeling of not feeling the way you want to feel.

9. Unidimensional, traditional treatments for obesity fail because they do not

a. address boredom in complying with food restrictions and exercise.
b. concurrently address the multiple bio-psycho-social and spiritual reasons for weight gain.
c. help motivate individuals to lose weight.
d. take a family systems approach to weight control.

10. A multidimensional treatment for overweight/ obesity is
    a. controlled dietary intake and exercise prescriptions.
    b. a psychotherapeutic model for stress eating.
    c. a cognitive–behavioral and aerobic exercise approach.
    d. holistic self-care for permanent weight control.

11. A basic principle of a multidimensional weight loss program is that
    a. clients must be in ultimate control of life changes since permanent weight loss takes a long time.
    b. stimulating all senses will maximize learning new eating habits.
    c. physicians, nurses, and nutritionists should all provide weight loss prescriptions.
    d. nurses' assessments, diagnoses, and prescriptions will be the primary driving force of a successful weight loss program.

12. Dieting as a means to lose weight
    a. can lower metabolic rate and cause feelings of deprivation that set clients up for failure.
    b. should be prescribed and monitored by a registered dietitian.
    c. must be the core of a total weight loss program.
    d. can be alternated with periods of time of higher caloric intake to avoid lowering metabolic rate.

13. A consistent, challenging exercise prescription that will eventually raise basal metabolic rate is
    a. aerobic exercise 5 to 7 days per week.
    b. brisk walk/run two times per week, alternating with 15 minutes of floor exercises two times per week.
    c. different aerobic exercises three to four times per week alternating with different types of weight lifting two to three times per week.
    d. strength training 6 to 7 days per week.

14. Cognitive restructuring, or positive self-talk, helps make permanent lifestyle changes that promote weight loss and maintenance because it
    a. replaces negative behaviors such as overeating to cope.

b. reprograms negative self-talk that causes unpleasant feelings that trigger overeating.

c. serves as a pneumonic device to replace negative self-talk.

d. reprograms by subliminal suggestions during relaxation training.

15. The four steps to stop overeating are as follows:

a. Eat only when your stomach growls, eat according to the food pyramid, eat consciously, and stop when you are satisfied.

b. Eat every 2 to 3 hours, eat small meals and snacks, eat according to behavior modification principles, and stop when you feel full.

c. Eat only 3 meals and 1 snack, eat a balanced diet with low fat, eat slowly, and stop when you feel nothing.

d. Eat only when hungry; eat exactly what your body wants; eat slowly, enjoying every bite; and stop when your hunger is gone.

Pause for a moment . . .

❑ *I will be physically rested by getting a good night's rest before the HNC examination.*

❑ *I am going to monitor my responsibilities the week of the HNC examination so that I arrive rested and free of worry.*

Situations 1–4

Situation 1: Ms. Smith, a 33-year-old woman, seeks help losing weight. She has an 8-year history of yo–yo dieting. She says, "Oh just tell me what to do, and I'll follow what you say exactly!"

Question 1: What basic assessments do you make if you subscribe to the holistic self-care model for permanent weight control?

Answer 1: Basic Responses   Optional Responses

_____

_____

_____

_____

Situation 2: Ms. Summers tells you that she used to run, swim, and be very physically fit until she had her two children and got so busy with her part-time job.

Question 2: What exercise prescriptions do you make with her, based on the holistic self-care model for permanent weight control?

Answer 2: Basic Responses   Optional Responses

_____

_____

_____

_____

Situation 3: Ms. Rolland, a 52-year-old woman, recently gained 20 pounds after she went on hormone replacement for menopause; she had never had a weight problem before. She relates having learned a lot about herself from the past 10 years in psychotherapy, and now she asks for help with weight control.

Question 3: Using the holistic self-care model, how do you set up a total program for Ms. Rolland?

Answer 3:   Basic Responses   Optional Responses

_____

_____

_____

Situation 4:   Mr. Harris, a 67-year-old, newly diagnosed Type II diabetic, seeks help with his stress eating. He relates that his weight gain has become worse since he retired 2 years ago.

Question 4:   What prescriptions can you make for Mr. Harris, based on the holistic self-care model?

Answer 4:   Basic Responses   Optional Responses

_____

_____

_____

_____

CHAPTER 28—SMOKING CESSATION

Pause for a moment . . .

❑ *I can imagine that today is the day of the HNC examination.*
❑ *I am arriving for the HNC examination physically and mentally prepared.*
❑ *I am proud of my accomplishments!*

Test Questions 1–15

1. Smoking is best defined as
   a. the use of tobacco.
   b. a natural means for reducing body weight.
   c. inhalation of tobacco burned in cigarettes for nicotine absorption.
   d. chewing tobacco leaves.
2. Smoking cessation is best defined as
   a. stopping the use of cigarettes, cigars, pipes, and all continuous tobacco intake.
   b. ceasing the use of tobacco in social situations only.
   c. throwing out all smoking paraphernalia.
   d. getting rid of cigarettes in automobiles.
3. Smoking is a factor in three of the five leading causes of death in the United States today. The three types of death associated with smoking include
   a. cancer, syphilis, meningomyelocele.
   b. HIV, cancer, AIDS.
   c. heart disease, cancer, inflammation of the abdomen.
   d. heart disease, cancer, chronic obstructive pulmonary disease.
4. Acute cardiovascular problems such as the following can affect smokers:
   a. Tachycardia.
   b. Increased blood pressure.
   c. Hypercholesterolemia.
   d. All of the above.
5. There is increased thrombotic potential in smokers because smoking
   a. increases platelet aggregation in the blood.
   b. enlarges the red blood cells.
   c. thickens the blood.
   d. decreases the oxygen transport capacity of red blood cells.
6. The addicting drug used in tobacco is
   a. acetylene.
   b. carbon monoxide.
   c. nicotine.
   d. nupreime.

7. Nicotine simulates an adrenergic state; thus,
   a. nicotine production from the adrenal glands increases.
   b. heart rate and cardiac contractility increase.
   c. production of insulin from the pancreas is enhanced.
   d. sputum output decreases.
8. An increase in low-density lipoproteins and a decrease in high-density lipoproteins can result in
   a. diabetes mellitus.
   b. Hashimoto's syndrome.
   c. hypercholesterolemia.
   d. Raynaud's disease.
9. Nicotine withdrawal symptoms generally include all of the following, except
   a. insomnia.
   b. conjunctivitis.
   c. headaches.
   d. constipation.
10. The "new vital sign" is
    a. blood pressure.
    b. circulatory status.
    c. smoking status.
    d. pulse oximeter.
11. The five stages of smoking cessation (behavioral change) include
    a. precontemplation, contemplation, preparation, action, and maintenance.
    b. precontemplation, contemplation, preparation, announcement, and maintenance.
    c. precontemplation, contemplation, programming, announcement, and maintenance.
    d. precontemplation, contemplation, programming, action, and maintenance.
12. At a minimum, a smoking diary should include
    a. date, time, cigarette brand.
    b. date, time, activity, perception of cigarette.
    c. date, time, activity, social support group.
    d. date, time, activity, perception of urgency for cigarette.
13. Guidelines relating intervention intensity to time factors include the following:
    a. Intervention should last at least 2 weeks.
    b. Sessions should last at least 20 to 30 minutes.
    c. There should be four to seven sessions at a minimum.
    d. All of the above.
14. The following factors contribute to continued smoking status:
    a. nicotine addiction.
    b. psychosocial reasons.
    c. habitual cues.
    d. all of the above.
15. Smokers are in the action stage of smoking cessation or behavioral change when they
    a. entertain thoughts about quitting.
    b. actively endeavor to promote smoking cessation and abstinence for at least 6 months.
    c. experience continued smoking abstinence beginning 6 months after cessation.
    d. are ready and open to advice about smoking cessation.

 Pause for a moment . . .

❑ *If I do not know an answer, I make a reasonable guess. "Intuition" and "hunches" are often correct answers.*
❑ *I understand that the HNC examination is based on the **AHNA Core Curriculum.***

Situations 1–4

Situation 1: Mr. Redford, a 45-year-old man, seeks help with smoking cessation. He has thought about quitting cigarettes and has even made two attempts, but resumed smoking after only 2 days in each case.

Question 1: How can you help him with more long-term smoking cessation and abstinence? Where is Mr. Redford in terms of the stages of smoking cessation/behavioral change? What are your suggestions for moving him into the next stage?

Answer 1:   Basic Responses   Optional Responses

Situation 2: Ms. Vines, a 23-year-old woman, requests a routine physical examination. She appears quite healthy, is single, and has no family. She has an odor of cigarette smoke about her person.

Question 2: What kind of assessment questions do you ask her? How can you begin to help her with smoking cessation?

Answer 2: Basic Responses   Optional Responses

_____

_____

_____

_____

Situation 3: Fred W., a 19-year-old high school student, has no plans, interests, or hobbies. He likes to hang out with the guys (mostly younger). He appears to be healthy but needs a physical examination for a part-time job. The assessment of smoking status as the new vital sign finds Fred to be a current, heavy smoker, smoking two packs per day.

Question 3: What is your assessment? How can you initiate interventions with Fred?

Answer 3: Basic Responses   Optional Responses

_____

_____

_____

_____

Situation 4: Ms. Stowe, a 58-year-old woman, is afraid to stop smoking. She smokes 15 cigarettes per day "to keep her weight down." Smoking also helps her concentrate on her job as a realtor, reduces her stress, and boosts her self-confidence.

Question 4: Has Ms. Stowe reached a particular stage for smoking cessation? How can you educate her and what interventions will she need to stop smoking?

Answer 4: Basic Responses   Optional Responses

_____

_____

_____

_____

CHAPTER 29—OVERCOMING ADDICTIONS

 Pause for a moment . . .

❑ *I answer the question before I look at the choices.*
❑ *I then look for the answer that is similar to the one that I generated.*

Test Questions 1–12

1. Addiction is characterized by
   a. loss of control over the use of alcohol and other drugs.
   b. periodic experimentation with drugs.
   c. frequent social use of alcohol.
   d. insight into the problems it creates.

2. Drug use usually continues in an individual when
   a. there is some curiosity about the drug.
   b. the drug taking produces a pleasurable effect.
   c. the drug has been forbidden by others.
   d. people make the drug available.

3. What percentage of the population is estimated to have a drug-related disorder?
   a. 1 to 9 percent.
   b. 15 to 25 percent.
   c. 25 to 50 percent.
   d. Less than 1 percent.

4. Which of the following is a risk factor for the development of addiction?
   a. Availability of multiple social networks.
   b. Involvement in extracurricular activities at school.
   c. Family chaos and inconsistency.
   d. High expectations and goal setting.

5. An example of a resiliency factor in the prevention of addiction-related problems is
   a. nonuse of illegal drugs.
   b. avoidance of cigarette smoking while drinking.
   c. fear of becoming an alcoholic "like Dad."
   d. a relationship with a caring adult role model.

6. Which of the following is not a protective/resiliency factor for prevention of addiction?
   a. Self-discipline.
   b. Sense of humor.
   c. Past history of alcohol abuse.
   d. Critical thinking skills.

7. Increasing resiliency factors to prevent addiction problems means
   a. avoiding harmful chemicals.
   b. treating the person before the use becomes abuse.
   c. helping develop healthy behaviors and support systems.
   d. identifying risk factors for addiction.

8. Which of the following theoretical models best explains the development of addiction as an outcome of repeated experiences in which addictive substances are used to solve stressful situations?
   a. Neurobiologic theory.
   b. Intraperson theory.
   c. Learning theory.
   d. Ultradian stress syndrome.

9. An effective screening tool specifically designed for adolescents is the
   a. CAGE.
   b. Trauma Scale.
   c. RAFFT.
   d. Brief MAST.

10. Which of the following would not be a priority during the detoxification phase?
    a. Provide opportunities to rehearse coping skills.
    b. Provide comfort measures.
    c. Assess patient thoroughly.
    d. Use acupuncture to minimize central nervous system responses.

11. Guided imagery of which type would be most likely to help a client reconnect with spiritual resources?
    a. Active images.
    b. End-state images.
    c. Healing images.
    d. Process images.

12. What would help a client who is in a 12-step recovery program deal with the stresses of everyday life?
    a. Expose the client to situations in which alcohol is present, so the client can get used to being around it without needing to drink.
    b. Teach the client to use rhythmic breathing, aromatherapy, and massage.
    c. Tell the client to sleep more than usual so he does not get physically sick.
    d. Let the client find his own ways of managing stress as he learns to use his recovery program strategies.

 Pause for a moment . . .

❑ *I look for key words in questions because these words give me clues to the correct answer.*
— *These are such words as "except," "not," or "but."*
— *Words such as "most," "next," or "first" indicate the order of steps or the priority.*

Situations 1–4

Situation 1:   Suzanne V., a 14-year-old girl, seeks your help in learning to manage headaches. She tells you that she is worried about her 19-year-old brother, who has started to experiment with cocaine. As she worries more about him, her headaches get more severe.

Question 1:   How can you assess Suzanne's risk and protective factors regarding her own potential for developing problems with addiction?

Answer 1:   Basic Responses   Optional Responses

_____

_____

_____

_____

Situation 2:   Mr. Logan, a 30-year-old sales representative, has asked you to help him learn to manage the stresses he feels in his job. He says he is particularly worried about himself, because his mother's alcoholism led to his parents' divorce.

Question 2:   What interventions would you carry out to help Mr. Logan develop healthy ways of coping with stress?

Answer 2:   Basic Responses   Optional Responses

_____

_____

_____

_____

Situation 3:   Mr. Martin, a 38-year-old man, has completed an inpatient detoxification process and a 4-week intensive outpatient treatment program for his addiction to alcohol, tobacco, and sedatives.

Question 3:   How can you help him with his recovery program to overcome his addictions?

Answer 3:   Basic Responses   Optional Responses

_____

_____

_____

_____

Situation 4:   Ms. Johnson, a 25-year-old registered nurse, has just acknowledged that she is dependent on narcotics.

Question 4:   How can you help her to overcome her addiction and return to work?

Answer 4:   Basic Responses   Optional Responses

_____

_____

_____

_____

CHAPTER 30—INCEST/CHILD SEXUAL ABUSE AND VIOLENCE

 Pause for a moment . . .

❑ *I do not read meaning into a question.*
❑ *I understand all the words in the question.*
❑ *I recognize when a word in a question is not familiar, and I try to figure out the meaning based on the context in which it appears in the question.*

Test Questions 1–14

1. Grounding is related to staying in the
   a. present.
   b. past.
   c. future.
   d. none of the above.
2. When having a flashback, the person
   a. forgets the present.
   b. remembers the abuse vividly.
   c. relives the abuse as it originally happened.
   d. understands what happened long ago.
3. The universal taboo against incest is supported by
   a. biologic arguments.
   b. economic arguments.
   c. sociologic arguments.
   d. all of the above.
4. Freud's retraction of his seduction theory resulted in
   a. widespread media attention to the problem of incest.
   b. loss of public knowledge about incest for half a century.
   c. increased interest by psychiatrists in incest.
   d. no effect on the problem of incest.
5. The current incidence data for incest is
   a. 1:7 girls and 1:10 boys.
   b. 1:4 girls and 1:7 boys.

   c. 1:4 girls and 1:10 boys.
   d. 1:7 girls and 1:4 boys.
6. The most common emotional/behavioral consequence of incest/abuse is
   a. anxiety.
   b. grief.
   c. depression.
   d. guilt.
7. Physical symptoms experienced by survivors are
   a. not usually too bothersome.
   b. a challenge to precise medical diagnosis.
   c. usually limited to one organ system.
   d. usually just psychosomatic in origin.
8. Sexual dysfunction, a physical consequence of incest/abuse, may manifest as
   a. sexual promiscuity.
   b. sexual abstinence.
   c. fear of physical touch.
   d. all of the above.
9. In assessing the client's condition, the nurse must
   a. wait for the client to introduce the subject of abuse.
   b. take the responsibility for moving the history taking quickly along.
   c. use good communication techniques.
   d. change the subject if the client seems uncomfortable.
10. The life domains useful for additional assessment data include
    a. social, spiritual, physical.
    b. physical, sexual, genetic.
    c. psychologic/emotional, familial, economic.
    d. sense of self, relation to men, relation to women.
11. The nursing diagnosis valuing relates to
    a. self-worth.
    b. spiritual well-being.
    c. coping.
    d. powerlessness.

12. The most important characteristic of the nursing plan is that it is
    a. co-created with the client.
    b. precisely written.
    c. neatly typed.
    d. no longer than 5 pages.
13. A sign that the client is dissociating is that he or she
    a. talks so rapidly it is difficult to understand him or her.
    b. stops talking in the middle of a sentence.
    c. has an animated effect.
    d. makes and holds eye contact.
14. Which of the following statements is not true about empowerment?
    a. Nurses should collaborate with the client in planning.

b. Nurses need not be experts in order to empower clients.
c. Disclosure of abuse is not a necessary step.
d. Teaching is an important part of empowering the client.

 Pause for a moment . . .

❑ *As I read the question, I understand that I am being asked to identify priorities, to determine the best intervention, or to evaluate outcomes.*
❑ *I read each question carefully. I do not rush.*
❑ *I develop my skills to understand the question being asked.*

Situations 1–4

Situation 1: Ms. Jones, a 30-year-old woman, is seeking help in dealing with recently recovered memories of incest. Her daughter has just celebrated her 5th birthday, the exact age at which Ms. Jones' abuse began at the hands of her father (a birthday "present"). Ms. Jones has told no one about her recovered memory, but she is sleeping poorly, having nightmares, and her husband is concerned.

Question 1: How would you go about preparing to plan Ms. Jones' care?

Answer 1: Basic Responses   Optional Responses

_____

_____

_____

Situation 2: Ms. Smith, a 50-year-old woman, is seeking help in dealing with her anger. She was sexually abused by her father from the time she was 9 years old until she left home for college. Although she never returned home, she has not forgotten the terror she lived in for so many years. She has been married and divorced four times. She has no children. Her father and mother were recently killed in an automobile accident. She says that she is frequently overcome by feelings of rage that leave her exhausted and ill. She is afraid that if this continues, she will be unable to retain her teaching position at a local high school.

Question 2: How can you help Ms. Smith deal with her anger?

Answer 2: Basic Responses   Optional Responses

_____

_____

_____

Situation 3: Laurie W. is a 19-year-old freshman in college who reports that she feels guilty all the time and is very worried about everything, especially her mother. She recently moved out of the family home into a small apartment, much to her mother's distress. She confided to you that she moved because her stepfather sexually abused her every day after school before her mother returned from work. This went on for more than 10 years. She says that she has met a young man at school who seems interested in her, and she just had to get away from her stepfather. Her mother does not know about the abuse. She says that she loves her mother and does not want to hurt her.

Question 3:   How can you empower this young woman so she can deal with this situation?

Answer 3:   Basic Responses   Optional Responses

_____

_____

_____

_____

Situation 4:   Mr. Jackson, a 36-year-old man, is seeking help in dealing with the emotional pain associated with sexual abuse by his older brother when he was in his early teens. He describes himself as gay and is in a loving relationship with a man about his own age. He is a talented writer, but feels that he has not lived up to his potential because of his inner turmoil and pain.

Question 4:   How can you help this man deal with his pain?

Answer 4:   Basic Responses   Optional Responses

_____

_____

_____

_____

Answers to Practice Examinations

Answers—Chapter 1

Answers to Test Questions 1–15

1. b	6. b	11. d
2. c	7. c	12. d
3. b	8. c	13. b
4. b	9. d	14. d
5. c	10. a	15. d

Answers to Situations 1–4

Question 1 Responses

Basic Responses (in any order)

A. AHNA Description of Holistic Nursing.
B. AHNA Standards of Holistic Nursing Practice.

Optional Responses (in any order)

1. Compare and contrast allopathic and holistic models.
2. Discuss the mind/body dilemma.
3. Explore the eras of medicine.
4. Discuss the mission and research of the Office of Alternative Medicine (OAM) at the National Institutes of Health (NIH).
5. Compare and contrast the bio-psycho-social model and the bio-psycho-social-spiritual model.
6. Explore the impact of meaning on an individual's response to well-being and illness.
7. Discuss other AHNA documents, such as the AHNA Position Statements on Holistic Ethics and A Healthy Environment.
8. Show videos that address holistic nursing.
9. Explore the integration of relationship-centered care.
10. Introduce the AHNA Position Statements on Holistic Ethics and A Healthy Environment.

Question 2 Responses

Basic Responses (in any order)

A. Compare and contrast allopathic and holistic models.
B. Discuss the mind/body dilemma.
C. Discuss the AHNA Description of Holistic Nursing.
D. Explain the AHNA Standards of Holistic Nursing Practice.

Optional Responses (in any order)

1. Explore the eras of medicine.
2. Discuss the mission and research of the Office of Complementary and Alternative Medicine (OCAM) at the National Institutes of Health (NIH).
3. Compare and contrast the bio-psycho-social model and the bio-psycho-social-spiritual model.
4. Explore the impact of meaning on an individual's response to well-being and illness.
5. Explore the integration of relationship-centered care.

Question 3 Responses

Basic Responses (in any order)

A. Determine which caring–healing modalities are accepted and covered by your state nurse practice act. Determine which caring–healing modalities are considered complementary and alternative therapies.
B. Explore the most common caring–healing modalities used by nurses.
C. Get a consensus of the caring–healing modalities that the staff wants to learn first.

Optional Responses (in any order)

1. Find out which nurses want to participate in the teaching process.
2. Invite staff nurses or guest speakers to describe the caring–healing modalities that they use in various clinical settings.
3. Explore various holistic nursing theorists and related research and the implications for clinical practice.
4. Analyze holistic nursing process.
5. Explore the psychophysiology of bodymind healing.
6. Analyze the components addressed in transpersonal human caring and healing, spirituality and healing, and energetic healing.
7. Invite nurse researchers to introduce their holistic research and its implications for clinical practice.
8. Introduce nurses to the AHNA position statements on holistic ethics and a healthy environment.
9. Start brown bag lunch sessions as a way to introduce different caring modalities.
10. Obtain AHNA Networker Guidelines and start a local AHNA Network in the community.
11. Provide nurses with ways to obtain additional holistic training through AHNA certificate courses and AHNA certification in holistic nursing.

Question 4 Responses

Basic Responses (in any order)

A. Encourage nurses to integrate caring–healing strategies in their own lives.
B. Empower nurses to take morning, lunch, and afternoon breaks during the workday.
C. Announce a date, time, and place for a brown bag lunch session to share holistic nursing practices and personal healing journeys.
D. Begin a local AHNA network in your community.
E. Encourage the exchange of caring–healing exemplars within the hospital.
F. Show videos that address holistic nursing.

Optional Responses (in any order)

1. Explore the three relationships addressed in relationship-centered care.
2. Discuss ways to develop patient–practitioner relationships.
3. Discuss ways to develop community–practitioner relationships.
4. Discuss ways to develop practitioner–practitioner relationships.
5. Explore different strategies for creating relationship-centered care.

ANSWERS—CHAPTER 2

Answers to Test Questions 1–15

1. d	6. d	11. d
2. a	7. c	12. c
3. b	8. a	13. a
4. d	9. b	14. d
5. d	10. b	15. b

Answers to Situations 1–4

Question 1 Responses

Basic Responses (in any order)

A. Center yourself in a healing, caring consciousness before and while you meet with him.
B. Discuss with him what he means by "winning the battle."
C. Assess what he is already doing for his care.
D. Determine if he makes any distinction between being cured of HIV infection and healing.
E. Ask him if he has specific ideas about how he wants you to help him.

Optional Responses (in any order)

1. Give Mr. Smith information about a variety of healing/caring modalities so that he can begin to make informed choices.
2. Offer him the opportunity to experience one or more of these (e.g., Therapeutic Touch, meditation, imagery).
3. Explain to him that you are not the "healer" but are eager to walk with him on his journey toward wholeness and healing.

Question 2 Responses

Basic Responses (in any order)

A. Center yourself in a healing, caring consciousness before and while you meet with her.
B. Explore with Ms. Jones her current understanding of "holistic."
C. Begin to explore with Ms. Jones her hopes and expectations from the use of a holistic approach.
D. Help correct any misunderstandings of the holistic model based on your knowledge of nursing and related theories.

Optional Responses (in any order)

1. Begin to explore the relationship that she has with her illness: Is she fighting it? Befriending it? Ignoring it?
2. Explore with her the concepts of wholeness and healing versus curing.
3. Determine if she makes any distinction between being cured of multiple sclerosis and healing.
4. Explain to her that you are not the "healer" but will be with her to help, support, and guide her on her journey.
5. Offer to do a Healing Touch or Therapeutic Touch treatment for her.

Question 3 Responses

Basic Responses (in any order)

A. Center yourself in a healing, caring consciousness before and while you meet with Ms. Lindsey.
B. Collect more data on her history of hypertension and any other approaches that she has tried or is currently using.
C. Explore her understanding of "energy work" and what she hopes to gain through it.
D. Correct any misunderstandings or unreasonable expectations of such approaches.

E. Explain that "energy work" and holistic nursing do not replace her standard care as prescribed by a physician or nurse practitioner.
F. Offer to do a Healing Touch or Therapeutic Touch treatment for her.

Optional Responses (in any order)

1. Assess her lifestyle, daily habits of exercise, diet, prayer, work, and family responsibilities.
2. Assess what self-care strategies she uses.
3. Review current literature on alternative and complementary therapies for hypertension.

Question 4 Responses

Basic Responses (in any order)

A. Center yourself in a healing, caring consciousness before and while you meet with Mr. Hines.
B. Maintain a safe, loving space for him to talk about his responses to the news.
C. Follow his lead in where and how his sharing unfolds, remembering that it is his process and you are only the midwife.
D. Let him know that while there may be no further medical options for treatment of his cancer, there is still something he can do for his healing.
E. Assure him that you will help him walk this path and will not abandon him.

Optional Responses (in any order)

1. Assess his beliefs about his illness, healing, and the difference between healing and curing.
2. Begin to explore potential healing/caring approaches that he may find useful.
3. Open up the discussion to include an exploration of his spiritual belief system and ways that it may help him to deal with this situation.
4. Offer to do Healing Touch or Therapeutic Touch for him as a nurturing and comforting measure.

ANSWERS—CHAPTER 3

Answers to Test Questions 1–20

1. d	8. c	15. c
2. b	9. d	16. d
3. a	10. b	17. a
4. a	11. a	18. d
5. b	12. b	19. b
6. c	13. a	20. c
7. d	14. b	

Answers to Situations 1–5

Question 1 Responses

Basic Responses (in any order)

A. Conduct a whole person assessment.
B. Refer family for counseling.

Optional Responses (in any order)

1. Suggest nutritional modifications, such as the elimination of sugar, red food dye, preservatives, natural sweeteners, and fruit juices.
2. Provide emotional support.
3. Use relaxation, imagery interventions.
4. Offer counseling for parents/family.
5. Educate the parents about smoking hazards for him.
6. Teach the family nurturing skills; demonstrate energy unruffling and balance.
7. Recommend physical activity, such as daily time outside with parents.

Question 2 Responses

Basic Responses (in any order)

A. Conduct a whole person assessment.
B. Make a referral to counselor.

Optional Responses (in any order)

1. Provide social support and family therapy.
2. Co-create realistic expectations and individual plan of care.
3. Provide emotional support.
4. Use relaxation and interventions.
5. Teach life management skills.

Question 3 Responses

Basic Responses (in any order)

A. Conduct a whole person/couple assessment.
B. Make a referral to holistic physician.

Optional Responses (in any order)

1. Teach life management skills.
2. Teach relaxation response and intellectual repatterning.
3. Provide energy balancing, healing touch, therapeutic touch.
4. Provide social support.
5. Encourage counseling to keep communication open.

Question 4 Responses

Basic Responses (in any order)

A. Provide support during the postoperative time.
B. Offer a referral to complementary practitioners.

Optional Responses (in any order)

1. Provide energy balancing, healing touch, therapeutic touch before surgery.
2. Offer nutritional counseling.
3. Use relaxation and imagery interventions.
4. Demonstrate breathing techniques and meditation.

Question 5 Responses

Basic Responses (in any order)

A. Conduct a whole person assessment.
B. Refer the patient to hospice.

Optional Responses (in any order)

1. Conduct a whole family assessment of attitudes and beliefs about the mother's condition.
2. Provide physical interventions; provide pain relief, using medications as appropriate.
3. Offer spiritual interventions, such as a ritual to help make this time of transition sacred.
4. Use energy balancing, massage.
5. Offer art therapy.
6. Ensure as natural an environment as possible.

ANSWERS—CHAPTER 4

Answers to Test Questions 1–20

1. d	8. c	15. c
2. f	9. b	16. c
3. e	10. c	17. c
4. c	11. a	18. c
5. a	12. c	19. a
6. g	13. c	20. b
7. b	14. b	

Answers to Situations 1–4

Question 1 Responses

Basic Responses (in any order)

A. Social support system.
B. Attitude, beliefs about health.

Optional Responses (in any order)

1. Willingness to seek health advice.
2. Willingness to accept health advice.
3. Perception of the seriousness of the injury.
4. Perception of susceptibility to harm and vulnerability because of the injury.
5. Perception of the benefits of better nutrition, exercise, and safety strategies regarding mobility.
6. Perception of the degree of interference with role function of new behaviors.

Question 2 Responses

Basic Response

A. Contemplation. Although in the past healthy behaviors have replaced problem behaviors for longer than 6 months past the action stage, Mr. Jones has suffered a relapse and is now in the contemplation stage again.

Optional Responses (in any order)

1. Efforts are directed toward moving into the action stage.
2. The process of change that might be useful at this stage is self-reevaluation.

Question 3 Responses

Basic Responses (in any order)

A. Health is defined as role performance and absence of disease.
B. Earl sees health-illness as on a continuum.

Optional Responses (in any order)

1. Cognitive theme is that health is manageable rather than unmanageable.
2. Health-illness has power/fear affective themes.
3. Health-illness changes to wellness-illness through body changes.

Question 4 Responses

Basic Responses (in any order)

A. Needs assessment or the needs of the employees.
B. Components of established programs that are successful.
C. Current health practices.
D. Research and program evaluation methods.
E. Marketing.
F. Health care reimbursement.

Optional Responses (in any order)

1. Ways to involve retired employees.
2. Ways to involve families and significant others.
3. Barriers to motivation:
   — Self-doubt and fear of the unknown.
   — Belief that higher priority projects leave too little time for learning or implementing the new behavior.
   — Dislike of the new behavior.
   — Previously unsuccessful attempts to change behavior.
   — Lack of confidence.
   — Cultural beliefs in conflict with the new behavior.
   — Lack of social support.

ANSWERS—CHAPTER 5

Answers to Test Questions 1–20

1. a	8. c	15. a
2. d	9. b	16. c
3. c	10. a	17. a
4. b	11. d	18. b
5. c	12. c	19. a
6. a	13. b	20. c
7. a	14. b	

Answers to Situations 1–4

Question 1 Responses

Basic Responses (in any order)

A. Assess what the doctor told the patient about his condition and what treatment she prescribed.
B. Ask him what he thinks raises his blood pressure.
C. Ask him what he would like to happen in regard to his blood pressure.
D. Explain that there are a variety of interventions to control blood pressure effectively.

E. Determine which approach to relaxation would be most suitable and provide an opportunity for him to experience its effects.
F. Have him describe a typical workday and help him find ways to incorporate relaxation into his schedule.
G. Develop a plan for both of you to evaluate the effectiveness of the interventions.

Optional Responses (in any order)

1. Help him become aware of events that tend to elevate his blood pressure.
2. Help him reframe situations to reduce their negative influence on his blood pressure.

Question 2 Responses

Basic Responses (in any order)

A. Assess her general sleep patterns, including what she identifies as the source of her problem.
B. Ask her to keep a sleep diary for 3 to 7 days, including a description of her sleep environment.
C. Identify which sleep practice may be adversely influencing her sleep.
D. Explain the pattern of the natural, biologic rhythms common to humans and their role in ensuring restful sleep.
E. Make appropriate suggestions for promoting restful sleep; have her test them and record the results in her sleep diary.

Optional Responses (in any order)

1. Have her also keep a food and activity diary for 3 to 7 days.
2. Examine the patterns as recorded in the diary with her and explore any changes that may promote restful sleep.
3. Affirm her efforts to adopt healthful practices.

Question 3 Responses

Basic Responses (in any order)

A. Assess her perception of the pain.
B. Determine the amount and time at which pain medication was last given.
C. Give her pain medication along with a relaxation exercise.
D. Lower the lights, give her a back rub, and listen to her comments.

E. Allow her to express her feelings about the cancer being out of remission, if she wishes to do so.

Optional Responses (in any order)

1. Ask, "What do you think is making your pain worse?"
2. Determine if there is a special person with whom she would like to talk.
3. Develop nursing interventions to return some control to Ms. Jones.
4. Assess what is most important to her at this time.

Question 4 Responses

Basic Responses (in any order)

A. Arrange to spend some time with Jimmy alone.
B. Acknowledge Jimmy's anger and pain and support him by telling him that his is a normal reaction.
C. Invite him to hit the pillow, cry, scream, or do anything else that will help him discharge his emotion in an acceptable manner.
D. Accept and encourage any and all of Jimmy's emotions.
E. Support his anticipatory grieving about the possibility of losing his leg.

Optional Responses (in any order)

1. Help Jimmy identify ways that he can maintain some control over his life.
2. Determine what it means to Jimmy to lose his leg.
3. At the appropriate time, provide information about rehabilitation and prostheses.
4. Provide movies and biographies of heroes who are physically challenged.

ANSWERS—CHAPTER 6

Answers to Test Questions 1–14

1. b	6. a	11. e
2. c	7. d	12. c
3. d	8. b	13. c
4. a	9. c	14. a
5. c	10. d	

Answers to Situations 1–4

Question 1 Responses

Basic Responses (in any order)

A. Be aware of your own spiritual perspective in response to Ms. George.
B. Offer her focused presence.
C. Ask her to tell you more about her grandchildren and share memories of times together.
D. Explore the factors related to her feeling that she will not see them again, perhaps concerns about death.
E. Noting the importance of these relationships, talk to family members about having the grandchildren visit.
F. Arrange for pictures or reminders of her family and cat to be brought to the hospital.
G. Note who visits her and talk to family members about her concerns.
H. Encourage her to tell her story.

Optional Responses (in any order)

1. Consider arranging a visit from her cat.
2. Explore other meaningful connections.

Question 2 Responses

Basic Responses (in any order)

A. Be aware of your own spiritual perspective in response to the patient.
B. Offer a listening presence.
C. Acknowledge the real demands of her life situation, reassure her that her feelings are OK, and explore ways of dealing with her feelings.
D. Ask her what she does to nurture herself and discuss ways that she may include these activities in her life more often.
E. Point out that she must be able to care for herself to be there for her family.
F. Explore important relationships and support in her life.
G. Explore the place of her church in her life and the effect of her beliefs on her perception of her role.

Optional Responses (in any order)

1. Teach her relaxation exercises, and plan how and when she can do these regularly.

2. Talk about different ways of centering (e.g., meditation, prayer, gardening), and explore what might work for her.
3. Explore the availability of resources in the church or community that may provide child care to allow for some "self-nurture" time.

Question 3 Responses

Basic Responses (in any order)

A. Be aware of your own spiritual perspective in response to the patient.
B. Take time to sit with him and listen to his concerns.
C. Explore what worries him most.
D. Discuss what "not being religious" means to him; ask what he values and believes.
E. Ask how he would pray if he could.
F. Explore whether there is a need for reconciliation with his brother and how this can take place.
G. Find out whether he wants anyone else there with him.

Optional Responses (in any order)

1. Consider helping him communicate with his brother directly or though imagery.
2. After determining his prayer style, consider praying with him if you are comfortable with this approach.
3. Ask whether he wants contact with the chaplain or someone from a particular religious group.

Question 4 Responses

Basic Responses (in any order)

A. Be aware of your own spiritual perspective in response to this family.
B. Talk to the father about his concerns for Joe.
C. Be aware of how you are reacting to the situation based on your beliefs and values.
D. In a nonjudgmental way, ask the father what he is doing and how he perceives its role in Joe's healing.
E. Explain to the father what you need to do and when for care, and ask him what time and space he needs so that you can support each other.
F. Provide sacred space as much as possible.
G. Stay centered when caring for Joe.

Optional Responses (in any order)

1. Ask how you can be of support to the father.
2. Explore the father's beliefs about illness and healing, if appropriate.

ANSWERS—CHAPTER 7

Answers to Test Questions 1–10

1. b	5. b	9. b
2. d	6. d	10. d
3. b	7. c	
4. b	8. a	

Answers to Situations 1–4

Question 1 Responses

Basic Responses (in any order)

A. Receive Healing Touch or another energetic touch therapy regularly.
B. At the consciousness level, develop a stress reduction routine.
C. At the transpersonal level, look at the dynamics of my psychologic experiences using counseling and meditation.

Optional Responses

(Any answer that reflects the material in the three levels of action of the Energetic Healing Modalities model is correct.)
Note: Optional responses will differ according to each nurse's personal experiences. Each answer must be in three parts, suggesting one action from each of the three levels of action of the Energetic Healing Modalities model.

1. At the body level:
   — Get a massage regularly.
   — Change my physical environment to a more soothing one.
2. At the consciousness level:
   — Discover what I can learn about my physical body through visualization and guided imagery.
   — Image a change in my physical body.
   — Determine the strength of my psychologic boundaries.

—Look at my life for physical and emotional addictions.
3. At the transpersonal, soul, spirit, seer level, evaluate my spiritual practices.

Question 2 Responses

Basic Responses (in any order)

A. At the body level, concentrate on avenues familiar to the clients (e.g., exercise, nutrition).
B. At the consciousness level, act from a caring perspective.
C. At the transpersonal, soul, spirit, seer level, determine the clients' willingness to discuss spiritual practices and beliefs. If they are open and interested, listen.

Optional Responses

(Any answer that reflects the material in the three levels of action of the Energetic Healing Modalities model is correct.)
1. At the body level:
   —Use standard allopathic nursing approaches.
   —Offer suggestions on ways to change the clients' living environment, such as adequate lighting to prevent falls.
2. At the consciousness level:
   —If they are open, teach them standard stress reduction techniques.
   —Use a role modeling approach to teach clients how to act in the situation with appropriate control.
   —Help clients to increase their own autonomy and personal physical and/or psychologic control over the situation.
3. At the transpersonal, soul, spirit, seer level, do not offer meditation or similar transpersonal exploring techniques or offer with sensitivity.

Question 3 Responses

Basic Responses (in any order)

A. At the body level, alter physical environment to maximize use of senses for healing.
B. At the consciousness level, offer guided imagery twice each day.
C. At the transpersonal, soul, spirit, seer level (if acceptable to the patients), teach meditation.

Optional Responses

(Any combination of modalities from the three levels of action from the Energetic Healing Modalities Model that will assist a patient to become more of his/her own healer is correct.)
1. At the body level:
   —Ask the Red Cross volunteers to develop a humor cart.
   —Arrange the physical environment for maximum patient use with staff comfort secondary.
2. At the consciousness level:
   —Teach relaxation techniques.
   —Teach stress reduction approaches.
   —Alter the psychologic environment so the patients are in control, as much as possible. For example, allow patients to wear their personal clothing if they wish.
   —Recommend appropriate counseling
   —Teach as much self-care as patients are willing/able to learn.
3. At the transpersonal, soul, spirit, seer level, teach self-hypnosis to those who are interested.

Question 4 Responses

Basic Responses (in any order)

A. At the body level, arrange the physical working environment so it is as conducive to positive sensory experiences as possible.
B. At the consciousness level, lead a 5-minute guided imagery session each day.
C. At the transpersonal level, teach and lead a simple meditation at staff meetings.

Optional Responses

(Any combination of modalities from the three levels of action from the Energetic Healing Modalities Model that will assist colleagues to become attuned to their own energetic healing is correct.)
1. At the body level, arrange for staff members to play and socialize together occasionally.
2. At the consciousness level:
   —Teach staff members relaxation techniques.
   —Teach staff members stress reduction techniques.
   —Have each staff member write a statement that begins with "I feel *x* (e.g., angry) when you do/say *y*." Use the responses to help staff members explore the level of unconscious-

ness operating in their responses and their own personal responsibility in the situation.
— Use role modeling theory to help staff gain insight.
— Ask the staff to accept group counseling weekly as part of the staff meeting.
3. At the transpersonal, soul, spirit, seer level, urge staff members to seek individual counseling.

ANSWERS—CHAPTER 8

Answers to Test Questions 1–10

1. d	5. b	9. d
2. c	6. a	10. b
3. d	7. d	
4. b	8. a	

Answers to Situations 1–3

Question 1 Responses

Basic Responses (in any order)

A. Rights of children.
B. Freedom and autonomy.
C. Rights of captive populations.
D. Standards of care.
E. Care of the whole person—body, mind, and spirit.

Optional Responses (in any order)

1. What is meant by the term *captive populations*?
2. How do the rights of children differ from the rights of adults?
3. Are there protective mechanisms that are available to the psychiatric patients to ensure "freedom"?
4. Does the nurse have a role in developing and implementing standards of care for the hospitalized psychiatric patient?
5. How are Don's spiritual needs being addressed?

Question 2 Responses

Basic Responses (in any order)

A. Definition of clinical death.
B. Description of extraordinary measures.
C. Death with dignity.
D. Euthanasia.
E. Care for the dying patient.

Optional Responses (in any order)

1. Do the criteria for clinical death vary from situation to situation?
2. What are the criteria for the initiation and discontinuation of life support measures?
3. What is the definition of passive euthanasia, and is it ever ethically justified?
4. How are the spiritual needs of dying patients met?

Question 3 Responses

Basic Responses (in any order)

A. Quality of life versus sanctity of life.
B. Extraordinary means.
C. Euthanasia.
D. Use of resources.

Optional Responses (in any order)

1. What is meant by and who determines the quality of life?
2. If we are spiritual as well as physical, mental beings, why do we cling to a compromised life on earth?
3. Where do we draw the line between euthanasia and allowing a natural death?
4. Is the nurse obligated to care for a patient when she feels that there is a moral compromise between her values and those of the client or situation?

ANSWERS—CHAPTER 9

Answers to Test Questions 1–13

1. d	6. a	11. b
2. a	7. a	12. b
3. d	8. d	13. a
4. c	9. d	
5. b	10. d	

Answer to Situation 1

Question 1 Responses

Basic Responses (in any order)

A. Present the client description.
B. Identify the theory to be used.
C. Present assessment data, using basic concepts and language of the theory.
D. Present the plan of care, using concepts and language of the theory.

Optional Responses (in any order)

1. Present assessment data, using detailed concepts from the theory.
2. Present plan of care, using detailed concepts from the theory.

ANSWERS—CHAPTER 10

Answers to Test Questions 1–8

1. a	4. c	7. d
2. b	5. d	8. d
3. c	6. b	

Answers to Situations 1–2

Question 1 Responses

Basic Responses

A. Determine the number of MRIs canceled because of anxiety from a retrospective chart audit over the past 6 months (or year).
B. When telephoning patients to schedule their MRI, ask if they would be interested in listening to soothing music during the procedure to cope with the stress of the experience.
C. Ask patients to bring a CD with soothing, relaxing music on the day of their MRI. If they do not have a CD, explain that they may choose a CD from the music library in the MRI center.
D. While the machine is being calibrated, spend a few minutes with the patient practicing deep breathing, doing muscle relaxation exercises, and focusing on the music.
E. During the MRI, encourage patients to focus all of their attention on the music. Explain that at times during the procedure, they will be unable to hear the music because of the noise from the machine. At such times remind patients to focus on their deep breathing and muscle relaxation.
F. Evaluate each patient's response to the therapy.
G. Determine the number of MRIs canceled because of anxiety among patients listening to music following 6 months (or 1 year) of the intervention.
H. Compare the number of cancelled MRIs among patients who have and those who have not received the music therapy intervention.

Optional Responses

1. Follow the approach described, but randomize half of the prospective patients to a music therapy intervention and half of the patients to the standard MRI protocol.

2. Compare the number of cancelled MRIs among patients who have and those who have not received the music therapy intervention.

Question 2 Responses

Basic Responses

A. Randomize half of the patients to the music therapy intervention and half to the standard conventional care group.
B. Guide the patients in the music therapy group twice a day, once in the morning and again in the afternoon, in a head-to-toe music therapy session for 20 minutes. Allow these patients to select the music of their choice from the unit's audiocassette library.
C. For patients in the standard conventional care group, monitor their psychophysiologic parameters specifically for the research study during two 20-minute sessions in which patients carry on with their normal CCU routines, once in the morning and once in the afternoon.
D. Before and after each session for the experimental and control group, measure the psychophysiologic parameters of heart rate, blood pressure, peripheral temperature, cardiac rhythm, and psychologic anxiety.
E. Continue the sessions twice daily until the patient is discharged from the CCU.
F. Compare the pre- and post-intervention scores on heart rate, blood pressure, peripheral temperature, cardiac rhythm, and psychologic anxiety between the experimental and control groups.

ANSWERS—CHAPTER 11

Answers to Test Questions 1–14

1. b	6. a	11. c
2. b	7. b	12. d
3. d	8. a	13. c
4. d	9. d	14. d
5. a	10. b	

Answers to Situations 1–4

Question 1 Responses

Basic Responses (In any order)

A. Focus on the therapeutic relationship.
B. Encourage Mr. Brown to participate actively in assessment.
C. Assess all or most of his human response patterns.

Optional Responses (in any order)

1. Use observation, measurement, and intuition.
2. Recognize the effect of one response pattern on another.
3. Use intuitive, scientific, personal, and esthetic knowing patterns.
4. Confer with other health professionals, if indicated.
5. Validate your impressions with the client.

Question 2 Responses

Basic Responses (in any order)

A. Specify the tools, tests, and observations necessary to accomplish desired outcomes.
B. Elicit appropriate goals in mutual process with Ms. Sullivan.

Optional Responses (in any order)

1. Avoid making assumptions without her collaboration.
2. Avoid rigid adherence to outcomes.
3. Try to ensure that she is acting from her own values and is not simply trying to please the nurse.
4. Discuss with Ms. Sullivan ways to increase her commitment to change.

Question 3 Responses

Basic Responses (in any order)

A. Prescribe nursing interventions (actions) that will foster the selected outcomes.
B. Prioritize actions according to what is of greatest health benefit.
C. Select interventions consistent with Ms. Gibson's values and beliefs.

Optional Responses (in any order)

1. Collaborate with her to identify needed referrals.
2. Communicate the plan to others involved in her care.

Question 4 Responses

Basic Responses (in any order)

A. Ensure that all interventions are safe.
B. Maintain her focus throughout the encounter.
C. Modify interventions as indicated by her response.

Optional Responses (in any order)

1. Acknowledge her humanness.
2. Elicit her feedback.
3. Incorporate art and humor into the encounter.
4. Encourage her active participation.

ANSWERS—CHAPTER 12

Answers to Test Questions 1–14

1. c	6. b	11. c
2. b	7. a	12. c
3. d	8. b	13. d
4. a	9. d	14. d
5. b	10. a	

Answers to Situations 1–14

Question 1 responses

Basic Response (best answer)

b

Optional Responses (in any order)

1. Listen carefully to Ms. King's feelings; especially focus on her current feelings about the situation.
2. Assist her to calm herself.
3. Explore what this means to her.
4. Focus on what she is learning from this event.
5. Find out if she has any goals or further needs around this situation.

Question 2 Responses

Basic Response (best answer)

d

Optional Responses (in any order)

1. Explore what this referral means to Billy.
2. Especially focus on his feelings.
3. See what his personal goals are around the referral.

Question 3 Responses

Basic Response (best answer)

d

Optional Responses (in any order)

1. Process her reaction to the feedback.
2. Find out if Ms. Parry chooses to do any further work on the purported goals or to set new goals.

Question 4 Responses

Basic Response (best answer)

b

Optional Responses (in any order)

1. As a troubleshooter, explore the problems.
2. Examine Ms. Becker's feelings, self-perceived limitations and other blocks.
3. Determine whether the planned steps in problem solving are too large for the client; if so, break them down.
4. With the client, draw up new plans with homework to facilitate action.
5. Continue providing support and honest feedback.

ANSWERS—CHAPTER 13

Answers to Test Questions 1–15

1. c	6. a	11. a
2. d	7. c	12. a
3. c	8. d	13. b
4. c	9. b	14. a
5. d	10. d	15. d

Answers to Situations 1–4

Question 1 Responses

Basic Responses (in any order)

A. Become aware of and accept cultural differences.
B. Become aware of her own beliefs and attitudes.
C. Understand the dynamic differences between cultures without promoting the superiority of any one.
D. Acquire basic knowledge about a specific patient's culture by reading and interacting with people from that culture.
E. Actively seek advice and feedback from patients and others of the specific culture in incorporating cultural understanding into practice.

Optional Responses (in any order)

1. Conduct a personal values clarification.
2. Recognize that the health care system is a culture.
3. Learn about the specific culture of each client.
4. Interact and intervene with cultural understanding.
5. Elicit feedback about the cultural understanding and interventions.

Question 2 Responses

Basic Responses (in any order)

A. Ask about Mr. Taylor's ethnic, religious, educational, family, and social background.
B. Ask about his daily patterns, eating, exercise, daily activities, and health practices.
C. Ask about traditions, beliefs, and coping mechanisms.
D. Explore what he thinks about his diagnosis and the meaning of the pain.
E. Explore various techniques for pain relief that may be acceptable to him.
F. Frequently reassess and discuss options for pain management.

Optional Responses (in any order)

1. Read the literature on African-American culture.
2. Use a cultural assessment guide from the literature.
3. Personalize the assessment by clarifying all issues and questions with him and/or his family.
4. Collaborate with him in designing some techniques to reduce pain.
5. Evaluate the efficacy of techniques and explore additional options with him and his family.

Question 3 Responses

Basic Responses (in any order)

A. Assess Ms. Lopez's explanatory models for the practices she uses and the specific herbs and foods she uses or avoids.
B. Determine which practices may be helpful, harmful, or neutral according to scientific perspectives.
C. Possibly involve her husband in prenatal education and decision making.
D. Employ cultural preservation strategies for helpful and neutral practices in use of prayer, massage, some of the teas.

E. Employ cultural accommodation to bridge the gap between the two cultures and to prepare her for the remainder of her pregnancy and delivery.

F. Employ cultural repatterning to help her change potentially harmful practices, such as some of her dietary practices.

Optional Responses (in any order)

1. Conduct a cultural assessment.
2. Research the explanatory models of Mexican-Americans.
3. Involve her husband in decision making, if needed.
4. Support and facilitate those practices that enhance the health of her pregnancy.
5. Use cultural understanding to work with her to adapt or repattern any other practices.
6. Offer additional techniques for comfort, stress, etc., such as imagery, touch, music; explore her response to these techniques.

Question 4 Responses

Basic Responses (in any order)

A. Explore Ms. Wilson's belief system and cultural background.
B. Assess what she has done to relieve the tension headaches.
C. Get more specific information about her support systems and sources of healing.
D. Discuss sources of tension.
E. Together, explore alternative approaches to stress reduction, pain relief, and healing.
F. Refer her to an appropriate practitioner.

Optional Responses (in any order)

1. Conduct a more thorough cultural assessment about her beliefs and use of nonbiomedical resources.
2. In collaboration with her, set up a plan to use a variety of techniques (e.g., touch, meditation).
3. Evaluate the efficacy, acceptability, and appropriateness of each modality.
4. Modify accordingly, working toward a program of self-care that intervenes at the source of the stress.

Answers—Chapter 14

Answers to Test Questions 1–15

1. d	6. d	11. b
2. c	7. a	12. d
3. a	8. c	13. b
4. b	9. d	14. c
5. c	10. a	15. d

Answers to Situations 1–4

Question 1 Responses

Basic Responses (in any order)

A. Nurse Norris' Adaptive Child responses.
B. Need to reach the supervisor at the Adult ego state.
C. Encourage him to explore his feelings about the feedback without agreeing with him or encouraging further gossip.

Optional Responses (in any order)

1. Redirect his playfulness toward insightful cartoons, a humor hotline, or other ways of supporting creativity.
2. Use nurturing parent transactions or adult agreements.
3. The psychological game from him might be called "I can fool the supervisor" or "I'm OK, but she's not."

Question 2 Responses

Basic Responses (in any order)

A. Lack of security by not getting paid may trigger Adaptive Child responses of fear and rejection in many, especially if they had dysfunctional parenting.
B. Asking employees for trust is an implied Child to Parent transaction although, in fact, the employer holds the position of authority.
C. Move to the negotiating table.

Optional Responses (in any order)

1. Hold the positive intent of employer and employees constant while issues of reasonable and timely payment for services are addressed.

2. If resolution cannot be found, consider legal action before all the "good" staff quietly resigns (Adaptive Child behavior).

Question 3 Responses

Basic Responses (in any order)

A. Explore a solution from each of the five ego states.
B. Examples: Nurturing Parent—"This is a tough time for you. Let's talk more about this."
Adult: "Something is wrong. Can you tell me more?"
Free Child: "Good for you! Let's goof off the schedule."
Adaptive Child: "You're making me late. I'll never get done with this blasted schedule to keep."

Optional Responses (in any order)

1. Explore a solution as warrior, healer, teacher, and visionary.
2. Explore the positive intent behind the patient's action.
3. Consider the positive intent behind the nurse's behavior.
4. Think of the most humorous approach that could be used.

Question 4 Responses

Basic Responses (in any order)

A. Consider that all change is threatening to the old order of established patterns. Bringing in any new idea may trigger the Adaptive Child or Critical Parent.
B. Access the Adult ego state with gradual exposure to information, allowing curiosity to build from within the organization rather than imposing change.

Optional Responses (in any order)

1. Consider ways that relationships are built through rapport, caring, mutuality, and agreement.
2. Consider negotiating so that the interest of others in a different project is honored and there is an exchange of ideas.
3. Bring in a friend who is unknown to speak of her experiences in a nonthreatening way.

ANSWERS—CHAPTER 15

Answers to Test Questions 1–15

1. a	6. a	11. b
2. b	7. d	12. d
3. a	8. c	13. a
4. c	9. b	14. d
5. d	10. c	15. c

Answers to Situations 1–3

Question 1 Responses

Basic Responses (in any order)

A. Explain to him as follows:
—The client is as comfortable as possible. Pain is managed, fear and anxiety are decreased or controlled.
—There is a feeling of integration of self and life. The individual knows who he or she is. One realizes that no one else would have lived life the same way.
—Goodbyes have been said.
—Important life goals have been met.
—The individual has achieved a kind of wisdom from the lessons of life.
—The individual's family is supported in the grief process.

Optional Responses (in any order)

1. The individual has been functional as long as possible.
2. The individual has enough energy to be able to "let go."
3. The family shares their grief.

Question 2 Responses

Basic Responses (in any order)

A. Provide a place or group in which families can share emotions safely (cry, get angry, laugh out loud).
B. Give information about the dying process as needed.
C. Help the family to hold hands with the dying person, or to touch him or her in some way during the dying process.

D. Suggest to family members that they can write letters to the one who has died to complete unfinished or unsaid things. Letters can be burned or floated in the ocean as a means of sending them to the universe.

E. Discuss with families the need to give away the things of a person who has died. Help them to make that time precious.

F. Celebrate anniversaries or birthdays as times to remember deceased loved ones with joy for their lives.

G. Identify signs of depression that require referral.

Optional Responses (in any order)

1. Help the family spend some time with their loved one after death.
2. Help the family make plans for burial or other final arrangements for the body.
3. Provide information about organ donation as provided by law in a sensitive manner.

Question 3 Responses

Basic Responses (in any order)

A. Massage or back rub.
B. Therapeutic Touch.
C. Heat.
D. Cold.
E. Accupuncture (within the legal constraints of the state practice act); or accupressure.
F. Transcutaneous Electrical Stimulation (if prescribed).

ANSWERS—CHAPTER 16

Answers to Test Questions 1–10

1. b	5. d	9. c
2. a	6. b	10. d
3. d	7. c	
4. e	8. b	

Answers to Situations 1–4

Question 1 Responses

Basic Responses (in any order)

A. Determine the client's current knowledge of nutrition.

B. Ask the client to keep food intake inventory forms for a week and use them as an assessment and education tool at the next session.

Optional Responses (in any order)

1. Provide the client with specific nutritional guidelines.
2. Give a general explanation of the way that nutrition affects the body-mind-spirit.

Question 2 Responses

Basic Responses (in any order)

A. Discuss and explain the following specific areas of emotional self-assessment:
   —Acknowledgment and acceptance of one's own feelings.
   —Acknowledgment and acceptance of other's feelings.
   —Ability to express feelings appropriately.
   —Perceptions of feelings.
   —Developmental tasks.
   —Role performance.
   —Situational stressors.
B. Evaluate the client's ability to assess his or her own mental state.

Optional Responses (in any order)

1. Teach the client the impact of nutrition, drugs, caffeine, and alcohol on mental state.
2. Explain that mental health cannot be assessed in isolation from physical and emotional health.
3. Teach relaxation, imagery, and breathing exercises.
4. Provide the client with mental self-assessment tool.

Question 3 Responses

Basic Responses (in any order)

A. Determine the client's current knowledge of exercise and its relationship to cardiovascular health.
B. Educate the client on the benefits of daily exercise.

Optional Responses (in any order)

1. Explain the difference and benefits of the various exercise systems.
2. Discuss with the client the potential effects of lack of exercise:

— Weak muscle tone and atrophied muscles.
— Increased blood sugar levels.
— Increased blood cholesterol levels.
— Decreased endurance for physical activities.
— Decreased cardiovascular tone.
— Decreased sense of well-being.
— Decreased ability to lose weight.

Question 4 Responses

Basic Responses (in any order)

A. Determine the client's current knowledge of holistic health.
B. Provide client with self-assessment tools.

Optional Responses (in any order)

1. Explain self-responsibility and its relationship to maximizing wellness.
2. Explore the area of self-confidence with the client.
3. Assess the client's assertiveness in self-care.
4. Assess the client's decision-making ability.
5. Discuss the client's openness to change.
6. Explore the client's willingness to be an active participant in the self-care process.

ANSWERS—CHAPTER 17

Answers to Test Questions 1–15

1. d	6. a	11. c
2. e	7. b	12. d
3. a	8. d	13. a
4. c	9. g	14. c
5. c	10. b	15. g

Answers to Situations 1–4

Question 1 Responses

Basic Responses (in any order)

A. Physical response: increased heart rate, blood pressure, rapid respirations, musculoskeletal tension (e.g., in the neck, shoulders, back, jaw), sweating (or any other signs of automatic nervous system arousal).
B. Feelings: anxiety, fear, frustration, anger, depression.
C. Automatic thoughts: Should take better care of myself. Always have to test the limits. Ought to get someone to do the yardwork. Never get help from the kids. Why always me. What if they find a serious blockage—will need surgery. What if they don't find a blockage—all in my head. What if they can't do anything—it's no use.
D. Cognitive distortions, irrational beliefs, silent assumptions: "It's not fair—did all the right things, but here I am with more pain"; all-or-nothing thinking; jumping to conclusions.
E. Reframing: stop–breathe–reflect–choose.

Optional Responses (in any order)

1. The nurse can facilitate this process by instructing the patient to stop, take a breath, release physical tension, and then guiding the patient through the process of cognitive appraisal and cognitive restructuring.
2. The nurse should continue to assess the client's response to the process.

Question 2 Responses

Basic Responses (in any order)

A. Physical response: increased heart rate, upset stomach, shallow breaths, muscle tension in her neck and shoulders; any other sign of autonomic nervous system arousal.
B. Automatic thoughts: I can't stand this! It'll never go away! I can't do anything! I'm useless! The doctors don't know what they are talking about!
C. Feelings: frustration, anger, depression, hopelessness.
D. Behaviors: Stop the swim therapy and medications that have been helping. Seek another medical opinion. Stop calling friends and family.
E. Cognitive distortions: all-or-nothing thinking, overgeneralization, labeling, emotional reasoning, magnification, jumping to conclusions.
F. Reframing: stop–breathe–reflect–choose.

Optional Responses (in any order)

1. The nurse can facilitate the process by guiding Ms. Havior in discovering some of the distortions related to the situation.
2. If Ms. Havior has trouble uncovering the automatic thoughts or underlying assumptions, coach her in the vertical arrow technique or ask her to journal about the stress as a homework assignment to help her uncover these thoughts and assumptions.

Question 3 Responses

Basic Responses (in any order)

A. Physical response: heart racing, rapid respirations, headache, muscle tension in his jaw and low back; any other autonomic nervous system response.
B. Automatic thoughts: I'll never fall asleep. I have to have 8 hours! I'll be too tired to do a good job tomorrow. I won't get my work done. I'll fall behind, and Fred will get the promotion. They will get rid of me because I can't do my job.
C. Feelings: fear, frustration, anger.
D. Behaviors: Toss and turn. Get out of bed, have another cigarette, and raid the refrigerator.
E. Cognitive distortions: all-or-nothing thinking, overgeneralization, jumping to conclusions (awfulizing and catastrophizing), magnification.
F. Reframing: stop–breathe–reflect–choose.

Optional Responses (in any order)

1. The nurse can facilitate the reframing process by helping Mr. Cross uncover some of his automatic thoughts and related behavior in response to his sleep disturbance.
2. Homework can include practicing his relaxation technique each night before going to bed and recording his physical, emotional, and cognitive response when he has difficulty falling asleep. These can be reviewed at his next appointment.
3. Keeping a sleep diary or journal may also be helpful.

Question 4 Responses

Basic Responses (in any order)

A. Physical response: musculoskeletal tension or any sign of autonomic system arousal.
B. Feelings: free-floating anxiety, sadness, loss, fear.
C. Automatic thoughts: Awful... Terrible... Worst possible... Won't get better... Will have to give up everything... Just like my mother... My father... Shouldn't have waited so long... Always at the worst time... Why me?
D. Cognitive distortions: jumping to conclusions; disqualifying the positive (i.e., ruled out myocardial infarction); magnification; personalization; awfulization.
E. Reframing: stop–breathe–reflect–choose.

Optional Responses (in any order)

1. The nurse can facilitate the reframing process by instructing the patient to stop, take a breath, release physical tension, and then guiding the patient through the process of cognitive appraisal and cognitive restructuring.
2. Because the patient is jumping to conclusions and magnifying the situation to the worse possible outcome, it is easy to become overwhelmed with feelings of hopelessness (depression) and, therefore, difficult to focus on teaching.
3. By addressing the underlying issue, the patient is more realistically able to appraise her situation and can, therefore, become a more active participant in discharge teaching, which may allow her to modify some of her health-risking behaviors.

ANSWERS—CHAPTER 18

Answers to Test Questions 1–17

1. d	7. d	13. b
2. a	8. a	14. c
3. b	9. a	15. d
4. a	10. b	16. c
5. d	11. b	17. d
6. d	12. b	

Answers to Situations 1-4

Question 1 Responses

Basic Responses (in any order)

A. Assess Mr. Love's knowledge of nutrition and cardiovascular disease.
B. Teach him nutrition guidelines for health promotion and prevention of cardiovascular disease.
C. Discuss other lifestyle factors that are associated with a healthy heart, including stress reduction and weight management.

Optional Responses (in any order)

1. Detail cardiovascular disease prevention programs, including
   —Low-fat/high-fiber diet.
   —Nutritional supplements for additional support.

—Stress reduction and relaxation techniques.
2. Guide him in creating a sample menu/diet plan.
3. Encourage him to use a wellness model and to view nutritional changes for health promotion as integral to achieving goals.

Question 2 Responses

Basic Responses (in any order)

A. Assess current diet and nutrient intake.
B. Teach Mr. Young the basic physiology involved in normal immune function.
C. Describe the connection between nutrition and immune function.
D. Give general explanations about nutrition's impact on health and quality of life.
E. Give patient nutritional guidelines for immune enhancement.

Optional Responses (in any order)

1. Encourage Mr. Young to keep a journal to learn how what he eats affects how he feels, with special attention on digestive symptoms.
2. Give specific dietary guidelines to prevent weight loss and wasting.
3. Guide him in nutritional supplementation of vitamins and minerals.
4. Increase awareness between digestive function and HIV as it relates to nutrient absorption.
5. Increase awareness of malabsorption and immunosuppression with a high-fat diet.
6. Increase awareness of the connection between a high-sugar diet and candidiasis.
7. Encourage him to monitor diet for lactose intolerance and any other food sensitivities.
8. Encourage him to develop an exercise program to maintain muscle mass and enhance immune function.

Question 3 Responses

Basic Responses (in any order)

A. Develop nutritional guidelines for health promotion and disease prevention.
B. Explore with Ms. Poe her fears about genetic predisposition and breast cancer.
C. Offer supportive strategies for strengthening immune function.
D. Encourage her to use positive imagery to replace her negative thoughts.

Optional Responses (in any order)

1. Guide Ms. Poe in a specific nutritional approach based on current research. For example, provide
   • Information on low-fat/high-fiber diet.
   • Antioxidant vitamin protocol.
   • Soy-based products.
   • Essential fatty acids and other nutritional supplements.
2. Increase her awareness of the connection of environmental cofactors and breast cancer (including pesticides and other chemicals in the food chain) as she moves toward a more natural whole foods diet.
3. Encourage her to develop a stress reduction program.
4. Encourage her to continue to develop healthy lifestyle strategies.

Question 4 Responses

Basic Responses (in any order)

A. Encourage Ms. Mead to keep an "eating/feeling" food journal.
B. Describe general dietary guidelines for weight management.
C. Guide her in developing a health plan that includes a nutritional approach, exercise plan, and stress reduction program.

Optional Responses (in any order)

1. Help Ms. Mead explore her feelings about her relationship to food and body image.
2. Assist her in designing a daily food plan based on emotional and physical well-being.
3. Encourage her to seek additional support systems.
4. Support her in developing an exercise program to incorporate into her wellness plan.
5. Guide her in reframing the relationship between food and health.

ANSWERS—CHAPTER 19

Answers to Test Questions 1–15

1. b	6. d	11. c
2. c	7. d	12. d
3. d	8. d	13. b
4. a	9. c	14. b
5. c	10. a	15. b

Answers to Situations 1–4

Question 1 Responses

Basic Responses (in any order)

A. Consider your preparation/state of being.
B. Clarify your intention.
C. Center yourself in whatever way is best for you.
D. Create a suitable environment for connection.
E. Identify a purpose (nursing diagnosis) for your time together.
F. Access relevant history: medical, body-mind-spirit, and therapeutic treatment.
G. Create opportunity for pattern recognition.
H. Mutually identify plan/intervention.
I. Identify the role of the nurse.
J. Identify the role of the client.

Optional Responses (in any order)

1. Identify patterns through
   — Interview.
   — Presence.
   — Dreamwork.
   — Body scan.
   — Inner advisor.
   — Meditation.
   — Holographic models (Ayurvedic, Rayid, and/or Chinese Five-Phase/Element).
2. Nurse serves as guide, facilitator, resource person, and supportive, caring partner.
3. Patient/Client: grants permission, co-participation, potential motivation and/or commitment.
4. Evaluate
   — Opportunity for reflection/mirroring
   — Mutual self-acknowledgement
   — Gratitude for shared experience

Question 2 Responses

Basic Responses (in any order)

A. Body-mind-spirit integration
B. Self-knowledge and self-reverence
C. Consciously work together with rhythms of self/earth (integrality)
D. Expression of spirit
E. Expression of movement is universal and diverse
F. Opportunity for reflection/mirroring

Optional Response

1. Expansions of specifics relevant to the basic responses

Question 3 Responses

Basic Responses (in any order)

A. Respect Mr. Chuen's cultural attitudes/values/beliefs.
B. Age.
C. Physical challenge.
D. Refer him to appropriate health care professionals, when necessary.

Optional Responses (in any order)

1. Refer to other health care professionals, when appropriate.
2. Use subtle energy expressions, such as touch, imagery, and music.

Question 4 Responses

Basic Response

A. The human/earth community functions as a whole: the movement of one is integral to the other.

Optional Responses (in any order)

1. Energy and matter are the same thing.
2. All matter, physical and subtle, has frequency.
3. The human is a pandimensional being within a universe of dynamic energy in many different frequencies and forms.
4. Physical expressions of energy patterns can be viewed as a process of constriction/dilation and building/releasing.
5. Consciouness is a form of energy.
6. Conscious thought participates in formation of reality.

ANSWERS—CHAPTER 20

Answers to Test Questions 1–15

1. b	6. b	11. a
2. d	7. b	12. a
3. d	8. c	13. b
4. a	9. d	14. c
5. c	10. a	15. b

Answers to Situations 1–4

Question 1 Responses

Basic Responses (in any order)

A. Give Ms. Marks your complete attention.
B. Listen to her story.
C. Avoid judgment.
D. Reassure her that, together, you can work out a plan to resolve the problem.

Optional Responses (in any order)

1. Involve Ms. Marks in some breath work to help relieve her tension.
2. Take an environmental exposure history.
3. Find out if anyone else is similarly affected.
4. Address the possibility of other sources of workplace stress (e.g., sexual harassment).
5. Ask her what she is doing to diminish her symptoms (e.g., fresh air breaks, medication).

Question 2 Responses

Basic Responses (in any order)

A. Determine who is responsible, institutionally, both for procurement and for waste disposal.
B. Confer with that person to determine if waste can be prevented initially, at the procurement end.
C. Be clear on what exactly belongs to the infectious waste category (red bag) and what constitutes solid waste.
D. Enlist assistance from at least one colleague in your unit.
E. Consider the possibility that the supplies and equipment need not be discarded at all, but may be donated to a clinic.
F. Learn whether or not the manufacturer plays, or is willing to play, any part in resolving this problem.

Optional Responses (in any order)

1. Confer with the institution's team on environment.
2. Find out what other institutions do with clean, disposable supplies and equipment.
3. Learn what possible outlets there may be for supplies, such as an inner city clinic.
4. Join the environment team so you can help address this as an institutional issue.

Question 3 Responses

Basic Responses (in any order)

A. Find a quiet place and time to reflect on and "be with" what you are seeing.
B. Be open to learning what path, for you, is most compatible with your needs, the needs of the environment, and those of your clients.
C. When a way becomes clear, enter it with focus and deliberation.
D. Be aware that, whatever course you take, you are making an important and singular contribution to the whole.

Optional Responses (in any order)

1. Learn who is knowledgeable about "tracking" one of the problems you see and confer with that person.
2. Investigate key literature about the problem.
3. Examine any regulations related to the problem.
4. Ask at least one person to share with you his or her experience with the problem.

Question 4 Responses

Basic Responses (in any order)

A. Basic health practices remain most important: handwashing, clean drinking water, avoiding exposures, vaccination.
B. It is important to strengthen the immune system through competent stress reduction management, nutrition, work, play, exercise, and nurturing relationships.
C. Each person has choices to make toward well-being and *has the ability* to make them.
D. Many environmental problems are "man-made," and humans can halt or reverse them.

Optional Responses (in any order)

1. Ask the young people what they consider to be problems.
2. Learn from them what they have done/are doing about the problems.
3. Show them visual evidence of a major health concern in the area; this part of the presentation may include an expert witness, human or nonhuman.
4. Share success stories.

ANSWERS—CHAPTER 21

Answers to Test Questions 1–12

1. c	5. d	9. b
2. b	6. d	10. a
3. c	7. a	11. c
4. c	8. b	12. c

Answers to Situations 1–4

Question 1 Responses

Basic Responses (in any order)

A. Reassure Mr. Jones that some anxiety is expected before surgery.
B. Explain that distracting a patient from an intense focus on frightening aspects of the illness can be helpful to relieve stress and relax the body.
C. Offer a list of humorous audiotapes, videotapes, and books that are available from the laughter library and arrange to have a volunteer deliver it to the patient.

Optional Responses (in any order)

1. Discuss with Mr. Jones the ability of humor to provide feelings of superiority and power while releasing tensions with laughter. Share a story of how another patient created humor or found a way to laugh about his or her situation.
2. Explore with him his favorite comedy performers and writers.
3. Review the list of choices available from the laughter library, and briefly describe those items that you feel may best match his preferred style.

Question 2 Responses

Basic Responses (in any order)

A. Ask Ms. Floyd to describe the playful activities she enjoyed as a child. Make a list of these.
B. Ask her family to bring in some of those toys, games, books, etc. Have them gas-sterilized.
C. Encourage her and her family to decorate her hospital room with funny posters and cards.
D. Ask family members to take pictures of themselves doing comical activities, making funny faces, or wearing amusing costumes. (Be sure to include the family pet.) Bring these in for her and place them nearby.

Optional Responses (in any order)

1. Provide Ms. Floyd with humorous tapes and books created by people who have struggled with cancer and managed to find a humorous perspective.
2. Place inspiring and amusing quotes in enlarged print on the walls and ceiling.
3. Create a list of funny TV programs, noting times and channels, and post this in a visible place.
4. During reverse isolation, decorate the surgical mask and cap in an amusing way, stick adhesive electrocardiogram leads (with the snap attachments) on the bottom of your shoes, and do a little tap dance and song when you enter the room.

Question 3 Responses

Basic Responses (in any order)

A. Prepare a new joke to tell Mr. Cornwall each visit.
B. Create a bulletin board with dietary cartoons.
C. Provide Mr. Cornwall and his fellow patients with a cartoon graphic, and ask them to create their own caption. Post these on the bulletin board.

Optional Responses (in any order)

1. Ask Mr. Cornwall to bring in a new joke to tell you each visit. Offer to tell him two for each one he shares.
2. With the help of Mr. Cornwall and the other patients, prepare a collection of "Murphy's Laws" about living with kidney disease.
3. Create a list of answers to "You know it's not on your diet if. . . ."

Question 4 Responses

Basic Responses (in any order)

A. Consult with the local librarian or hospital Child Life Specialist for advice on age-appropriate humor.
B. Provide Jennifer with a riddle book so that she can quiz the staff.
C. Wear amusing hats or costume accessories and use oversized props when caring for Jennifer.
D. Perform magic tricks at the bedside.

Optional Responses (in any order)

1. Provide Jennifer with a squirt gun to protect herself from staff who want to interrupt her play time or TV shows for therapy.

2. Schedule a hospital or community clown to visit Jennifer twice a week. If she responds positively, try to have the clown arrive during the mother's visit.
3. Teach Jennifer some simple magic tricks to entertain her family and staff.

ANSWERS—CHAPTER 22

Answers to Test Questions 1–12

1. b	5. d	9. a
2. c	6. b	10. d
3. a	7. c	11. a
4. c	8. b	12. d

Answers to Situations 1–4

Question 1 Responses

Basic Responses (in any order)

A. Inviting Ms. James to tell her story.
B. Encouraging her to use a form of art (drawing, sculpting, painting, writing) to identify and illustrate her patterns of person-environment interaction.

Optional Responses (in any order)

1. Listening to her identify strengths and resources.
2. Using a values clarification exercise.
3. Teaching her assertiveness skills.
4. Encouraging her to listen to the rhythms of the world around and within her.

Question 2 Responses

Basic Responses (in any order)

A. Billy has not yet resolved his identity.
B. Billy does not have a private area in which to practice self-reflection.

Optional Responses (in any order)

1. Billy does not have the support of his parents.
2. The nurse may not see Billy more than once.
3. Billy does not have a strong social support network.
4. Billy is not currently connected with school or other activities that could provide structure and meaning for his identity crisis.

5. Billy has not yet adapted to the culture of living on the street.

Question 3 Responses

Basic Responses (in any order)

A. Journaling, letter-writing, and keeping a scrapbook.
B. Life review using a photograph album to reminisce.
C. Drawing pictures and sculpting forms with clay.

Optional Responses (in any order)

1. Reflecting on their past experiences and feelings.
2. Identifying persons and events that were important to them.
3. Physical activities of a creative nature.

Question 4 Responses

Basic Responses (in any order)

A. Strengthening cognitive awareness by providing simple facts.
B. Providing diagrams and simple illustrations of anatomy and physiology.
C. Simple descriptions of how chemotherapy works.
D. Spending time with him and reflecting his feelings.

Optional Responses (in any order)

1. Bibliotherapy—assigning him to read about cancer.
2. Connecting him with a support group to explore feelings.
3. Helping Mr. Smith to identify things that he really enjoys doing.
4. Encouraging him to express his feelings.
5. Encouraging him to ask questions about his body, cancer, and cancer treatments.

ANSWERS—CHAPTER 23

Answers to Test Questions 1–16

1. b	7. d	13. a
2. a	8. c	14. a
3. d	9. a	15. b
4. b	10. b	16. b
5. c	11. c	
6. a	12. d	

Answers to Situations 1–4

Question 1 Responses

Basic Responses (in any order)

A. Assess what Ms. Hampton knows about the relaxation process.
B. Assess her anxiety level to determine whether she is able to learn at this time; if anxiety is too high for learning to occur, initiate breathing exercises to help her become more comfortable.
C. Describe briefly several types of relaxation approaches.
D. Explain the role of breathing in relaxation.
E. Describe basic breathing exercises.
F. Give a general explanation of the effect of relaxation.
G. Lead her through several breathing exercises.
H. Teach her basic physiology involved in the relaxation response.
I. Teach her the importance of positive expectation of desired outcomes.

Optional Responses (in any order)

1. Be aware of Ms. Hampton's response to breathing exercises to be able to move toward desired outcomes.
2. Encourage her to describe her experience after each breathing exercise.
3. Ask her what she wishes to gain from the session.
4. Focus on her baseline feelings to guide the session.
5. Be aware of the importance of rapport, trust, and empathy in the nurse–client encounter, and examine your own feelings.

Question 2 Responses

Basic Responses (in any order)

A. Begin by guiding Mr. Adams through a basic breathing relaxation exercise.
B. Observe for visual cues of relaxation from him, such as a change from slower, deep breaths to slow, somewhat shallower breathing as relaxation deepens; easing of jaws' tightness; and release of emotions (e.g., tears, deeper faster breathing).
C. Introduce a brief, imagery exercise of being in a safe place. Ask for feedback concerning his ability to respond to the imagery. Have the client respond with a finger movement and make changes as necessary.
D. Move into a meditation exercise of the type John has been learning.
E. Allow time for discussion of the experience.

Optional Responses (in any order)

1. Explore Mr. Adam's feelings about his evaluation and help him develop a plan to deal with the situation.
2. Help him develop a positive expectation of what he desires to see as the solution. Build this into his meditation practice.
3. Assign homework; practice breathing exercises 10 minutes a day and meditation for 20 minutes at a different time.

Question 3 Responses

Basic Responses (in any order)

A. Can you describe what this experience was like for you?
B. Was the background music pleasant or distracting?
C. In what ways do you feel different, if any, from how you felt at the beginning of the session?
D. Can you suggest anything that would improve the experience for you?

Optional Responses (in any order)

1. Do you need more practice here before you will be able to practice the exercises at home?
2. What physical sensations, if any, were changed by the exercises?
3. What emotional feelings, if any, were changed by the exercises?

Question 4 Responses

Basic Responses (in any order)

A. Assess what Mr. Stratman knows about meditation.
B. Ask him what influenced his decision to begin meditating.
C. Explain the common aspect of various types: concentration on a repetitive focus in order to experience an inner peaceful quietness.
D. Briefly review several types of meditation.
E. Give a general explanation of the effect of relaxation and meditation.
F. Describe the four major routes to the meditative state.
G. Teach him how to deal with distracting self-talk: note it, let it go, and return to the focus.

Optional Responses (in any order)

1. Avoid overloading Mr. Stratman with too much information.
2. Whenever possible, give short experiential exercises (e.g., asking him to chant the OM mantra after you as you introduce him to mantra meditation).
3. Suggest reading material.
4. Explain to him that to grasp the meaning and benefit of meditation fully requires practice, practice, and more practice. Give homework for the next session.

ANSWERS—CHAPTER 24

Answers to Test Questions 1–19

1. a	8. b	15. d
2. c	9. b	16. c
3. c	10. a	17. d
4. a	11. c	18. b
5. c	12. c	19. c
6. b	13. a	
7. d	14. c	

Answers to Situations 1–4

Question 1 Responses

Basic Responses (in any order)

A. Assess what Ms. Smith knows about the imagery process.
B. Describe basic imagery exercises.
C. Explain that the choice of words can cause the body-mind-spirit to respond in a negative or positive manner.
D. Give a general explanation of the ways that relaxation and imagery affect the body-mind spirit.
E. Describe receptive imagery as "just bubbling up" or an inner thought just being received.
F. Describe active imagery as what occurs when a person focuses on the conscious formation of an image.

Optional Responses (in any order)

1. Discuss receptive imagery and ways to change receptive imagery to active imagery in order to move toward desired outcomes.

2. Find out what experiences she wishes to gain from session. Work with eyes open or closed.
3. Use reframing techniques.
4. Focus on baseline feelings of client to guide the session.
5. Have client develop a positive expectation of what is desired.

Question 2 Responses

Basic Responses (in any order)

A. Encourage him to use imagery skills 20 minutes twice a day, as well as to hold "mini-practice" sessions every day.
B. Teach him the basic physiology involved in the normal immune function and the healing process.
C. Begin with several minutes of relaxation such as abdominal breathing exercises.
D. Develop images of the following:
   — The problem/disease.
   — Inner healing resources (strengths, belief systems, and coping strategies).
   — External healing resources (treatments, medication, tests, and surgery).
   — Final healed state or the desired state of well-being.

Optional Responses (in any order)

1. Guide him in the use of words/phrases to empower his imagery process, such as metaphors, truisms, embedded commands, linkage, therapeutic double-bind, synesthesia, and reframing.
2. Help him explore his images, colors, symbols, and meanings in relationship to his belief system.
3. Assist him with imagery as he deepens his practice.
4. Explore drawing with him and help him to assess his imagery process:
   — Disease or disability: the vividness of the client's views of the disease, illness, or disability; if the process is ongoing, its strength or ability to overcome health or focus on the reverse—the ability of the client to stop the process.
   — Internal healing resources: the vividness of the client's perception of the healing ability and effectiveness of this ability/action to combat the disease.
   — External healing resources: the vividness of the treatment description and the effectiveness of some positive mechanism of action.

Question 3 Responses

Basic Responses (in any order)

A. Help him to form correct biologic images of the normal evolution from myocardial injury to myocardial integrity.
B. Encourage him to image as he takes his daily medication how the medication is helping in the healing process.
C. Encourage him to continue cardiac rehabilitation and make a commitment to a healthy lifestyle.

Optional Responses (in any order)

1. Describe in detail the normal evolution from myocardial injury to myocardial integrity (e.g., health lattice network of good new blood flow around the damaged area; solid scar formation at site of myocardial injury).
2. Use specific words to empower placebo effects of healing.
3. Add specifics about cardiac rehabilitation (e.g., low-fat diet, exercise, stress management, no smoking, family and support groups).

Question 4 Responses

Basic Responses (in any order)

A. Introduce Jane to subjective experiences: what is to be felt, heard, or seen before, during, or after the cast removal: hearing buzz of saw, feeling vibrations or tingling, seeing chalky dust, feeling warmth on leg as saw cuts cast, feeling stiffness in leg after cast removal, feeling lightness in leg after cast removal.
B. Give Jane information about objective experiences: where the cast will be removed, when the surgeon will remove the cast, what information will be discussed after cast removal.

Optional Responses (in any order)

1. Obtain Jane's perception of the procedure/treatment/test to be experienced.
2. Choose words that have meaning for Jane.
3. Use synonyms that have less emotional impact, such as "discomfort" instead of "pain."
4. Give Jane specific examples of helpful experiences rather than abstract experiences.
5. Help Jane reframe negative imagery if any are elicited in the previous steps.

ANSWERS—CHAPTER 25

Answer to Test Questions 1–15

1. b	6. d	11. c
2. a	7. c	12. c
3. c	8. a	13. a
4. a	9. d	14. a
5. b	10. d	15. c

Answers to Situations 1–4

Question 1 Responses

Basic Responses (in any order)

A. Assess his fears and concerns about the procedure.
B. Assess his knowledge and experience with relaxation techniques.
C. Guide him in a general head-to-toe relaxation session followed by 20 minutes of music of his choice.
D. Record the session so that he can use the tape at home as a music therapy guide.
E. Encourage Mr. McGee to practice music therapy twice a day for 20 minutes each day before the MRI.

Optional Response

1. Encourage Mr. McGee to take his tape and recorder with him so that he can immerse himself in the music and relaxation while waiting for the MRI. Because some MRI machines have built-in audiocassette or CD players, have him call the MRI Center to determine whether it is possible to listen to his own tape or CD during the procedure. Be sure he understands that at times he will be unable to hear the music because of the noise from the machine. During these times, suggest that he focus his attention on deep breathing and head-to-toe relaxation.

Question 2 Responses

Basic Responses (in any order)

A. Explore with him what he means when he says the therapy is "not working."
B. Explain to him that there are no right or wrong ways to participate in a music therapy session and that the experiences vary with each session.

C. Explain that the outcomes of relaxation and music therapy are a function of practice; the more one practices, the better the skills become.
D. Encourage him to continue his participation in music therapy for a few more sessions before drawing any conclusion that the therapy is "not working."

Optional Responses (in any order)

1. Assess his fears and determine his understanding of bodymind unity (i.e., how his emotional stress and fear can affect his physiologic status).
2. Determine what his expectations of the session are.
3. Find out whether he believes another type of music might be more effective or soothing for his sessions.
4. Discuss the range of emotions, feelings, sensations, and images that people can experience during a session, while emphasizing that sometimes none of these experiences occur.
5. Respect his wishes not to participate in further sessions. Explore with him other options such as guided relaxation sessions, imagery, or touch.

Question 3 Responses

Basic Responses (in any order)

A. Suggest that she practice some relaxation and music therapy following her return home from work each day.
B. Recommend that she start each session with some deep breathing and muscle relaxation exercises.
C. Encourage her to start her sessions with a 2- to 3-minute musical selection that resonates with her stressful mood and then add more soothing music to relax her (i.e., iso-principle).
D. Encourage her to experiment with different types of music for relaxation. Explain also that the appropriate type of music will likely vary, depending on her bodymind state for that day.

Optional Responses (in any order)

1. Recommend that she try the Music Bath script to prepare for her stressful day before leaving for work.
2. Encourage her to take short breaks during her day at work.
3. Suggest that she remember to do diaphragmatic breathing during stressful encounters at work.

Question 4 Responses

Basic Responses (in any order)

A. When phoning patients to schedule their surgery, ask if they would be interested in listening to soothing music following their surgery as a way to help them recover from their anesthesia.
B. Ask patients to bring a soothing, relaxing tape, recorder, and headset with them the morning of surgery.
C. Preoperatively, spend a few minutes guiding the patient on how to breathe deeply, relax muscles, and focus on the music.
D. Following surgery, place the headset on the patient and turn on the music.
E. As the patient begins to wake up, orient him or her to time, place, and person, and remind the patient to practice deep breathing, relax, and focus on the music.
F. Evaluate each patient's response to the therapy.

Optional Responses (in any order)

1. Have several tape recorders, headsets, and different types of music available for patients who wish to participate in the music therapy, but who do not have this equipment available.
2. Ask the patient to choose the music on the morning of surgery.

ANSWERS—CHAPTER 26

Answers to Test Questions 1–12

1. d	5. c	9. d
2. b	6. c	10. b
3. d	7. b	11. a
4. c	8. d	12. c

Answers to Situations 1–12

Question 1 Responses

Basic Responses (in any order)

A. Give a general explanation of the ways that touch therapies affect the body-mind-spirit.
B. Help her to release pent up emotions.
C. Encourage deep breathing to induce emotional release.

D. Allow music and atmosphere to help her feel nourished.
E. Provide a safe place for her to articulate her loss.
F. Provide touch to support her as she has lost her primary touch partner.
G. Provide ongoing stable nurturance through the time of loss.

Optional Responses (in any order)

1. Determine what her identified needs are.
    — Support her in seeking out this information.
    — Use intuitive skills and sensitive listening.
    — Experiment with other gentle touch/healing modalities, while also using familiar ones.
2. Add energy healing to balance entire field.
3. Stay centered and set intent on making energy available to activate her inner healer.
    — Trust in her innate power to heal self.
    — Work with all available senses.
4. Support Ms. Quigley's deep relaxation physically, emotionally, and spiritually.
5. Acknowledge the increasing importance of touch in her healing process.
    — Seek input from her prior to working.
    — Help her to identify needs through focusing.
    — Add imagery to touch therapies and music.
6. Encourage her to use all available resources.

Question 2 Responses

Basic Responses (in any order)

A. Invite the mother to come in for a consultation.
B. Find a space conducive to learning/teaching.
C. Assess the mother's potential for centering.
    — Teach the mother the basic concepts of therapeutic touch.
    — Help her to set intent on the child's behalf.
    — Help her to keep herself calm.
D. Teach the mother the basic therapeutic touch maneuvers and steps.
E. Have the mother practice in your presence.

Optional Responses (in any order)

1. Encourage the child to become involved. Perhaps make it a game for him to figure out how to identify his needs immediately and to calm himself.
2. Teach the child about centering and setting intent.
    — Use terminology that he can relate to, perhaps images and descriptions that he himself developed.

— Have the child practice in your presence, using your expanded energy field to help him become aware of his own field.
3. Teach mother and child to work together as a team.
4. Help them to identify the most vulnerable times and ways to avert a full-blown crisis.
5. Teach the child to work with imagery to minimize fear response.
6. Create a variety of outlets for the child to explore the personal meaning of his condition, including art projects, music or dance, movement.
7. Encourage the child to teach other children how to help him when this occurs. Get friends and teachers involved to minimize panic responses in his immediate environment.

ANSWERS—CHAPTER 27

Answers to Test Questions 1–15

1. b	6. c	11. a
2. a	7. a	12. a
3. d	8. d	13. c
4. b	9. b	14. b
5. c	10. d	15. d

Answers to Situations 1–4

Question 1 Responses

Basic Responses (in any order)

A. Assess Ms. Smith's physical measures of body mass index, percentage of body fat, resting heart rate, blood pressure, physical fitness (submaximal bicycle ergometer), and strength.
B. Examine her psychologic profile (i.e., biographic inventory and dieting history, Bulit scale, body image, Daily Tension Stress Scale).
C. Discuss the successes and failures of weight loss approaches that she has used in the past.
D. Determine her willingness to learn about biopsycho-social and spiritual reasons for weight gain.
E. Assess her willingness to stop overeating, do consistent and challenging physical exercise, and do cognitive restructuring based on reversal theory.

F. Ask her to keep daily calendar recordings of exercise and overeating to detect patterns toward which interventions may be targeted.

Optional Responses (in any order)

1. Assess Ms. Smith's blood profile (i.e., cholesterol, lipoproteins, sugar).
2. Measure percentage of body fat using hydrostatic weighing.
3. Measure body circumferences (upper arm, chest/bust, waist, abdomen, hips, legs).

Question 2 Responses

Basic Responses (in any order)

A. Explain to Ms. Summers how to complete the personal daily calendar for 1 week to collect data about usual exercise, overeating, and tension stress patterns.
B. Make individualized nursing diagnoses and client outcomes with her while discussing the patterns revealed in her daily calendar.
C. Help her complete her daily calendar 1 week in advance to plan exercise and target homework about how to stop overeating; to get regular, challenging exercise; and to change negative self-talk. Give her audiocassette on how to stop overeating (*Diets Don't Work* by B. Schwartz (Chicago: Nightingale-Court) and *Fit or Fat Woman: Solutions for Women's Unique Concerns* by C. Bailey and L. Bishop (Boston: Houghton Mifflin Co., 1989) and relate it to the homework schedule.
D. Review with her the calendar pages and assignments for next week, and negotiate an individualized plan related to how to stop overeating, get regular exercise, and change self-talk.
E. On her return visit, analyze together her patterns of overeating, deterrents from getting regular exercise, and problematic self-talk related to overeating triggers. Develop strategies for countering problem areas according to cognitive restructuring based in reversal theory.

Optional Responses (in any order)

1. Ask Ms. Summers to take her resting heart rate before getting out of bed in the morning three times in the next week and calculate the target heart range.
2. Ask her to give a return demonstration of how to monitor heart rate during exercise and do warm-up and cool-down stretches.

3. Discuss appropriate clothes and shoes for exercise sessions.
4. Ask her to explain the food pyramid in relation to her preferences.

Question 3 Responses

Basic Responses (in any order)

A. Perform a full assessment and develop an individualized program for all three areas: stopping overeating; getting regular, challenging exercise; and changing negative self-talk that triggers overeating.
B. Assess Ms. Rolland's use of hormone replacement therapy.

Optional Responses (in any order)

1. Ask Ms. Rolland to explain the holistic self-care program to her regular physician and convey her intent to participate in the program to determine whether the physician recommends any special precautions.
2. Offer to talk with the physician if she desires.

Question 4 Responses

Basic Responses (in any order)

A. Perform a full assessment and develop an individualized program for all three areas: stopping overeating; getting regular, challenging exercise; and changing negative self-talk that triggers overeating.
B. Assess Mr. Harris' knowledge of diabetes mellitus.

Optional Responses (in any order)

1. Ask Mr. Harris to explain the holistic self-care program to his regular physician.
2. By conveying his intent to participate in the program, he will learn of any risks and necessary precautions.
3. Offer to talk with the physician if he desires.
4. Pay special attention to his cardiovascular condition to participate in aerobic and strength training exercises.
5. Evaluate his prescribed diet to ensure that six small meals and snacks are spaced evenly according to proposed activities and exercises. Make suggestions for dietary adjustments to allow natural hunger to drive his eating as much as possible.
6. Keep strict food records in the beginning to ensure optimal control of his diabetes. Adjust the

daily calendar pages to accommodate entry of daily intake and space to write prescribed blood glucose self-monitoring results.

Answers—Chapter 28

Answers to Test Questions 1–15

1. c	6. c	11. a
2. a	7. b	12. d
3. d	8. c	13. d
4. d	9. b	14. d
5. a	10. c	15. b

Answers to Situations 1–4

Question 1 Responses

Basic Responses (in any order)

A. Assess what Mr. Redford knows about the health effects of smoking and smoking cessation.
B. Have him do a self-assessment of why he smokes (i.e., smoke diary).
C. Have him list the reasons that he wants to quit and benefits of quitting.
D. Depending on his priority reasons for smoking, select the appropriate interventions.
E. Use the Fagerstrom Nicotine Tolerance Test to determine if he is addicted to nicotine; if so, recommend nicotine gum.
F. Since he is thinking seriously about cessation and has made a few attempts, consider him in the contemplation to preparation stages of change.
G. Provide him with interventions that can move him beyond the nicotine withdrawal and promote long-term lifestyle change, such as weight control through exercise and stress management techniques.
H. Encourage him to seek support from family, friends, and co-workers.

Optional Responses (in any order)

1. Assess smoking status as a new vital sign.
2. Assess actual motivation for quitting cigarettes.
3. Provide guidance concerning relapse prevention.

Question 2 Responses

Basic Responses (in any order)

A. Assess smoking status as the new vital sign to determine if your sense of smell is correct. If Ms. Vines is a current smoker, assess
— the amount of smoking, smoking rate (number of cigarettes per day).
— her reasons for smoking.
— the health effects of smoking.
B. Ask her if she would like to have some help with cessation.

Optional Responses (in any order)

1. Assess Ms. Vines' motivation for quitting (if any is present at this point).
2. Begin subtle discussion, counseling, and interventions.
3. Remember the four "Rs" (i.e., relevance, risks, rewards, and repetition) in working with her.

Question 3 Responses

Basic and Optional Responses (in any order)

A. Recognize that Fred is probably at the precontemplation stage of behavioral change, and it will be a challenge to motivate him to quit smoking.
B. Determine whether Fred's lack of plans and interests indicates that he lives for the present moment and is not inclined to think about his health in the future.
C. At first, use smoking cessation interventions with a "shock" value to get Fred in touch with the adverse effects of smoking and to help him learn about the dangers of smoking.
D. Try to apply peer pressure and support to help Fred quit smoking. The challenge will be to find nonsmoking friends and family who are respected by Fred and who are willing to provide that support.
E. Use the Fagerstrom Nicotine Tolerance Test to determine whether Fred is already addicted to nicotine because he is a heavy smoker.

Question 4 Responses

Basic and Optional Responses (in any order)

A. Consider that Ms. Stowe is at the contemplation stage for smoking cessation; however, it will take some time and effort to help her move into the preparation stage where her motivation and commitment to stop smoking may increase.

B. Educate her about the adverse effects of smoking so that she will view smoking in a less positive light. Once she is convinced that smoking is harmful, she may become more interested in moving into the action and maintenance stages of smoking cessation.

C. Persuade her to exercise actively and watch her diet in order to maintain her weight.

D. Institute interventions for stress reduction and confidence building (e.g., imagery, relaxation, self-affirmations) to substitute for smoking.

E. Help her to seek support from friends and family.

F. Follow up to build a sense of self-confidence and help with observing the long-term health benefits from smoking cessation.

ANSWERS—CHAPTER 29

Answers to Test Questions 1–12

1. a	5. d	9. c
2. b	6. c	10. a
3. a	7. c	11. c
4. c	8. c	12. b

Answers to Situations 1–4

Question 1 Responses

Basic Responses (in any order)

A. Ask Suzanne if she currently uses alcohol, tobacco, or other drugs.

B. Ask if there is any history of alcohol or other drug problems in her family.

C. Ask her about her relationships with the members of her family.

D. Assess the degree of substance use among Suzanne's peer group.

E. Ask how Suzanne does in school and what activities she participates in.

F. Ask Suzanne what goals she has set for herself.

G. Have Suzanne tell you about her neighborhood.

H. Find out if Suzanne attends any church activities.

I. Ask Suzanne to describe herself, her positive qualities.

Optional Responses (in any order)

1. Assess what Suzanne already knows about the problematic use of psychoactive substances.

2. Discuss Suzanne's perceptions of her school and her relationships with her teachers.

3. Ask what parenting style Suzanne's parents use.

4. Determine Suzanne's general state of physical and mental health.

Question 2 Responses

Basic Responses (in any order)

A. Teach Mr. Logan general relaxation and imagery exercises with a focus on helping him to be more in tune with his body's responses to stress.

B. Teach him to reframe stressful situations, to see the positive learning aspects of the situation rather than the negative ones.

C. Encourage him to keep a journal or get involved in some expressive hobby, such as painting or sculpting.

D. Develop a written contract for health, including healthy nutrition, regular exercise, regular practice of relaxation and imagery techniques, and healthy recreation.

E. Help him build a support system, including members of his family and friends who do not have problems with addictive substances.

F. Encourage him to strengthen his connections to his spirituality.

G. Teach him to complete daily affirmations, focusing on inner strengths and positive qualities.

H. Screen him for actual or potential problems with addictive substances.

Optional Responses (in any order)

1. Teach Mr. Logan about the components of a healthy lifestyle.

2. Strengthen family interactions by helping him to resolve any conflicts that may remain in his family; suggest family therapy if these conflicts are severe.

3. Provide information about prevention services available to him in his workplace and community.

4. Increase his sense of empowerment and self-responsibility.

5. Provide anticipatory guidance if he is contemplating major changes.

6. Help him identify outlets that would relieve boredom.

Question 3 Responses

Basic Responses (in any order)

A. Create a relationship with Mr. Martin so that he feels safe talking about issues and feelings.
B. Teach him general relaxation and imagery techniques.
C. Teach him specific imagery techniques, including cleansing images, protective shield images, images of what it will be like to be drug-free and sober, healing images.
D. Help him to visualize himself handling stressful situations in a constructive way.
E. Teach him to recognize negative thinking and to replace it with positive thinking.
F. Encourage him to ask his family and friends for support and acceptance in his efforts at recovery.
G. Determine what spirituality means to him, and encourage him to strengthen his spiritual connections.
H. Ask him to tell his personal story.
I. Encourage him to attend Alcoholics Anonymous and Narcotics Anonymous meetings at least daily for the next 3 months.
J. Talk about any resistance that he has to the spiritual component of 12-step meetings.
K. Have him identify high-risk situations that may trigger an urge to use alcohol or drugs again, and rehearse strategies for dealing with those urges.

Optional Responses (in any order)

1. Assess what Mr. Martin knows about the health consequences of addiction, and provide information to fill in any gaps in knowledge.
2. Teach him to complete daily affirmations, focusing on positive qualities and inner resources.
3. Assess his compliance with other parts of his recovery plan.
4. Assess the degree of craving, and collaborate with other professional health care providers regarding management of the cravings.

Question 4 Responses

Basic Responses (in any order)

A. Help Ms. Johnson to describe how her dependence on narcotics has interfered with her work and the rest of her life.
B. Convey respect and compassion, as well as hope that she will transform her life into a healthy one.
C. Provide information about treatment options and settings.
D. Encourage her to take responsibility for entering treatment through a detoxification program.
E. Reinforce the concept that narcotic dependence is a treatable illness.

Optional Responses (in any order)

1. Involve any members of Ms. Johnson's support system that she may identify as helpful.
2. Teach her about addiction and its consequences.
3. Conduct a personal inventory to determine if personal use or attitudes about addictive substances may interfere with your ability to help this colleague.

ANSWERS—CHAPTER 30

Answers to Test Questions 1–14

1. a	6. c	11. b
2. c	7. b	12. a
3. d	8. d	13. b
4. b	9. c	14. c
5. b	10. d	

Answers to Situations 1–4

Question 1 Responses

Basic Responses (in any order)

A. Consider your own comfort about working with an adult survivor of incest.
B. Identify your attitudes about incest/child sexual abuse.
C. Use references and other written materials to address any gaps in knowledge.

Optional Responses (in any order)

1. Consult with a clinician who is an expert in this area.
2. Refer Ms. Jones to a colleague if you feel unable to assess her condition competently because of your comfort level, attitudes, or knowledge base.

Question 2 Responses

Basic Responses (in any order)

A. First realize that a client's inability to express, or fear of expressing, anger/rage is a learned response.

B. Help Ms. Smith understand that
   — Her feelings of anger/rage are appropriate and understandable in light of her early incest experiences.
   — She has repressed those feelings for years.
   — She has probably expressed them in disguised form, affecting her ability to maintain a long-term intimate relationship.
   — The recent death of her parents has released the feelings, especially since she can no longer confront them about what they did to her.
C. Begin work with her to identify ways in which she can express her anger safely that would be comfortable for her and consistent with her lifestyle.

Optional Responses (in any order)

1. Assist Ms. Smith to "dose" her anger, using a 30-second to 3-minute timer to indicate the time period that a safe amount of anger can be expressed.
2. Instruct her to record on tape the expression of anger during the predetermined time (30 seconds to 3 minutes) and bring the tape to the next session to play and review.
3. Instruct her to experiment with various suggested means of expressing anger, and bring a report of their effectiveness to the next session.

Question 3 Responses

Basic Responses (in any order)

A. Realize that Laurie has many strengths as demonstrated by her ability to get away from the abusive situation, enroll in college, and develop a relationship with a young man.
B. Collaborate with the client to identify desired outcomes and set goals.
C. Provide opportunity for and support Laurie during full disclosure.
D. Teach her about appropriate family function, including roles and responsibilities, to provide an alternative way of understanding what has happened to her and how she has been functioning in an adult/spousal role with her stepfather.

E. Explore new or alternative behaviors that Laurie could try that will allow her to continue her relationship with her mother without returning to the abusive situation.

Optional Responses (in any order)

1. Help Laurie realize and believe that she is the only "true expert" in this situation and that she has the information to lead her to the best decision for her life.
2. If Laurie shows any sign of dissociation during her disclosure, teach her grounding skills that she can use to stay in the present.

Question 4 Responses

Basic Responses (in any order)

A. Start with the technique of writing (journaling and letter writing).
B. Suggest that Mr. Jackson begin keeping a daily journal, recording thoughts, feelings, dreams, nightmares, etc.
C. Emphasize the importance of privacy to write and the security of what is written. If necessary, help him find ways to ensure privacy/security so that he can express himself without censorship.
D. Instruct him to bring the journal with him to his next appointment so you can assist him in recognizing the source and expression of his pain.
E. Use the journal entries to guide "homework" assignments, such as rewriting the story of his abuse the way he would like it to come out.

Optional Responses (in any order)

1. Have Mr. Jackson write an uncensored letter to his brother, telling him how he feels about the abuse and how it has affected his life.
2. Have him bring the letter to the next appointment and read it aloud.
3. Help him to analyze the letter, his emotional responses and/or release in writing and/or reading, and, if indicated, identify next steps.

Standards of Holistic Nursing Practice

American Holistic Nurses' Association (AHNA) Standards of Holistic Nursing Practice

Part I:	**Discipline of Holistic Nursing Practice**
Concept I.	Holistic Philosophy
Concept II.	Holistic Foundation
Concept III.	Holistic Ethics
Concept IV.	Holistic Nursing Theories
Concept V.	Holistic Nursing and Related Research
Concept VI.	Holistic Nursing Process

Part II:	**Caring and Healing of Clients and Significant Others**
Concept VII.	Meaning and Wholeness
Concept VIII.	Client Self-Care
Concept IX.	Health Promotion

AHNA Standards of Holistic Nursing Practice

Part I: Discipline of Holistic Nursing Practice

Concept I. Holistic Philosophy

Standards of Care:

1. Holistic nurses shall be committed to the development of the art and science of holistic nursing practice.
2. Holistic nurses shall actively participate in professional activities to promote competency in practice and to assure quality of care to clients.

Standards of Practice:

A. Holistic nurses shall participate in the continuing education of nursing, holistic disciplines, holistic history, and theories.

Source: Reprinted with permission from the American Holistic Nurses' Association, 4101 Lake Boone Trail, Suite 201, Raleigh, NC 27607. Phone 1-800-278-AHNA, Fax 919-787-4916. Copyright © 1994, Revised 1997.

B. Holistic nurses shall support, share, and recognize nursing expertise.
C. Holistic nurses with expertise shall mentor others in professional growth (from novice to expert) in areas of holistic development.
D. Holistic nurses shall develop competency in practice to facilitate a sense of sacredness about their work.
E. Holistic nurses shall explore and develop the state of "nurse as healing environment."

Concept II. Holistic Foundation

Standard of Care:

1. Holistic nurses shall be committed to personal development of holism.

Standards of Practice:

A. Holistic nurses shall continue their own personal development to ensure expertise in holistic nursing practice and interventions.
B. Holistic nurses shall be optimistic that they can participate in improving the client's situation.
C. Holistic nurses shall have clear intent to care and possess a sense of balance between what they give to self and others.
D. Holistic nurses shall consciously participate in the evolutionary holistic process recognizing that crisis can equal opportunity.
E. Holistic nurses shall mentor and support others in reaching personal goals.

Concept III. Holistic Ethics

Standards of Care:

1. Holistic nurses shall adhere to a professional ethic of caring and healing that seeks to preserve the dignity and wholeness of the person who is receiving care.
2. Holistic nurses shall participate in establishing and promoting conditions in society where holistic health can be achieved.
3. Holistic nurses shall actively participate in professional activities to assist in responding to changes occurring in the practice environment.

Standards of Practice:

A. Holistic nurses shall adhere to the integration of caring and healing that seeks to preserve the dignity and wholeness in various practice environments of the clients and significant others.
B. Holistic nurses shall become aware of local, state, national, and international nursing organizations and actively focus on health issues at various levels.
C. Holistic nurses shall become politically active on issues that impact health from a holistic perspective.
D. Holistic nurses shall be proactive on issues that impact their professional practice in holistic nursing.

Standard of Care:

4. Holistic nurses shall participate in the ethics of caring and identify a linkage of caring to public policy.

Standards of Practice:

A. Holistic nurses shall become involved in holistic health care reform and policy development.
B. Holistic nurses shall go beyond advocacy to deal with the pressing issues of health care delivery itself, and work with the sociocultural world or industry of health care to bring about needed change.

Standards of Care:

5. Holistic nurses shall participate in holistic ethics by a commitment to practices that respect, nurture, and enhance an integral relationship with the earth's functioning.

6. Holistic nurses shall act politically to protect, foster, and advocate for the interspecies of life on the planet.
7. Holistic nurses shall teach, share, and serve as resources in considering the holistic nature of the universe.

Standards of Practice:

A. Holistic nurses shall value and promote mutually enhancing activities, industries, and policies for the human and natural world.
B. Holistic nurses shall advocate for the well-being of the global community's economy, education, and ethical norms.

Concept IV. Holistic Nursing Theories

Standard of Care:

1. Nursing theory shall provide the framework for documenting professional nursing practice.

Standards of Practice:

A. Holistic nurses shall identify a nursing theory or theories upon which to base their nursing practice.
B. Information relevant to client care shall be gathered according to the theoretical framework.
C. Client problems/patterns/needs or opportunities to enhance health and well-being shall be identified based on the theoretical framework.
D. Nursing actions shall be derived from the theory.
E. Care shall be documented and evaluated in the language of the theory.
F. Clients' records shall be written from within the framework of the nursing theory.

Concept V. Holistic Nursing and Related Research

Standards of Care:

1. Clients and significant others shall receive advice on nursing interventions and holistic therapies based on research findings.
2. Clients and significant others shall receive care by nurses who deliver nursing care grounded in a nursing theory/conceptual model.

Standards of Practice:

A. Holistic nurses shall create an environment conducive to systematic inquiry into clinical problems by engaging in nursing research, and/or supporting and utilizing the research of others.
B. Holistic nursing interventions and recommendations shall be based on research.
C. Holistic nursing care shall be grounded in one of the many theories of nursing practice.

Concept VI. Holistic Nursing Process

Standard of Care:

1. Clients shall be assessed holistically and continually.

Standards of Practice:

A. Holistic nurses shall collect data in an organized, systematic fashion to ensure completeness of assessments.
B. Holistic nurses shall utilize appropriate physical examination techniques.
C. Holistic nurses shall demonstrate competency in communication skills.
D. Holistic nurses shall gather pertinent bio-psycho-socio-spiritual data from the client, significant others, and other health team members.

E. Holistic nurses shall collect pertinent data from previous client records.
F. Holistic nurses shall also use intuition as a means of gathering data from a client and significant others. Intuitive knowledge may be validated with the client and significant others.
G. Holistic nurses shall collaborate with other health team members to collect data.
H. Holistic nurses shall review the database as new information is available.
I. Holistic nurses shall document all pertinent assessment data in the client's record.

Standard of Care:

2. Client actual and high-risk problems/patterns/needs and opportunities to enhance health and well-being, and their priorities shall be identified based upon collected data.

Standards of Practice:

A. Holistic nurses shall utilize collected data to establish a list of actual and high risk problems/patterns/needs and opportunities to enhance health and well-being.
B. Holistic nurses shall collaborate with the client, significant others, and health team members in identification of actual and high risk problems/patterns/needs and opportunities to enhance health and well-being.
C. Holistic nurses shall utilize collected data to formulate hypotheses as to the etiologic bases for each identified actual or high-risk problem/pattern/need and opportunity to enhance health and well-being.
D. Holistic nurses shall utilize nursing diagnoses for the actual or high risk problems/patterns/needs and opportunities to enhance health and well-being that nurses, by virtue of education and experience, are able, responsible, and accountable to treat.
E. Holistic nurses shall establish the priority of problems/patterns/needs according to the actual or high-risk threats to the client. Opportunities to enhance health and well-being shall also be included.
F. Holistic nurses shall reassess the list and priorities as the database changes.
G. Holistic nurses shall record identified actual or high risk problems/patterns/needs and opportunities to enhance health and well-being and indicate priority in the client's record.
H. Holistic nurses shall document client situations that provide opportunities to enhance and support growth, development, and movement toward recognizing wholeness.

Standards of Care:

3. Client's actual or high-risk problems/patterns/needs or opportunities to enhance health and well-being shall have appropriate outcomes specified and revised as appropriate.
4. Client's outcomes will reflect a concern of persons as a total system and a view of health that identifies both internal and external environments which maximizes the client's potential for functioning within the environment.

Standards of Practice:

A. Holistic nurses shall specify one or more measurable client outcomes for each actual or high-risk problem/pattern/need or opportunity to enhance health and well-being in collaboration with others. Each outcome shall specify something that should or should not occur, the time at which it should occur, who it should be accomplished by, and the expected results.
B. Holistic nurses shall record outcomes, communicate to others, and revise as needed.

Standards of Care:

5. Clients shall have an appropriate plan of holistic nursing care formulated focusing on health promotion or health maintenance activities.
6. Clients and significant others shall be told the degree to which information is known or not known regarding all nursing recommendations for care.

Standards of Practice:

A. Holistic nurses shall develop the plan of care in collaboration with the client, significant others, and other health team members.

B. Holistic nurses shall determine nursing interventions for each problem/pattern/need or opportunity to enhance health and well-being.

C. Holistic nurses shall develop the plan of care based on the client's genetic predisposition and mental and emotional capacities.

D. Holistic nurses shall incorporate interventions that communicate acceptance of the client's and significant others' values, beliefs, culture, religion, and socioeconomic background.

E. Holistic nurses shall identify areas for education of the client and significant others.

F. Holistic nurses shall develop appropriate client goals for each problem/pattern/need or opportunity to enhance health and well-being in collaboration with the client, significant others, and other health team members.

G. Holistic nurses shall organize the plan to reflect the priority of identified problems/patterns/needs and opportunities to enhance health and well-being.

H. Holistic nurses shall revise the plan of care to reflect the client's current status.

I. Holistic nurses shall communicate the plan to those involved in the client's care.

J. Holistic nurses shall incorporate the plan of nursing care on the client record.

Standards of Care:

7. Client's plan of holistic nursing care shall be implemented according to the priority of identified problems/patterns/needs or opportunities to enhance health and well-being.

8. Client's plan of holistic nursing care shall be implemented within the context of assisting the individual to progress forward and upward toward a higher potential of functioning.

Standards of Practice:

A. Holistic nurses shall implement the plan of nursing care in collaboration with the client, significant others, and other health team members.

B. Holistic nurses shall support and promote client participation in care.

C. Holistic nurses shall participate in care in an organized and compassionate manner.

D. Holistic nurses shall integrate current scientific knowledge with nursing care.

E. Holistic nurses shall integrate the intuitive art of nursing with the scientific knowledge and technical competencies.

F. Holistic nurses shall provide care in a timely manner and in a way as to prevent complications and life-threatening situations.

G. Holistic nurses shall coordinate care delivered by other health team members.

H. Holistic nurses shall document interventions in the record.

Standard of Care:

9. Client's response to holistic nursing care shall be continuously evaluated.

Standards of Practice:

A. Holistic nurses shall ensure the relevance of nursing interventions to identified client problems/patterns/needs or opportunities to enhance health and well-being.

B. Holistic nurses shall collect data for evaluation within an appropriate time interval after intervention.

C. Holistic nurses shall compare the client's response with expected outcomes.

D. Holistic nurses shall base the evaluation on data from pertinent sources.

E. Holistic nurses shall collaborate with the client, significant others, and other health team members in the evaluation process.

F. Holistic nurses shall attempt to determine the cause of any significant deviation between the client's response and the expected outcomes.

G. Holistic nurses shall review the plan of care and revise it based on evaluation outcomes.

H. Holistic nurses shall document evaluation and outcomes in the client record.

Part II: Caring and Healing of Clients and Significant Others

Concept VII. Meaning and Wholeness

Standards of Care:

1. Clients and significant others experience the presence of the nurse as a shared humanness that includes a sense of connectedness and attention to them as unique persons.

2. Clients and nurses experience a sense of valued interchange (authenticity).

Standards of Practice:

A. Holistic nurses shall focus care on the whole client and significant others, not merely the current presenting symptoms or tasks to be accomplished.

B. Holistic nurses shall respect the client's and significant others' rights and choices and act as an advocate for the client and significant others.

C. Holistic nurses shall make decisions about how to proceed with nursing care based on a comprehensive assessment of relevant areas and on holistic understanding of the client and significant others.

Standards of Care:

3. Clients and significant others shall receive care consistent with their cultural backgrounds, health beliefs, and values.

4. Clients' and significant others' cultural diversity and its importance to the global community will be respected, protected, and enhanced.

Standards of Practice:

A. Holistic nurses shall gain knowledge of cultural practices of clients and significant others in their care, and integrate this knowledge in practice.

B. Holistic nurses shall assess meaning of health, illness, risk behaviors, and the management of care for each client and significant others.

C. Holistic nurses shall make use of appropriate community resources and experts to validate knowledge and practices of different cultural groups.

D. Holistic nurses shall recognize the critical nature of diversity to the global community.

Standards of Care:

5. Clients and significant others shall receive care that is consistent with their values and beliefs.

6. Clients shall be cared for as whole, spiritual beings.

7. Clients and significant others shall receive support for their spiritual growth.

Standards of Practice:

A. Holistic nurses shall assess the client's values and beliefs, and plan individualized care.

B. Holistic nurses shall provide an environment conducive to reflection, prayer, and spiritual growth.

C. Holistic nurses shall actively support the client's and significant others' search for meaning and purpose in life, illness, and death.

D. Holistic nurses shall actively support the client's and significant others' search for relationship with self, others, the environment, and a higher power.

Concept VIII. Client Self-Care

Standards of Care:

1. Clients and significant others shall be facilitated and supported in managing self-care to maximize quality of life (e.g., treatments and side effects, activities of daily living, changes in relationships, and lifestyle).
2. Clients and significant others shall have the information and resources needed for ongoing holistic health care.
3. Clients shall receive care aimed at empowering them to accept responsibility for their own health and well-being.

Standards of Practice:

A. Holistic nurses shall plan with clients and significant others for self-care by assisting with identification and facilitation of their desired level of physical, psychological, sociological, and spiritual potential.
B. Holistic nurses shall provide information on nursing and multidisciplinary resources available in the clinic, hospital, or community including home health services.
C. Holistic nurses shall initiate referrals and facilitate access to health care resources for clinic appointments, client admissions, or financial counseling or to community agencies for psychological counseling, allied health services, social service support, or educational assistance in a school setting.
D. Holistic nurses shall provide phone numbers and the name of person(s) to contact with questions/concerns or for urgent/emergent situations that include daytime and after-hours numbers.
E. Holistic nurses shall maintain contact as necessary with clients and significant others, and other health team members involved in the client's care.

Standards of Care:

4. Clients and significant others shall receive care in an environment that is safe.
5. Clients and significant others shall receive care in an environment that is respectful and healing.
6. Clients and significant others shall be cared for in as healthy an environment as possible (e.g., clean air and water, nutritious food, and with environmentally "friendly" life sustaining practices).

Standards of Practice:

A. Holistic nurses shall practice according to policies and procedures in relation to environmental safety and emergency preparedness.
B. Holistic nurses shall respect privacy, confidentiality, and environments conducive to experiencing wholeness and harmony.
C. Holistic nurses shall recognize that the well-being of the ecosystem of the planet is a prior determining condition for the well-being of the human.

Concept IX. Health Promotion

Standards of Care:

1. Clients and significant others possess the knowledge they want and need in order to be involved in decisions about health care, work, home life, and recreation.
2. Clients and significant others receive health care based on priorities of care that contribute to desired outcomes.
3. Clients and significant others are active partners in health care planning and decision making based on individual desires.

Standards of Practice:

A. Holistic nurses shall use the principles of teaching and learning; they shall provide ongoing assessment, education, and evaluation of clients' and significant others' knowledge in relation to illness, diagnostic and treatment plans, anticipated outcomes, and self-care activities.

B. Holistic nurses shall collaborate with other health care providers; they shall give timely information related to preparation for procedures and results of tests.

C. Holistic nurses shall engage the client and significant others in mutual planning for goals, diagnostic tests, treatments, home-care, and follow-up care.

D. Holistic nurses shall be persistent in responding to environmental barriers to the delivery of holistic goal-oriented care; they can take risks, if necessary, to advocate for the client and significant others.

E. Holistic nurses shall support the clients' sense of personal responsibility and assist clients to achieve their desired outcomes.

F. Holistic nurses shall be flexible, willing, and be able to give up control of routines, information, "knowing what is best," and so forth in order to participate in client-centered care.

G. Holistic nurses shall engage clients and significant others in problem solving discussions in relation to living with changes secondary to illness and treatment.

Standards of Care:

4. Clients and significant others shall recognize patterns that place them at risk for health problems (e.g., personal habits, personal and family health history, age-related risk factors).

5. Clients and significant others shall practice preventive measures (e.g., immunizations, breast self exam, fitness/exercise programs, belief practices [prayer]).

Standards of Practice:

A. Holistic nurses shall provide and access information to and from clients and significant others in relation to primary, secondary, and tertiary nursing interventions.

B. Holistic nurses shall assist and support clients and significant others to identify ways to incorporate health promotion or health maintenance activities in their lifestyles.

Inventory of Professional Activities and Knowledge of a Holistic Nurse (IPAKHN) Survey

INTRODUCTION

The American Holistic Nurses' Association (AHNA) is conducting a national survey entitled **Inventory of Professional Activities and Knowledge of a Holistic Nurse (IPAKHN)**. The **IPAKHN Survey** will ensure adequate content validity for the **AHNA Certification Examination**.

In an effort to ensure the highest quality, AHNA, in collaboration with the National League for Nursing, will develop a valid and reliable certification examination that will certify a registered nurse in holistic nursing for various practice settings.

DESCRIPTION OF HOLISTIC NURSING

Holistic nursing embraces all nursing practice that has healing the whole person as its goal. Holistic nursing recognizes that there are two views regarding holism: that holism involves studying and understanding the interrelationships of the bio-psycho-social-spiritual dimensions of the person, recognizing that the whole is greater than the sum of its parts; and that holism involves understanding the individual as an integrated whole interacting with and being acted upon by both internal and external environments. Holistic nursing accepts both views, believing that the goals of nursing can be achieved within either framework.

Holistic practice draws on nursing knowledge, theories, expertise, and intuition to guide nurses in becoming therapeutic partners with clients in strengthening the clients' responses to facilitate the healing process and achieve wholeness.

Practicing holistic nursing requires nurses to integrate self-care in their own lives. Self-responsibility leads the nurse to a greater awareness of the interconnectedness of all individuals and their relationships to the human and global community, and permits nurses to use this awareness to facilitate healing.

ORGANIZATION OF IPAKHN SURVEY

The **AHNA Standards of Holistic Nursing Practice** adopted by the AHNA in 1994 serve as the blueprint for the **IPAKHN Survey**. This blueprint defines the dimensions of holistic practice, professional activities and knowledge that are required of a registered nurse in various practice environments. The **AHNA Standards of Holistic Nursing Practice** are divided into two major parts and nine categories as follows:

Source: Reprinted with permission from the American Holistic Nurses' Association, 4101 Lake Boone Trail, Suite 201, Raleigh, NC 27607. Phone 1-800-278-AHNA, Fax 919-787-4916. Copyright © 1994, Revised 1997.

Part I: Discipline of Holistic Nursing Practice

Concept I.   Holistic Philosophy
Concept II.   Holistic Foundation
Concept III. Holistic Ethics
Concept IV.   Holistic Nursing Theories
Concept V.   Holistic Nursing and Related Research
Concept VI.   Holistic Nursing Process

Part II: Caring and Healing of Clients and Significant Others

Concept VII. Meaning and Wholeness
Concept VIII. Client Self-Care
Concept IX.   Health Promotion

INSTRUCTIONS

Each statement should be rated for its importance to knowledge (**Column #I**), for frequency of performance (**Column #II**), and for its importance to practice (**Column #III**). Use a ruler to focus on the correct line. Those responsibilities that rank highest in terms of knowledge, frequency, and importance will be more fully represented in the AHNA examination blueprint.

Column #I—Knowledge: Using this scale, indicate how important each statement is to your knowledge base as a holistic nurse:

Not important: This knowledge is *not* required for holistic nursing.
Slightly important: This knowledge is required *from time to time,* but my performance could be acceptable without it.
Important: This knowledge is *generally* required in order for me to perform satisfactorily as a holistic nurse. Without it, my performance could be marginal.
Very important: This knowledge is *one of the key* requirements for my work in holistic nursing.

Fill in the appropriate box that corresponds to your rating as to the importance of knowledge in Column #I.

Column #II—Frequency: Using the following scale, select the response that most closely matches the number of times a week you perform the activity:

Less than once per week
1–5 times per week
6–10 times per week
Over 10 times per week

Fill in the appropriate box beside each activity that you perform to indicate how frequently you do it in the course of one week.

Column #III—Professional Activity: Indicate how important each activity is to your success as a holistic nurse:

Not important: This activity is only a trivial part of my overall duties.
Slightly important: This is among the least important activities of my job.
Important: This is among the more important activities of my job.
Very important: This is one of the most critical activities of my job.

Fill in the appropriate box beside each activity you perform to indicate its relative importance to your successful performance as a holistic nurse.

PART 1: DISCIPLINE OF HOLISTIC NURSING PRACTICE

Concept I. Holistic Philosophy

	I Knowledge				II Frequency of Activity					III Professional Activity			
	Not important	Slightly important	Important	Very important	Do not perform	Less than 1 per week	1–5 per week	6–10 per week	Over 10 per week	Not important	Slightly important	Important	Very Important
1. Use the AHNA Standards of Holistic Nursing Practice to guide nursing practice, professional education, and personal development.	❑	❑	❑	❑	❑	❑	❑	❑	❑	❑	❑	❑	❑
2. Explore health as a process by which individuals attain and sustain a sense of wholeness and function in the face of changes in themselves and the environment.	❑	❑	❑	❑	❑	❑	❑	❑	❑	❑	❑	❑	❑
3. Be a therapeutic, caring presence in all interactions.	❑	❑	❑	❑	❑	❑	❑	❑	❑	❑	❑	❑	❑
4. Identify relationship as the foundation of any therapeutic or healing activity.	❑	❑	❑	❑	❑	❑	❑	❑	❑	❑	❑	❑	❑
5. Release personal attachment from outcome of client's process.	❑	❑	❑	❑	❑	❑	❑	❑	❑	❑	❑	❑	❑
6. Empower the client's personal process and decision making in achieving health goals and outcomes.	❑	❑	❑	❑	❑	❑	❑	❑	❑	❑	❑	❑	❑
7. Continually develop understanding of holistic philosophy, theory, practice, and caring/healing modalities.	❑	❑	❑	❑	❑	❑	❑	❑	❑	❑	❑	❑	❑
8. Use mentoring in areas where needed to further holistic philosophy, theory, and practice.	❑	❑	❑	❑	❑	❑	❑	❑	❑	❑	❑	❑	❑
9. Achieve balance between what is given to self and to others.	❑	❑	❑	❑	❑	❑	❑	❑	❑	❑	❑	❑	❑
10. Recognize that crisis can be an opportunity in the growth of self and change.	❑	❑	❑	❑	❑	❑	❑	❑	❑	❑	❑	❑	❑
11. Care for self (e.g., exercise, nutrition, relaxation, relationships, spiritual development, etc.) to model personal health, well-being, and balance.	❑	❑	❑	❑	❑	❑	❑	❑	❑	❑	❑	❑	❑
12. Mentor others in areas of holistic development and modalities in service to the whole.	❑	❑	❑	❑	❑	❑	❑	❑	❑	❑	❑	❑	❑

Concept II. Holistic Foundation

	Not important	Slightly important	Important	Very important	Do not perform	Less than 1 per week	1–5 per week	6–10 per week	Over 10 per week	Not important	Slightly important	Important	Very Important
13. Approach human beings as integrated, open, living, energy systems rather than arrangement of parts; any disturbance in one area reflects a disturbance in the whole system.	❑	❑	❑	❑	❑	❑	❑	❑	❑	❑	❑	❑	❑
14. Identify spiritual, mental, and emotional distress as issues that influence a person's body-mind-spirit unity and well-being.	❑	❑	❑	❑	❑	❑	❑	❑	❑	❑	❑	❑	❑
15. Integrate steps towards preventing illness by a healthy lifestyle that leads toward wholeness, well-being, and more effective coping with illness or crisis.	❑	❑	❑	❑	❑	❑	❑	❑	❑	❑	❑	❑	❑

	I Knowledge				II Frequency of Activity					III Professional Activity			
	Not important	Slightly important	Important	Very important	Do not perform	Less than 1 per week	1–5 per week	6–10 per week	Over 10 per week	Not important	Slightly important	Important	Very Important
16. Identify healing as a process where a person's natural ability to heal can be strengthened. …	☐	☐	☐	☐	☐	☐	☐	☐	☐	☐	☐	☐	☐
17. Use multiple healing approaches as agreed by nurse, client, and significant others. ……	☐	☐	☐	☐	☐	☐	☐	☐	☐	☐	☐	☐	☐
18. Collaborate with others to integrate resources to provide the best plan of care for the client and significant others. ……	☐	☐	☐	☐	☐	☐	☐	☐	☐	☐	☐	☐	☐
19. Use natural, safe methods that mobilize the individual's healing resources in a manner that complements traditional therapies. ……	☐	☐	☐	☐	☐	☐	☐	☐	☐	☐	☐	☐	☐
20. Offer choices of natural, low-risk methods as the first intervention when appropriate. ……	☐	☐	☐	☐	☐	☐	☐	☐	☐	☐	☐	☐	☐
21. Achieve holistic consciousness and intentionality to evolve a state of being authentically present in the moment. ……	☐	☐	☐	☐	☐	☐	☐	☐	☐	☐	☐	☐	☐
22. Integrate modalities that assist with spiritual evolution in areas of meaning, purpose, inner strength, and interconnections (self, others, and the universe). ……	☐	☐	☐	☐	☐	☐	☐	☐	☐	☐	☐	☐	☐

Concept III.   Holistic Ethics

	I Knowledge				II Frequency of Activity					III Professional Activity			
23. Adhere to a professional ethic of caring and healing that seeks to preserve the dignity and wholeness of the person who is receiving care. ……	☐	☐	☐	☐	☐	☐	☐	☐	☐	☐	☐	☐	☐
24. Increase awareness of care of the community as a system to support individual well-being and wholeness. ……	☐	☐	☐	☐	☐	☐	☐	☐	☐	☐	☐	☐	☐
25. Identify the spectrum of support necessary to provide whole person care and to help access necessary resources based on client identified priorities. ……	☐	☐	☐	☐	☐	☐	☐	☐	☐	☐	☐	☐	☐
26. Improve the environment for different practitioners to work together, by fostering a sense of community and collaboration. ……	☐	☐	☐	☐	☐	☐	☐	☐	☐	☐	☐	☐	☐
27. Integrate holistic nursing practices in collaborative approaches with other community practitioners and agencies when appropriate. ……	☐	☐	☐	☐	☐	☐	☐	☐	☐	☐	☐	☐	☐
28. Participate in activities as an advocate for wholeness and well-being of diverse populations. ……	☐	☐	☐	☐	☐	☐	☐	☐	☐	☐	☐	☐	☐
29. Participate in local, state, national, and international nursing organizations. ……	☐	☐	☐	☐	☐	☐	☐	☐	☐	☐	☐	☐	☐
30. Actively focus on health issues at various levels. ……	☐	☐	☐	☐	☐	☐	☐	☐	☐	☐	☐	☐	☐
31. Stay informed of political issues and activities that influence health care reform and policy development. ……	☐	☐	☐	☐	☐	☐	☐	☐	☐	☐	☐	☐	☐

	I Knowledge				II Frequency of Activity					III Professional Activity			
	Not important	Slightly important	Important	Very important	Do not perform	Less than 1 per week	1–5 per week	6–10 per week	Over 10 per week	Not important	Slightly important	Important	Very Important
32. Advocate for the pressing issues of health care reform and health care delivery.	❑	❑	❑	❑	❑	❑	❑	❑	❑	❑	❑	❑	❑
33. Promote sustainable strategies, activities, industries, and policies to improve the human and environment conditions.	❑	❑	❑	❑	❑	❑	❑	❑	❑	❑	❑	❑	❑
34. Advocate for the well-being of the global community's wholeness, economy, and education.	❑	❑	❑	❑	❑	❑	❑	❑	❑	❑	❑	❑	❑

Concept IV. Holistic Nursing Theories

	I Knowledge				II Frequency of Activity					III Professional Activity			
35. Recognize how nursing theories complement and contribute to nursing practice.	❑	❑	❑	❑	❑	❑	❑	❑	❑	❑	❑	❑	❑
36. Identify holistic nursing theory upon which to base nursing practice.	❑	❑	❑	❑	❑	❑	❑	❑	❑	❑	❑	❑	❑
37. Use nursing theory to guide nursing actions and professional approaches to care decisions.	❑	❑	❑	❑	❑	❑	❑	❑	❑	❑	❑	❑	❑
38. Use holistic nursing theory to guide one's intentional focus on caring presence and healing.	❑	❑	❑	❑	❑	❑	❑	❑	❑	❑	❑	❑	❑
39. Use holistic nursing theory to help integrate one's knowing, doing, and being in nursing practice.	❑	❑	❑	❑	❑	❑	❑	❑	❑	❑	❑	❑	❑
40. Use nursing theory for nursing practice and nursing research.	❑	❑	❑	❑	❑	❑	❑	❑	❑	❑	❑	❑	❑
41. Identify client problems/patterns/needs or opportunities to enhance health based on the nursing theoretical framework.	❑	❑	❑	❑	❑	❑	❑	❑	❑	❑	❑	❑	❑
42. Derive nursing actions from the nursing theory.	❑	❑	❑	❑	❑	❑	❑	❑	❑	❑	❑	❑	❑
43. Document and evaluate care in the language of the nursing theory.	❑	❑	❑	❑	❑	❑	❑	❑	❑	❑	❑	❑	❑

Concept V. Holistic Nursing and Related Research

	I Knowledge				II Frequency of Activity					III Professional Activity			
44. Create an environment conducive to systematic inquiry of health and health care practices (e.g. the experience of living with HIV infection).	❑	❑	❑	❑	❑	❑	❑	❑	❑	❑	❑	❑	❑
45. Integrate specific research recommendations when possible into nursing practice.	❑	❑	❑	❑	❑	❑	❑	❑	❑	❑	❑	❑	❑
46. Inform clients and significant others of the information about options in treatment.	❑	❑	❑	❑	❑	❑	❑	❑	❑	❑	❑	❑	❑

Concept VI. Holistic Nursing Process

	I Knowledge				II Frequency of Activity					III Professional Activity			
47. Utilize the nursing process to enhance client's and significant others' care.	❑	❑	❑	❑	❑	❑	❑	❑	❑	❑	❑	❑	❑

	I Knowledge				II Frequency of Activity					III Professional Activity			
	Not important	Slightly important	Important	Very important	Do not perform	Less than 1 per week	1–5 per week	6–10 per week	Over 10 per week	Not important	Slightly important	Important	Very Important

Assessment

48. Collect bio-psycho-social-spiritual data incorporating scientific and intuitive approaches. .... ❏ ❏ ❏ ❏ ❏ ❏ ❏ ❏ ❏ ❏ ❏ ❏ ❏

49. Validate intuitive insights with the client and significant others. .... ❏ ❏ ❏ ❏ ❏ ❏ ❏ ❏ ❏ ❏ ❏ ❏ ❏

50. Assess state of energy field and meaning to the client when energy field disturbances are present. (Use if appropriate) .... ❏ ❏ ❏ ❏ ❏ ❏ ❏ ❏ ❏ ❏ ❏ ❏ ❏

51. Use appropriate physical examination techniques. .... ❏ ❏ ❏ ❏ ❏ ❏ ❏ ❏ ❏ ❏ ❏ ❏ ❏

52. Use therapeutic communication skills. .... ❏ ❏ ❏ ❏ ❏ ❏ ❏ ❏ ❏ ❏ ❏ ❏ ❏

53. Identify stages of change and readiness to learn. .... ❏ ❏ ❏ ❏ ❏ ❏ ❏ ❏ ❏ ❏ ❏ ❏ ❏

54. Collect pertinent data from previous client records. .... ❏ ❏ ❏ ❏ ❏ ❏ ❏ ❏ ❏ ❏ ❏ ❏ ❏

55. Collaborate with other health team members to collect data if appropriate. .... ❏ ❏ ❏ ❏ ❏ ❏ ❏ ❏ ❏ ❏ ❏ ❏ ❏

56. Incorporate new information into holistic assessment. .... ❏ ❏ ❏ ❏ ❏ ❏ ❏ ❏ ❏ ❏ ❏ ❏ ❏

57. Document all pertinent data in the client's record. .... ❏ ❏ ❏ ❏ ❏ ❏ ❏ ❏ ❏ ❏ ❏ ❏ ❏

Client problems/patterns/needs

58. Use collected data to establish a list of the client's and significant others' strengths, problems/patterns/needs. .... ❏ ❏ ❏ ❏ ❏ ❏ ❏ ❏ ❏ ❏ ❏ ❏ ❏

59. Collaborate with the client and significant others, and health team members in identification of priority strengths, problems/patterns/needs and opportunities to enhance health. .... ❏ ❏ ❏ ❏ ❏ ❏ ❏ ❏ ❏ ❏ ❏ ❏ ❏

60. Use collected data to formulate hypotheses as to the etiologic bases for each identified actual or high-risk problems/patterns/needs and opportunity to enhance health .... ❏ ❏ ❏ ❏ ❏ ❏ ❏ ❏ ❏ ❏ ❏ ❏ ❏

61. Use nursing diagnoses for strengths, problems/patterns/needs and opportunities to enhance health. .... ❏ ❏ ❏ ❏ ❏ ❏ ❏ ❏ ❏ ❏ ❏ ❏ ❏

62. Reassess priorities as the database changes. ....

63. Record identified problems/patterns/needs/opportunities to enhance health. .... ❏ ❏ ❏ ❏ ❏ ❏ ❏ ❏ ❏ ❏ ❏ ❏ ❏

Outcomes

64. Identify outcomes created with client and significant others, and other health care practitioners. .... ❏ ❏ ❏ ❏ ❏ ❏ ❏ ❏ ❏ ❏ ❏ ❏ ❏

65. Specify one or more measurable client outcomes for each problem/pattern/need or opportunity to enhance health in collaboration with others. .... ❏ ❏ ❏ ❏ ❏ ❏ ❏ ❏ ❏ ❏ ❏ ❏ ❏

	I Knowledge				II Frequency of Activity					III Professional Activity		
	Not important	Slightly important	Important	Very important	Do not perform	Less than 1 per week	1–5 per week	6–10 per week	Over 10 per week	Not important	Slightly important	Important	Very Important

Plan

66. Develop appropriate client goals for each need in collaboration with the client and significant others, and other health care practitioners. .... ❏ ❏ ❏ ❏ ❏ ❏ ❏ ❏ ❏ ❏ ❏ ❏ ❏

67. Co-create a plan of self-care using personal resources. .... ❏ ❏ ❏ ❏ ❏ ❏ ❏ ❏ ❏ ❏ ❏ ❏ ❏

68. Co-create plan of care that facilitates health and wellness using modalities that enhance the body's innate healing abilities to balance and harmonize. .... ❏ ❏ ❏ ❏ ❏ ❏ ❏ ❏ ❏ ❏ ❏ ❏ ❏

69. Determine nursing interventions for select needs to enhance the health of the client and significant others. .... ❏ ❏ ❏ ❏ ❏ ❏ ❏ ❏ ❏ ❏ ❏ ❏ ❏

70. Determine interventions/holistic modalities that communicate acceptance of the client's and significant others' values, beliefs, culture, religion, and socioeconomic background. ...... ❏ ❏ ❏ ❏ ❏ ❏ ❏ ❏ ❏ ❏ ❏ ❏ ❏

71. Identify with the client and significant others areas for holistic education and health maintenance. .... ❏ ❏ ❏ ❏ ❏ ❏ ❏ ❏ ❏ ❏ ❏ ❏ ❏

72. Organize the plan of care to reflect the priority of identified client and significant others' needs and opportunities to enhance health. .... ❏ ❏ ❏ ❏ ❏ ❏ ❏ ❏ ❏ ❏ ❏ ❏ ❏

73. Revise the plan of care to reflect the client's current status or ongoing changes. .... ❏ ❏ ❏ ❏ ❏ ❏ ❏ ❏ ❏ ❏ ❏ ❏ ❏

74. Communicate the plan of care to those involved in the client's care. .... ❏ ❏ ❏ ❏ ❏ ❏ ❏ ❏ ❏ ❏ ❏ ❏ ❏

75. Record the plan of care in the client record as indicated. .... ❏ ❏ ❏ ❏ ❏ ❏ ❏ ❏ ❏ ❏ ❏ ❏ ❏

Indicate Caring-Healing Complementary Modalities Used in Clinical Practice

76. Acupressure .... ❏ ❏ ❏ ❏ ❏ ❏ ❏ ❏ ❏ ❏ ❏ ❏ ❏
77. Addictions Counseling .... ❏ ❏ ❏ ❏ ❏ ❏ ❏ ❏ ❏ ❏ ❏ ❏ ❏
78. Art Therapy .... ❏ ❏ ❏ ❏ ❏ ❏ ❏ ❏ ❏ ❏ ❏ ❏ ❏
79. Biofeedback .... ❏ ❏ ❏ ❏ ❏ ❏ ❏ ❏ ❏ ❏ ❏ ❏ ❏
80. Cognitive Therapy .... ❏ ❏ ❏ ❏ ❏ ❏ ❏ ❏ ❏ ❏ ❏ ❏ ❏
81. Deathing/Death/Grief Counseling .... ❏ ❏ ❏ ❏ ❏ ❏ ❏ ❏ ❏ ❏ ❏ ❏ ❏
82. Environmental Counseling .... ❏ ❏ ❏ ❏ ❏ ❏ ❏ ❏ ❏ ❏ ❏ ❏ ❏
83. Exercise/Movement .... ❏ ❏ ❏ ❏ ❏ ❏ ❏ ❏ ❏ ❏ ❏ ❏ ❏
84. Goal Setting/Contracts .... ❏ ❏ ❏ ❏ ❏ ❏ ❏ ❏ ❏ ❏ ❏ ❏ ❏
85. Healing Touch .... ❏ ❏ ❏ ❏ ❏ ❏ ❏ ❏ ❏ ❏ ❏ ❏ ❏
86. Holistic Self-Assessments .... ❏ ❏ ❏ ❏ ❏ ❏ ❏ ❏ ❏ ❏ ❏ ❏ ❏
87. Humor/Laughter .... ❏ ❏ ❏ ❏ ❏ ❏ ❏ ❏ ❏ ❏ ❏ ❏ ❏
88. Imagery .... ❏ ❏ ❏ ❏ ❏ ❏ ❏ ❏ ❏ ❏ ❏ ❏ ❏
89. Journaling .... ❏ ❏ ❏ ❏ ❏ ❏ ❏ ❏ ❏ ❏ ❏ ❏ ❏
90. Massage .... ❏ ❏ ❏ ❏ ❏ ❏ ❏ ❏ ❏ ❏ ❏ ❏ ❏
91. Meditation .... ❏ ❏ ❏ ❏ ❏ ❏ ❏ ❏ ❏ ❏ ❏ ❏ ❏
92. Music/Sound Therapy .... ❏ ❏ ❏ ❏ ❏ ❏ ❏ ❏ ❏ ❏ ❏ ❏ ❏

	I Knowledge				II Frequency of Activity					III Professional Activity			
	Not important	Slightly important	Important	Very important	Do not perform	Less than 1 per week	1–5 per week	6–10 per week	Over 10 per week	Not important	Slightly important	Important	Very Important
93. Nutrition Counseling	❏	❏	❏	❏	❏	❏	❏	❏	❏	❏	❏	❏	❏
94. Therapeutic Touch	❏	❏	❏	❏	❏	❏	❏	❏	❏	❏	❏	❏	❏
95. Play Therapy	❏	❏	❏	❏	❏	❏	❏	❏	❏	❏	❏	❏	❏
96. Relationship Counseling	❏	❏	❏	❏	❏	❏	❏	❏	❏	❏	❏	❏	❏
97. Self-Reflection	❏	❏	❏	❏	❏	❏	❏	❏	❏	❏	❏	❏	❏
98. Sexual Abuse Counseling	❏	❏	❏	❏	❏	❏	❏	❏	❏	❏	❏	❏	❏
99. Spirituality Counseling	❏	❏	❏	❏	❏	❏	❏	❏	❏	❏	❏	❏	❏
100. Smoking Cessation	❏	❏	❏	❏	❏	❏	❏	❏	❏	❏	❏	❏	❏
101. Violence Counseling	❏	❏	❏	❏	❏	❏	❏	❏	❏	❏	❏	❏	❏
102. Weight Management	❏	❏	❏	❏	❏	❏	❏	❏	❏	❏	❏	❏	❏
103. Wellness Counseling	❏	❏	❏	❏	❏	❏	❏	❏	❏	❏	❏	❏	❏
104. Others	❏	❏	❏	❏	❏	❏	❏	❏	❏	❏	❏	❏	❏
_____	❏	❏	❏	❏	❏	❏	❏	❏	❏	❏	❏	❏	❏
_____	❏	❏	❏	❏	❏	❏	❏	❏	❏	❏	❏	❏	❏
_____	❏	❏	❏	❏	❏	❏	❏	❏	❏	❏	❏	❏	❏

Implementation

	I Knowledge				II Frequency of Activity					III Professional Activity			
105. Implement the plan of care with the client, significant others, and other health care practitioners.	❏	❏	❏	❏	❏	❏	❏	❏	❏	❏	❏	❏	❏
106. Promote client participation in care.	❏	❏	❏	❏	❏	❏	❏	❏	❏	❏	❏	❏	❏
107. Provide a supportive, therapeutic presence of wholeness.	❏	❏	❏	❏	❏	❏	❏	❏	❏	❏	❏	❏	❏
108. Integrate the intuitive art of nursing with scientific information and technical competencies.	❏	❏	❏	❏	❏	❏	❏	❏	❏	❏	❏	❏	❏
109. Provide safe care that prevents complications and life-threatening situations.	❏	❏	❏	❏	❏	❏	❏	❏	❏	❏	❏	❏	❏
110. Document interventions in the client record.	❏	❏	❏	❏	❏	❏	❏	❏	❏	❏	❏	❏	❏

Evaluation

	I Knowledge				II Frequency of Activity					III Professional Activity			
111. Collect data for evaluation.	❏	❏	❏	❏	❏	❏	❏	❏	❏	❏	❏	❏	❏
112. Evaluate outcomes based on attainment of client's personal goals.	❏	❏	❏	❏	❏	❏	❏	❏	❏	❏	❏	❏	❏
113. Assess effectiveness of nursing interventions to achieve client outcomes and opportunities to enhance health.	❏	❏	❏	❏	❏	❏	❏	❏	❏	❏	❏	❏	❏
114. Reference the plan from pertinent sources clarifying rationale for intervention.	❏	❏	❏	❏	❏	❏	❏	❏	❏	❏	❏	❏	❏
115. Collaborate with the client, significant others, and other health care practitioners in the evaluation process.	❏	❏	❏	❏	❏	❏	❏	❏	❏	❏	❏	❏	❏
116. Determine factors that contribute to deviations between the client's response and the identified outcomes.	❏	❏	❏	❏	❏	❏	❏	❏	❏	❏	❏	❏	❏
117. Ongoing revision of the plan of care as the evaluation indicates a need for change.	❏	❏	❏	❏	❏	❏	❏	❏	❏	❏	❏	❏	❏
118. Recognize that all measurable outcomes may not be immediate but are a process of becoming.	❏	❏	❏	❏	❏	❏	❏	❏	❏	❏	❏	❏	❏
119. Document evaluation and outcomes in the client record.	❏	❏	❏	❏	❏	❏	❏	❏	❏	❏	❏	❏	❏

PART 2: CARING AND HEALING OF CLIENTS AND SIGNIFICANT OTHERS

Concept VII. Meaning and Wholeness

	I Knowledge				II Frequency of Activity					III Professional Activity			
	Not important	Slightly important	Important	Very important	Do not perform	Less than 1 per week	1–5 per week	6–10 per week	Over 10 per week	Not important	Slightly important	Important	Very Important
120. Focus care on the client's and significant others' body-mind-spirit.	☐	☐	☐	☐	☐	☐	☐	☐	☐	☐	☐	☐	☐
121. Identify the client's and significant others' perceptions in regard to health maintenance and well-being.	☐	☐	☐	☐	☐	☐	☐	☐	☐	☐	☐	☐	☐
122. Base care on a comprehensive assessment of the client and significant others.	☐	☐	☐	☐	☐	☐	☐	☐	☐	☐	☐	☐	☐
123. Preserve the client's dignity and rights by respecting personal choices, achieving mutual consensus.	☐	☐	☐	☐	☐	☐	☐	☐	☐	☐	☐	☐	☐
124. Advocate for the client and significant others.	☐	☐	☐	☐	☐	☐	☐	☐	☐	☐	☐	☐	☐
125. Assess meaning of health, illness, and treatment of each client and significant other.	☐	☐	☐	☐	☐	☐	☐	☐	☐	☐	☐	☐	☐
126. Gain understanding of cultural practices that impact the care outcomes of clients and significant others.	☐	☐	☐	☐	☐	☐	☐	☐	☐	☐	☐	☐	☐
127. Integrate client's cultural beliefs and needs in planning and implementation.	☐	☐	☐	☐	☐	☐	☐	☐	☐	☐	☐	☐	☐
128. Use appropriate community resources to gain understanding of health care practices and beliefs of different cultural groups.	☐	☐	☐	☐	☐	☐	☐	☐	☐	☐	☐	☐	☐
129. Appreciate the critical nature of diversity in the global community.	☐	☐	☐	☐	☐	☐	☐	☐	☐	☐	☐	☐	☐
130. Assess the client's and significant others' values and beliefs.	☐	☐	☐	☐	☐	☐	☐	☐	☐	☐	☐	☐	☐
131. Plan individualized care incorporating client's and significant others' values.	☐	☐	☐	☐	☐	☐	☐	☐	☐	☐	☐	☐	☐
132. Assist the client and significant others to identify ways to support a sacred environment conducive to reflection, prayer, and spiritual growth.	☐	☐	☐	☐	☐	☐	☐	☐	☐	☐	☐	☐	☐
133. Provide opportunities to support the client and significant others in their search for a relationship with self, others, the environment, and a higher power.													

Concept VIII. Client/Self-Care

	Not important	Slightly important	Important	Very important	Do not perform	Less than 1 per week	1–5 per week	6–10 per week	Over 10 per week	Not important	Slightly important	Important	Very Important
134. Develop with clients and significant others self-care strategies to enhance their desired level of physical, psychological, sociological, vocational, and spiritual well-being.	☐	☐	☐	☐	☐	☐	☐	☐	☐	☐	☐	☐	☐
135. Initiate referrals and facilitate access to health care resources (e.g., clinic appointments, patient admissions, community agencies, schools, financial counselors).	☐	☐	☐	☐	☐	☐	☐	☐	☐	☐	☐	☐	☐

	I Knowledge				II Frequency of Activity					III Professional Activity			
	Not important	Slightly important	Important	Very important	Do not perform	Less than 1 per week	1–5 per week	6–10 per week	Over 10 per week	Not important	Slightly important	Important	Very Important
136. Develop a plan with clients to track self-care and to identify self-care opportunities across the lifespan.	□	□	□	□	□	□	□	□	□	□	□	□	□
137. Assist client to create sacred space within one's self, as well as in the home and workplace.	□	□	□	□	□	□	□	□	□	□	□	□	□
138. Practice environmental safety and emergency preparedness.	□	□	□	□	□	□	□	□	□	□	□	□	□
139. Promote environments conducive to experiencing wholeness and harmony.	□	□	□	□	□	□	□	□	□	□	□	□	□
140. Recognize that the well-being of the ecosystem of the planet and the well-being of the human are co-created.	□	□	□	□	□	□	□	□	□	□	□	□	□

Concept IX. Health Promotion

	I Knowledge				II Frequency of Activity					III Professional Activity			
141. Teach clients and significant others that healing is a process of learning.	□	□	□	□	□	□	□	□	□	□	□	□	□
142. Use teaching and learning principles with all holistic health education.	□	□	□	□	□	□	□	□	□	□	□	□	□
143. Provide ongoing body-mind-spirit assessment, and evaluation of client's and significant others' knowledge in relation to wellness, illness, diagnostic tests, treatments, anticipated outcomes, and self-care activities.	□	□	□	□	□	□	□	□	□	□	□	□	□
144. Empower the client and significant others in co-creating a mutual plan for goals, diagnostic tests, treatments, resource identification, health development, homecare, and follow-up care.	□	□	□	□	□	□	□	□	□	□	□	□	□
145. Identify environmental barriers to the integration of holistic care.	□	□	□	□	□	□	□	□	□	□	□	□	□
146. Take risks (depending on circumstances), if necessary, to advocate for the client and significant others.	□	□	□	□	□	□	□	□	□	□	□	□	□
147. Support the client's sense of personal responsibility and ability to achieve desired health outcomes.	□	□	□	□	□	□	□	□	□	□	□	□	□
148. Assist clients and significant others in problem-solving discussions regarding how to live with changes secondary to illness and treatment.	□	□	□	□	□	□	□	□	□	□	□	□	□
149. Assist the clients and significant others to access health information and to choose health promotion strategies that lead toward desired outcomes.	□	□	□	□	□	□	□	□	□	□	□	□	□
150. Utilize change theory to assist clients and significant others to integrate health promotion strategies.	□	□	□	□	□	□	□	□	□	□	□	□	□
151. Support clients and significant others in the discovery of their health pattern behaviors.	□	□	□	□	□	□	□	□	□	□	□	□	□

AHNA Member #
_____

AHNA
American Holistic Nurses' Association
4101 Lake Boone Trail, Suite 201
Raleigh, North Carolina 27607
(800) 278-AHNA
FAX (919) 787-4916

If address is incorrect, please note corrections in space below.

_____
_____
_____
_____

Please take a moment to review the demographic information listed **on both sides.**
Please indicate your current information on the form and return it to AHNA in the envelope provided.
Your support of AHNA is vital to the accomplishment of our goals and the advancement of holistic nursing.

MARK ONLY ONE RESPONSE UNLESS INSTRUCTED OTHERWISE

1. GENDER
❏ Male
❏ Female

2. ANNUAL HOUSEHOLD INCOME
❏ $24,999 or below ❏ $55,000–74,999
❏ $25,000–39,999   ❏ $75,000+
❏ $40,000–54,999

3. AGE GROUP
❏ Between 18–24   ❏ Between 45–49
❏ Between 25–29   ❏ Between 50–54
❏ Between 30–34   ❏ Between 55–60
❏ Between 35–39   ❏ Between 61–65
❏ Between 40–44   ❏ Over 65

4. RACE-ETHNIC ORIGIN
❏ African-American
❏ Asian or Pacific Islander
❏ Caucasian
❏ Hispanic
❏ American Indian or Alaskan Native
❏ Other _____
          Please specify

5. MARITAL STATUS
❏ Divorced/Separated
❏ Domestic Partner
❏ Married
❏ Single
❏ Widowed

6. LANGUAGES SPOKEN FLUENTLY
(mark all that apply)
❏ Chinese   ❏ Spanish
❏ English   ❏ Sign Language
❏ French   ❏ Other _____
                      Please specify
❏ German

7. DO YOU HAVE A MILITARY OR FEDERAL AFFILIATION?
❏ Yes
❏ No

8. LICENSE
❏ RN

STATE(S) IN WHICH YOU CURRENTLY PRACTICE _____

STATE NURSING LICENSE/S # _____
_____

9. DO YOU HOLD AN ADVANCED PRACTICE NURSING LICENSE IN YOUR STATE?
❏ Yes
❏ No

10. EMPLOYMENT STATUS
❏ Full Time
❏ Not Employed
❏ Part Time
❏ Retired
❏ Seeking Work

11. HOW MANY HOURS PER WEEK DO YOU WORK AS A NURSE?

10	20	30	40	50	60	70	80	90	HOURS
❏	❏	❏	❏	❏	❏	❏	❏	❏	

12. HIGHEST NURSING DEGREE/ CREDENTIAL
❏ Associate   ❏ MA
❏ BS   ❏ MEd
❏ BSN   ❏ MN
❏ Diploma   ❏ MS
❏ DNS   ❏ MSN
❏ DNSc   ❏ PhD
❏ DSN   ❏ N/A
❏ EdD   ❏ Other _____
                    Please specify

13. YEAR GRADUATED FROM BASIC NURSING PROGRAM

_____

14. HIGHEST ACADEMIC DEGREE HELD OUTSIDE NURSING
❏ AA   ❏ EdD   ❏ JD   ❏ MS
❏ BA   ❏ MD   ❏ MA   ❏ Other _____
❏ BS   ❏ PhD   ❏ MBA   Please specify

15. HONORARY DISTINCTIONS
❏ FACC   ❏ FAAN
❏ FCCM   ❏ Other _____
                  Please specify

16. NUMBER OF YEARS AS AN RN:

<1	<2	<3	<4	<5	<6	<7	<8	<9	YEARS
❏	❏	❏	❏	❏	❏	❏	❏	❏	
<10	<15	<20	<25	<30	<35	<40	<45	<50	
❏	❏	❏	❏	❏	❏	❏	❏	❏	

17. NUMBER OF YEARS AS A HOLISTIC NURSE:

<1	<2	<3	<4	<5	<6	<7	<8	<9	YEARS
❏	❏	❏	❏	❏	❏	❏	❏	❏	
<10	<15	<20	<25	<30	<35	<40	<45	<50	
❏	❏	❏	❏	❏	❏	❏	❏	❏	

Over

18. HOLISTIC NURSING EDUCATION
(mark all that apply)
❑ Formal Education
❑ Seminars/Workshops
❑ Extended Programs in Specific
   Modalities

19. DO YOU USE THE FOLLOWING TO ACCESS HOLISTIC INFORMATION OR HOLISTIC CONNECTIONS?
❑ E-Mail   ❑ Internet   ❑ Computers

20. WHAT HOLISTIC MODALITIES HAVE YOU STUDIED?

_____ ❑ >1 ❑ >5 ❑ >10 ❑ >15 ❑ >20 YEARS

_____ ❑ >1 ❑ >5 ❑ >10 ❑ >15 ❑ >20 YEARS

_____ ❑ >1 ❑ >5 ❑ >10 ❑ >15 ❑ >20 YEARS

_____ ❑ >1 ❑ >5 ❑ >10 ❑ >15 ❑ >20 YEARS

---

21. PRIMARY POSITION HELD (mark all that apply)
❑ Academic Faculty
❑ Clinical Dir./Administrator/VP
❑ Clinical Nurse Specialist
❑ Consultant
❑ Corporate Executive

❑ Direct Care/Bedside/Staff Nurse
❑ Healing Touch Practitioner
❑ Independent Practice
❑ Inservice/Staff Dev. Instructor
❑ Manager

❑ Massage Therapist
❑ Nurse Midwife
❑ Nurse Practitioner
❑ Nurse Therapist/Healer
❑ Nurse Researcher
❑ Other _____
                    Please specify

---

22. TYPE OF FACILITY IN WHICH EMPLOYED (mark all that apply)
❑ Clinic
❑ Collaborative Practice
❑ College/University
❑ Community Hospital (Nonprofit)
❑ Community Hospital (Profit)
❑ County Hospital
❑ Federal Hospital
❑ HMO/Managed Care
❑ Health Center
❑ Home Health
❑ Hospice
❑ Military Hospital

❑ Non-Academic Teaching Hospital
❑ Physician's Office
❑ Private Industry
❑ Registry
❑ School Nurse
❑ Private Practice (Self-Employed)
❑ State Hospital
❑ Travel Nurse
❑ University Medical Center
❑ Other _____
            Please specify

23. NUMBER OF BEDS IN FACILITY:
❑ under 100   ❑ 300–499
❑ 100–299   ❑ 500 or more

---

24. AREA EMPLOYED (mark all that apply)
❑ Chemical Dependency
❑ Critical Care/ICU _____
                    Please specify
❑ Community/Public Health
❑ Corporate Industry
❑ Emergency Department
❑ Hemodialysis Unit
❑ Holistic Center

❑ Home Care
❑ Hospice
❑ Long-Term Care
❑ Obstetrics/Gynecology
❑ Oncology Unit
❑ Operating Room
❑ Orthopedics
❑ Pain Management

❑ Pediatrics
❑ Psychiatric/Mental Health
❑ Recovery Room/PACU
❑ Research Nurse _____
                    Specify area
❑ Telemetry
❑ Other _____
            Please specify

---

25. PROFESSIONAL SPECIAL INTEREST
(mark all that apply)
❑ CNS/Advanced Practice
❑ Clinical Practice
❑ Education
❑ Ethics
❑ Gerontology
❑ Management
❑ Military
❑ Research
❑ Transcultural
❑ Rehabilitation _____
                    Please specify
❑ Other _____
            Please specify

26. CLINICAL SPECIALTIES
(please specify)

27. PROFESSIONAL CERTIFICATIONS
(please specify)

28. OTHER ASSOCIATION MEMBERSHIPS (please specify)

Thank you for taking the time to fill out this survey.

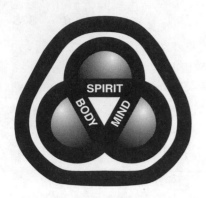

Index